Special Recreational Services
Therapeutic and Adapted

Special Recreational Services
Therapeutic and Adapted

JAY S. SHIVERS, Ph.D.
Professor
Department of Sport and Leisure Studies
University of Connecticut
Storrs, Connecticut

HOLLIS F. FAIT, Ph.D.
Late Professor
Department of Sport and Leisure Studies
University of Connecticut
Storrs, Connecticut

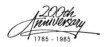

Lea & Febiger   1985   Philadelphia

Lea & Febiger
600 Washington Square
Philadelphia, Pa. 19106-4198
U.S.A.
(215)922-1330

Library of Congress Cataloging in Publication Data
Shivers, Jay Sanford, 1930–
    Special recreational services.
    Bibliography: p.
    Includes index.
    1. Recreational therapy. 2. Handicapped—Services for. 3.
Handicapped—Recreation. I. Fait, Hollis F. II. Title.
RM736.7.S538   1985   615.8'5153   84-14329
    ISBN   0-8121-0964-3

PRINTED IN THE UNITED STATES OF AMERICA

Print Number: 3   2   1

To all of those who are afflicted and to those who provide the services for relief.

Homo sum; humani nihil a me alienum puto.

Preface

This book is designed as a comprehensive, yet easily understood, text for students and practitioners in the recreational service field whose employment requires providing services for clients with special needs as the consequence of their illness or disability. The book's title reflects the purpose of the book: to prepare recreationists to offer programs of that special nature which most benefits clients whose conditions necessitate participation in activities of therapeutic benefit and/or of adaptation to their unique needs. A wide range of conditions that require special recreational services is presented: physical disabilities, mental retardation, learning disabilities, mental disturbances, aging, and social deviation. Programming for clients with these conditions is discussed as it functions in various types of treatment centers and community settings.

To ensure that the text offers the kinds of information needed by recreationists to serve ill and disabled clients effectively, the authors have drawn upon a wide range of literature from allied fields and related disciplines. As a result the book offers a broad basic background in the clinical aspects of disabling diseases and injuries; a good foundation for development of sympathetic understanding of the psychologic problems imposed by disabilities; and a wealth of practical "know how" for adaptation of recreational activities to serve the special needs of clients. The relevance of the book's content is further enhanced by the inclusion of personal techniques, methods, and evaluation tools developed during our long and varied experiences working with ill and disabled people in treatment centers and in community and educational settings.

Matters of particular professional concern to recreationists receive due discussion in the book. The differences as well as the many similarities in providing special recreational services in treatment centers and community settings are detailed. Particular attention is given to the way in which the therapeutic recreationist works with personnel in the various medical and therapeutic disciplines. Emphasis is also directed toward the provision of adapted and mainstreamed recreational programs for ill and disabled clients in the community.

In development of the book, recognition has been made of the influence of federal legislation and adjudication on the provision of recreational services for those who are ill and disabled. Not only have the opportunities for participation been increased for these individuals, but the dimensions of service by recreationists have been expanded to include educational settings. Ways in which the recreationist can assist the schools in meeting their mandate to identify and provide recreational skill development for handicapped students with deficiencies are presented throughout the book.

The goal of recreation is the re-creation of human energy and enthusiasm through an infinite variety of pleasurable pursuits. The goal should be as readily attainable by those who are ill and disabled as by any others in our society. That this is not so gives added significance to the need for developing good special recreational programs and providing well-trained, compassionate personnel to staff them. Deep awareness of the need and dedication to the task of fulfilling it inspired this book. Our hope is that those who study from it will likewise become aware and dedicated.

Jay S. Shivers
Hollis F. Fait

Storrs, Connecticut

Acknowledgments

We are indebted to many people who, in generously sharing with us their experiences, observations, and knowledge, have greatly enhanced the content of this book. We particularly wish to acknowledge the assistance of many ill and disabled clients in providing information that only they can offer. Likewise, we wish to recognize the unique contributions of those who have sat in our classes over the years. Also greatly appreciated are the ideas, information, and suggestions offered by colleagues and professional friends.

Several individuals offered specific help in their areas of expertise, and we wish to express our gratitude to them: Dr. Bernard Thorne, Brattleboro (VT) Retreat, for reviewing the chapter on assessment and evaluation; Dr. Earl F. Hoerner, University of Connecticut, for reviewing the chapter on special programming considerations; Dr. John M. Dunn, Oregon State University, for assistance with the chapter on mental retardation and learning disabilities; Dr. Charles C. Bullock, University of North Carolina, for contributions to the development of materials on recreational education in the schools; and Paul A. Roper, doctoral candidate at the University of Connecticut and teacher of the handicapped, for reviewing the chapter on games, sports, and exercise.

Also, to Gladene Hansen Fait, former community recreational director, for valuable suggestions and assistance in editing and rewriting, and Laurel Millix, secretary, for typing the manuscript and greatly facilitating the preparation of the manuscript by her kind and generous ways.

Appreciation is expressed to Paul A. Roper, photographer, and all others who loaned or granted permission for the use of photos, illustrations, and other materials.

Contents

Section 1. FOUNDATIONS AND FUNDAMENTALS

Chapter 1: Introduction 3
   Understanding the Terminology 3
   The Nature of Therapeutic and Adapted Recreational
      Services 7
   Values of Recreational Activities 9
   Historic Foundations 13
   Recent Federal Legislation 17
   Other Therapeutic and Educational Modalities 17

Chapter 2: Professional Development and
Responsibilities 21
   Roles and Responsibilities 21
   Competencies 23
   Professional Preparation 26
   Attributes 28
   Professional Ethics 29
   Certification and Licensing 30
   Continuing Education 31
   Professional Organizations 31
   Promotion of the Profession and Public Relations 33

Chapter 3: Theories, Processes, and Instruments 35
   The Rehabilitative Process 35
   Homeostasis 36
   Motivation 37
   Psychoanalysis 40
   Psychotherapy 41
   Group Therapy 41

Therapeutic Milieu and Milieu Therapy 43
Prescription 43
Sensory or Perceptual Training 45
Relaxation 46
Exercise and Physical Fitness 47
Activity Analysis 49
Kinetic or Skill Analysis 50
Leisure Counseling and Leisure Education 51
Normalization and Mainstreaming 52

Chapter 4: Special Recreational Service in Treatment Centers
           and Community Settings 55
Therapeutic Recreational Service in Treatment Centers . . 55
  Nature of Therapeutic Recreational Service 56
  Organizational Structure 58
Adapted Recreational Service in Community Settings . . 65
  Nature of Adapted Recreational Service 65
  Number in the Special Population to Be Served 66
  Departmental Organization for Community Adapted
  Recreational Service 68
  Clients in Other Programs 70
  Transportation Services 73
  Facilities and Equipment 74
  Scheduling in Treatment Centers 75
  Scheduling in Community Settings 76
  Participant Planning 76
  Use of Volunteers 78

Chapter 5: Understanding Problems of Adjustment Caused by
           Illness and Disability 80
Attitudes toward Disability 80
Attitudes toward Self 82
Psychology of Acute Illness 83
Psychology of Physical Disability 85
Social Problems of Disablement 87
Personality Characteristics of the Impaired 89

Chapter 6: Determining Status and Progress: Assessment and
           Evaluation 90
Evaluation and Legal Requirements of PL 94-142 90
Administrative Evaluation and Assessment
  Requirements 92
Basic Types of Instruments of Assessment and
  Evaluations 93
Developing Goals and Objectives 103
Assessment and Evaluation Models and Systems 105

Section 2. CONDITIONS OF ILLNESS, DISABILITY, SOCIAL MALADJUSTMENT

Chapter 7: Physical Disabilities 111
  Orthopedic and Neurologic Problems 112
    Orthopedic Disabilities 112
    Neurologic Disorders 124
    Programming Recreational Activities 129
  Cardiac and Pulmonary Disorders 135
    Cardiopathic Disorders 135
    Pulmonary Diseases 140
    Programming Recreational Activities 143
  Auditory and Visual Impairments 144
    Auditory Disabilities 144
    Visual Disabilities 146
    Programming Recreational Activities 148

Chapter 8: Mental Retardation and Learning Disabilities . . 152
  Mental Retardation 152
    Nature of Intelligence 153
    Measuring Mental Capacity 153
    Causes of Mental Retardation 156
    Selecting or Setting the Environment 159
    Programming Recreational Activities 159
  Learning Disabilities 161
    Perceptual-Motor Learning 162
    Perceptual-Motor Learning Problems and Activities . . 163

Chapter 9: Mental Disturbances 172
  Classification in Psychiatry 172
  Diagnosis 179
  Attitudes Toward Mental Disturbances 179
  Treatment Methods 182
  Developing the Therapeutic Program 183
  Programming Recreational Activities 185

Chapter 10: Aging 192
  The Process of Aging 192
  The Social Dimensions of Aging 195
  Recreational Services for the Elderly 198

Chapter 11: Socially Deviant Behavior 201
  The Criminal Justice System 201
  Therapeutic Program 202
  Diversional or Regular Program 203
  Programming Recreational Activities 204
  Suggested Activities 207

Secion 3. ACTIVITIES—SELECTION AND ADAPTATION

Chapter 12: Special Considerations in Programming 215
Prescription Versus Diversional Activities 215
Mobility As a Factor in Programming 216
Tolerance Level 229
Age and Interests 230
Side Effects of Medication 232
Rights of Ill and Disabled People 233

Chapter 13: Graphic and Performing Arts 235
Graphic Arts 235
Factors Which Determine Adaptation 235
Selecting Arts and Crafts Activities 237
Functional Considerations in Craft Activities 238
Art as a Therapeutic Adjunct 240
Performing Arts 242
Dance: Program Considerations and Adaptations . . . 243
Music: Program Considerations and Adaptations . . . 244
Drama: Program Considerations and Adaptations . . . 246

Chapter 14: Games, Sports, and Exercises 251
Sport and Game Activities 251
Competitive Sport Teams 272
Exercise and Conditioning 273

Chapter 15: Horticulture, Animal Husbandry, and Culinary
Arts 287
Horticulture 288
Unique Therapeutic Benefits 288
Horticultural Therapy 289
Adapting Activities 290
Animal Husbandry 292
Unique Therapeutic Benefits 292
Pet Therapy 293
Adapting Activities 293
Culinary Arts 294
Unique Therapeutic Benefits 295
Adapting Activities 296

Chapter 16: Social and Service Activities and Passive
Entertainment 300
Social Activities 300
Value of Social Activities As a Therapeutic Tool 301
Selecting Social Activities 302
Developing Social Activity Prescription 303

Service Activities   304
    Value of Service Activities As a Therapeutic Tool . . .   304
    Identifying Service Possibilities   306
Passive Entertainment Activities   307
    Value of Passive Entertainment As a Therapeutic
    Tool   307
    Structuring Passive Entertainment Events   308
    Preparing Patients and Clients for Entertainment
    Events   309
    Passive Games   310
    Special Events in Treatment Centers   310

Chapter 17: Camping and Nature-Oriented Activities   313
    Camping As a Therapeutic Adjunct   314
    Types of Camps   318
    The Program   320
    Adaptation of Camping and Nature-Oriented
    Activities   321
    Adapting Conditions to Meet Community Needs   322

Appendices   325

Index   349

Section 1

Foundations and Fundamentals

Chapter 1

Introduction

Recreational activity has had a significant role in human existence since its beginning. Participation in recreational outlets is a recognized need, providing as it does a balance in a life of tension, stress, obligations, and demands. There has always been a segment in society whose needs for such balance is greatest but the fulfillment of which has been least. Society's recognition and acceptance of this sad fact in recent decades has given impetus to the development of recreational services especially for those incapacitated by illness or disability.

From a small beginning as a facet of existing recreational programs, the "special" recreational services experienced especially vigorous and rapid growth. Not only was the value of providing such service recognized by hospitals and institutions, but communities, too, became aware of the vast unmet recreational needs. The rapid expansion of programs increased the demand for trained personnel. Colleges and universities throughout the country responded by developing new training programs or expanding existing ones. Courses, like the one for which this book is intended, were established with the objective of developing a true professional: one equipped with the understanding and knowledge to enable those with special needs to enjoy the benefit and satisfaction to experience the balance of participation in recreational activities.

UNDERSTANDING THE TERMINOLOGY

As new areas of endeavor develop, a special vocabulary is required to express the concepts for which no terminology exists. Entirely new terms may be created, but just as frequently old words are given new or added meaning to make them applicable in the new situation. Hence, until there is general acceptance of precise definitions of the special vocabulary, the words are often used slightly differently by people in the field. To some extent this is the case with the profession under discussion in this textbook; therefore, to prevent any misunderstanding of the concepts presented here, the terms used in the discussion are defined in the following paragraphs.

Recreation

Authorities in the field have traditionally defined recreation as a procedure, that is, a pastime, diversion, or exercise affording relaxation and enjoyment, which is performed in one's leisure. Shivers regards this conventional definition as too restrictive because recreation is, in his view, more than a process; it is also a concept. Accordingly, he sees recreation simply as a "nondebilitating consummatory experience." [1] Therefore, any activity in which one participates that is completely engaging and produces no deleterious results for the individual or society is recreation. The more encompassing nature of recreation is also reflected in the definitions of other writers; an example is this statement by Gray and Grebin that recreation ". . . is characterized by feelings of masterly, achievement, exhilaration, acceptance, success, personal worth, and pleasure." [2] Regardless of the particular choice of words used in the broader definitions of recreation, inherent in them all is the idea the recreational activity is undertaken voluntarily during leisure for the participant's personal pleasure and satisfaction.

Recreational Service

Given the meaning of recreation, described above, the word is used inappropriately when applied to the organization, planning, and conduct of recreational activities by recreational personnel for others. Such work is more properly referred to as service, service being defined as all of the work undertaken by an agent to benefit or enhance the condition, status, or situation of another by provision of certain opportunities, exposure, or activities. Thus the work performed by those who assist people to lead more satisfying lives by enhancing their physical, mental, social, and cultural capacities by active or passive involvement in recreational experiences is service.

Recreationist—Recreator

Two terms are used to describe the professionally trained individual who is involved with providing recreational service: recreationist and recreator. Preference is given by the authors to use of recreationist since the suffix "ist" denotes a practice—the exercise or pursuit of a profession, while the suffix "or" denotes who or that which does something. A recreator, therefore, can be one who participates as a client in recreational activities as well as the one who conducts the program. There is no such ambiguity with the term recreationist that by definition applies only to one who conducts the recreational service. Further, the definition signifies the professional nature of the work being done by recreational service personnel, an element that is lacking in the term recreator.

Special

The word *special,* when used in this text in connection with recreational services, indicates unique provisions in the program for any individual who cannot participate to his or her advantage or cannot benefit from the regular program of recreational activities. Conditions that can produce special needs and necessitate special programming include illness, disability, delinquency, and alcoholic and drug abuse. Some authorities refer to groups of people who need special services because of conditions as *special populations.*

Special Programs

Recreational programs that serve special populations have been identified by various names over the years. Among the most common are *hospital recreation, medical recreation, recreation therapy, therapeutic recreation,* and *adapted recreational services.* Hospital recreation is an older term used to indicate the recreational services provided for patients in a treatment center. The term medical recreation is infrequently used in the place of therapeutic recreation and implies programs that are conducted under the close supervision of medical personnel. Recreation therapy is a term used in the job description of the U. S. Civil Service. The term is generally understood to mean the use of recreational services as therapy designed to treat or cure a specific illness. This is in contrast to therapeutic recreational programs which utilize recreational activities for purposive intervention in some problem of a physical, mental, or social nature. (A fuller discussion follows later in the chapter.) Adapted recreational service, a much newer term than the others, refers to recreational programming in which the activities, facilities, and / or equipment are modified to meet the needs of the clients being served.

People with Special Needs

Various terms are used to describe those people who have special needs arising from medical conditions. Generally, persons with problems attributable to aging or delinquency are not included among those to whom the terms are applied.

There are slight distinctions among the definitions of the terms. Ill refers to a condition in which the individual has a disease or is in poor health; a temporary state of the condition is implied. Impaired denotes a pronounced organic or functional disorder, while disabled is used to describe those who because of impairment are incapacitated or are limited or restricted in executing some skills or participating in some activity.

The Federal Government in Public Law 94-142, the Education of the Handicapped Act, identifies those who are handicapped as persons who are: mentally retarded, hard of hearing, deaf, speech impaired, visually handicapped, seriously emotionally disturbed, orthopedically impaired, other health impaired, deaf-blind, multi-handicapped, or specific learning disabled.[3]

The American Alliance for Health, Physical Education, Recreation and Dance recommends the use of the word handicapped be limited to refer to individuals who are adversely affected psychologically, emotionally, or socially by their disability and that other terms such as impaired and disabled be applied only to those persons who have a physical disorder but have made a satisfactory adjustment.[4]

Other words used to identify the individual for whom special recreational services are offered are *client* or *participant* and *patient.* Client or participant refers to anyone who is receiving the services; patient is used only for the person who is under direct medical care and treatment due to illness or injury.

Therapeutic

Confusion about the meaning of the word *therapeutic* sometimes occurs due to the different ways in which the parent word *therapy* is used. In the medical situation, therapy refers to the treatment of disease; there is the connotation of intervention, a stopping of the process of deterioration or debilitation with the hope of effecting recovery and rehabilitation. In general usage, however, therapy is applied to any act, hobby, task, program, etc. that relieves tension and provides for the general well being of the individual. By this definition, all recreational experiences are therapeutic for those who are healthy and able as well as those who are ill and disabled. But in the view of some authorities, only those recreational activities that are medically prescribed, i.e., recommended on the basis of knowledge of the patient's condition and attitude, can be called therapeutic.

Adapted

The word *adapted* refers to adjustment or modification of an activity to allow an individual with limitations due to illness or disability to participate in the activity. The modifications may be in the way the movement of the activity is executed; in the tool, instrument, or equipment used in the activity; or in the environment and standards or rules and regulations that normally apply to the activity.

Adaptations are made by the recreationist for the individual client, although some clients develop highly personalized adaptations through experimentation on their own. Appropriate adaptations are the result of analysis based on knowledge of the movements required and an understanding of the limitations of the client. Adaptations are not medically prescribed, although discussions with medical personnel may be necessary to make a competent analysis and to ensure the safety of the patient.

THE NATURE OF THERAPEUTIC AND ADAPTED RECREATIONAL SERVICES

When the term *therapeutic recreation* was first used, which is thought to have been in the federal legislation creating the Works Progress Administration (WPA) in 1938,[5] it referred to any recreational activity that was participated in by those who were ill or disabled. With the growth of recreational programs in hospitals and institutions, the activities came more and more to be based on recommendations or prescriptions by medical personnel; and "therapeutic recreation" became the term applied to programs of prescribed recreational activities as well as to those programs in which persons with illnesses or disabilities participated.

This development prompted Witt to comment on the inappropriateness of the word therapeutic when used to describe recreational programs designed for individuals who require adapted or modified leisure services because of physical or mental limitations.[6] Other authorities have felt a need to make a distinction between the two types of clients served and the kind of recreational service provided each. O'Morrow identifies the two approaches to providing recreational activities for ill and disabled clients as clinical and nonclinical.[7] The clinical approach focuses on the use of recreational service in the treatment of illness or disability while the nonclinical centers on the broader concept of recreation, the subjective enjoyment and enrichment of the clients' living experience.

There is obvious difficulty in drawing a hard and fast line between the clinical and nonclinical approaches since the two often exist in combination, i.e., in the treatment for one who is ill or disabled the recreational experience, by all probability, enriches the client's daily life in addition to aiding in the treatment. We have chosen to distinguish between the two approaches by labeling all recreational activities that are medically prescribed as therapeutic and using the term adapted for all those activities offered as recreational experience and modified to meet the needs of clients with mental, emotional, or physical problems.

Prescription is the essential element that transforms recreational experience into a therapeutic modality. Through recreational activities selected for that purpose the recreationist consciously directs the client toward a behavioral change that will effect improvement in the client's physical or mental condition. This is in contrast to non-prescriptive recreational experience in the regular program of recreational activities where the client is exposed to a variety of activities from which he or she makes a choice and receives assistance from the recreationist only when it is needed to ensure optimum enjoyment from the experience. The values and benefits come about indirectly; they are not deliberately planned for and directly sought.

The prescription evolves from the diagnosis by the patient's physician or therapist of the pathologic condition of the patient and from the recommendations on ways in which the patient's specific needs may best be met in the recreational experience to be provided. Evaluations of needs and recommendations may also be received from other hospital personnel who have been closely involved with the patient. Based on all the information made available, the recreationist selects appropriate activities and develops a program for the individual patient.

Recreation infers an element of voluntary participation; however, therapeutic recreational service is prescriptive. Therefore, in developing activities for established needs, like those in the example above, effort must be made to provide opportunities to the clients for selection of activities to the extent of their competence to make choices that will satisfy the prescription. The recreationist does not necessarily permit a completely undirected choice but guidance is provided to assure that the clients participate in those activities that lead to satisfying the requirements of the prescription. A structured environment is maintained; otherwise it becomes difficult to adhere to the prescribed program and fulfill the diagnosed needs.

A structured environment although sometimes necessary for those with physical illnesses and disabilities, is particularly important when working with those with mental disabilities and emotional problems. Without structure, patients may very well do absolutely nothing or, in the case of the mentally ill, dwell on their own illnesses excessively. In the latter instance the patient is not being helped and, in fact, such permissiveness or nonstructured environment may actually contribute to deterioration since the pathologic behavior may reinforce itself and bring about further decline. A prescription may call for active relationship with one or more people, social contact, physical activity, or negation of inferiority or guilt feelings. The recreationist must then develop a program, having a variety of opportunities, from which the patient may select one or more for participation. The scope of a program might very well include everything from conversation to role-playing in a psychodrama, from swimming to oil painting, limited only by need, interest, knowledge, talent, or capacity to perform.

Adapted Recreational Activities

Adapted recreational activities are those in which the usual means of participation is altered or modified to accommodate the limitations of ill and disabled clients to enable them to experience the values and benefits inherent in recreational activities. It is recognized that prescribed recreational activities may also need to be modified to meet the special needs of the clients, but the total program is regarded as therapeutic because it is prescribed. It is expected that when recreationists adapt activities for the ill and disabled clients, they are also concerned that the recreational experience should help alleviate the physical, mental, or emotional problem(s) of the participant.

It is essential, of course, that the community provide opportunities for rehabilitated clients who are re-entering the community to utilize and expand the skills and talents that have been developed in the therapeutic recreational service program of the treatment center. Communication should occur between treatment center and community recreational services personnel so that the latter can be alerted when clients are returning to the community and be apprised of the abilities, interests, and special needs of each client. In many cases, the returning client will be able to participate in the community program with no special accommodation, but in other cases adaptations will need to be made. The adaptations may be in the way the skills of an activity are performed, in the equipment or facilities utilized for the activity, or in the nature of the activity itself. In general, they will be the same as or similar to modifications made by the therapeutic recreationist in the treatment center. Nearly all of the techniques and methods of serving clients in the therapeutic recreational services program of the treatment center can be used equally effectively in providing recreational services in the community setting for those with special needs arising from a disabling illness or injury.

Leisure Education and Recreation Participation

Leisure education and *recreational participation* are terms long utilized by the profession, but they have taken on new significance as the result of their being identified by the National Therapeutic Recreation Society (NTRS) as two specific areas of professional endeavor which together with a third area, therapy, provide a continuum of recreational services to ill and disabled clients.[8] The society describes leisure education as a service that provides opportunities for the acquisition of skills, knowledge, and attitudes relating to leisure involvement. "Recreation participation" is defined as a service that provides opportunities which allow voluntary client involvement in recreational interests and activities. The area of recreational participation is basic to community recreational programs but not to therapeutic recreation in treatment centers, where client involvement is not necessarily voluntary at least initially. Both types of programs engage in leisure education to some extent, the amount being determined by the specific objectives of the programs.

VALUES OF RECREATIONAL ACTIVITIES

The values of participation in recreational activities are the same for individuals who are ill and disabled as for those who are healthy and able bodied; but because the needs of the former are greater, the benefits are also greater. The benefits are many and varied; but for purposes of overview, they may be classified in these general categories: physical and motor fitness, mental health, social adjustment, and enjoyment. The categories are not mutually exclusive but rather overlap one another: factors that operate in one category may well influence the development or deterioration of the beneficial effects in the others.

Physical and Motor Fitness

The benefits of vigorous physical recreational activity are well documented. Regular participation in certain gross motor activities (sports, games, dance, and exercises) contributes to functional powers and stamina and has a positive effect on the physiologic structure of the muscular-skeletal system and specific organs of the body. These desirable results are due to improved physical fitness, specifically the development of several of the various components of physical fitness; muscular strength, flexibility, and cardiorespiratory and muscular endurance.[9] Also effected by strenuous physical activity, although not considered a physical fitness component, is body composition or body fat. Both of these terms refer to the percentage of total body weight that is fat. Achievement and maintenance of optimum body weight is facilitated through regular, vigorous exercise.

In addition to its contributions to physical fitness, participation in physical recreational activities develops motor fitness, i.e., improvement in the skills of motor performance. Commonly involved are such elements or components as eye-hand or eye-foot coordination, balance, and agility.[10] They are acquired through practice of motor skills which emphasize their use. Recreational activities that utilize fine and gross motor skills offer the opportunity to increase motor skills, and, hence, motor fitness.

Mental Health

Mental health refers to a mental state free from mental and emotional stress. Although not substantial, there is some evidence to demonstrate that a beneficial relationship exists between participation in recreational activities and good mental health. Among the evidence is a research study that indicates vigorous muscular activity provides a release from the anxiety and tension often experienced by individuals working in sedentary jobs.[11]

Kraus reports that the strongest support of the value of recreational activities' contribution to mental health comes from the psychiatrists.[12] Their research has established that the well-adjusted person has greater interest and engages more extensively in recreational activities than one with mental health problems. The first sign of recovery for the latter is often the return to participation in recreational activities. Although the exact effects of recreation upon the recovery of those with mental illnesses is not known, it has been established that a mentally healthy person utilizes recreational activities to satisfy needs.[13] It can, therefore, be surmised that specific needs of mentally ill individuals are also served to a satisfying degree by recreational activities and that in so doing, the return to normalcy is assisted.

Social Adjustment

Participation in recreational activities, because it necessitates a certain amount of social interaction, has value in promoting personal social adjustment. It is true that some activities, such as listening to music or stamp collecting, are by virtue of their self-involvement not highly social. Nevertheless, when undertaken in a recreational setting, the participant in this type of activity is encouraged to share his or her pleasure and enthusiasm with others who also enjoy the activity. All other recreational pursuits that involve group participation, which may be anything from play production to sports participation, require considerable social interaction in the form of giving and following directions, exchanging ideas, offering and responding to criticism, and reacting to the experience.

As individuals participate in a recreational activity, a basis is created for the development of new social skills or for rejuvenating or expanding old skills that have been lost or have grown "rusty" through disuse. The process of learning or of relearning is often painful and frustrating. But in a recreational setting, there are always people (recreational personnel and/or clients) present to offer encouragement and assistance. This is a particularly significant factor in achieving social adjustment.

Participation in recreational activities offers many opportunities for working together and sharing with others and for making friends and learning to adjust to the complex relationships that society imposes. The atmosphere is usually one of geniality because people are coming together in enjoyable activities. For many ill and disabled individuals, participation in the recreational program is one of the few opportunities they have for social interaction on an equal basis and for experiencing the warmth and congeniality of groups engaged in pleasing activity.

Enjoyment

Individuals engaging in recreational activities enjoy themselves. Participation, whether active or passive, promotes a feeling of pleasure in individuals because of their complete absorption in an interesting and satisfying experience. Enjoyment is felt even when the activity is laborious and fatiguing. Experiencing joy serves the ill or disabled person as a counterbalance to periods of pain and stress, so that enjoyment has significance in achieving and maintaining the emotional equilibrium necessary for well-being.

There is also evidence that enjoyment has positive effects on the physiologic functions of the body. That emotions influence the way the body responds has been well established by scientific study. Mind-sets of happiness and unhappiness have been shown to positively or negatively affect the digestive process, especially the digestion of fats. Fear and anxiety are known to cause the increased flow of adrenaline, which influences possibly adverse conditions or rapid heart rate and muscular tension. There is also recent evidence that points to the influence of affirmative feelings on the development of endorphin, a hormone in the pituitary gland that has an inhibiting effect on pain. The conclusion can be drawn from these examples that a happy, relaxed, positive state of mind produces certain desirable physiologic responses that favorably influence the health of the body. This relationship suggests enjoyment is equally as important to physical health as to mental health.

The enjoyment to be found in participation is one of the greatest benefits of recreation. Its value to those who are ill and disabled is inestimable.

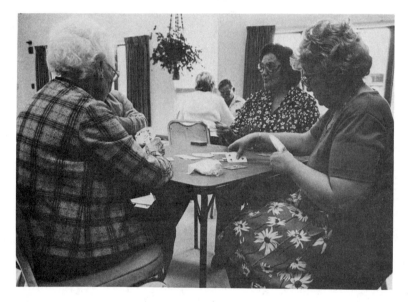

Fig. 1-1 Enjoyment is one of the great benefits of participation in recreational activity for special clients.

Attaining the Values

It must be recognized that the values of recreational services to the individual are not automatically realized through the act of participation. Only the potential for the development of the benefits is inherent in the recreational activities. Positive individual reaction to the program as well as circumstances appropriate to the development of the values must be present. This can be illustrated by an obvious example in the category of physical and motor fitness, where the personal commitment to regular exercise and the need for a program of increasingly strenuous workouts are essential for the values to be attained.

Individual differences also affect the degree of benefit received from recreational activities. Although basically all persons respond physiologically in a similar way to participation in physical recreational activities, the rate and degree of physical and motor fitness development are highly individualized. In contrast, the responses to situations of socialization tend to be different for different individuals, depending on their basic natures and experiences. The same observation might also be applied to the mental health aspect. Responses are affected, also, by other people: the mere presence of others can have a significant effect on individuals' intellectual and motor performance as well as their social reactions.[14]

In most cases, for recreational experiences to be of greatest value, they must be planned and tailored to the individual. This is particularly true if the individual has special needs due to illness or disability. Hence, the *raison d'etre* of therapeutic and adapted recreational services.

HISTORIC FOUNDATIONS

It is useful for the recreationist to have some knowledge of the historic development of recreational services for those who are ill and disabled. Information about the past helps to put modern day services for these persons in perspective and aids in the decision making process by furnishing a broader background. The presentation here is not intended to provide a complete discussion of the progress of therapeutic and adapted recreational services through the ages; rather, the intent is to provide an overview that will indicate, to those interested in reading further, the history of the periods and subject areas that will prove most fruitful for investigation. Sources of additional information are listed among the references found at the end of the chapter.

Treatment of mental and physical health problems through recreation has long been practiced. Historic evidence is not sufficiently precise to indicate when recreational activities were first used in therapy or when adaptations were first made to enable those with illness or injury to participate in the activities. However, ancient writings make frequent reference to the therapeutic use of recreational activities; and it is logical to assume that when the patient had difficulty engaging in an activity due to restrictions imposed by the condition, adaptations were devised and applied.

Primitive Civilizations

Specific evidence that primitive peoples utilized recreational activities for treating ailments is lacking. However, archaeologic findings do reveal that the campfire was a center of socialization as well as serving the utilitarian purposes of cooking and warmth. It is not too difficult to imagine that physically injured and mentally weary men and women, during such times as they were free to sit around the fire and talk and tell stories, experienced the "therapeutic" effect of the fire's heat and friendship's warmth.

Early Civilizations

As human society progressed, more systematic care and treatment for illness and injury developed. Although in various periods of early civilization, the attitude toward those who were sick and disabled was often one of complete rejection or benign neglect, there were also times and places where considerable humanitarian concern was manifested. Evidence indicates that the early societies of Egypt, Greece, Rome, and China all had well organized systems of care and treatment for their afflicted people.

Recognition of the therapeutic value of recreational activities by these ancient societies is apparent in their writings. Egyptians who were ill were advised by an unknown medical writer to walk in the gardens, take planned exercise, dance, and listen to concerts. The Greeks were urged by Pythagorus, a famous mathematician and teacher of the healing arts, to use music in conjunction with gymnastics and dancing to relieve mental disorders. A Roman physician prescribed recreational activities to help achieve relaxation of the body and mind, and in Roman hospitals patients were encouraged to walk in the sun to assist their recuperation.[15]

Evidence from the ancient societies of the Orient and India also indicates early recognition of the value of various forms of recreational activities in promoting the health of the mind and body of those with illnesses and injuries. In the fifth century a series of medical exercises called Cong Fu, which had been practiced in China since 2600 B.C., were recorded by a priest. These exercises when included with breathing exercises had as their purpose prolonging life and ensuring immortality. Another form of exercise, Tai Chi Chuan, also developed in ancient China, stressed slow, controlled, rhythmic movements that help to reduce the physical and mental stress that often prevents achieving the beneficial effects of exercise. Yoga, another therapeutic exercise, originated in ancient India. It was a system of mental and physical discipline by which the participant sought to attain union with an "ultimate principle."

Middle Ages and the Renaissance

Following the fall of the Roman Empire, the treatment and rehabilitation of ill and disabled people regressed in the general decline of intellectual and humanitarian endeavors of the Middle Ages. Treatment of mentally ill and physically disabled persons was almost universally unsympathetic and harsh. The former were often beaten and tortured to "drive out their madness" and to relieve them of the manifestations of their illness. Those with physical disabilities were socially shunned and often excluded from the work and affairs of the community. The hospitals of that day were devoid of any rehabilitative services; and since the morality of the times held play and leisure to be evil, any recreational activity was strictly forbidden.

The flowering of the humanistic spirit in the Renaissance reversed the earlier severe attitude and treatment of ill and disabled people. With the renewed interest of Renaissance scholars in early Greek culture, emphasis was again focused on the values of recreational activities as therapeutic tools.

The Period from 1600 to 1900

Over the succeeding centuries, recreational activities progressed slowly but steadily toward acceptance in the rehabilitative process for those receiving hospital care. Likewise, the distrust and reserve exhibited by the general public toward those with illnesses and disabilities gradually diminished. In these circumstances it was possible for a movement to be initiated for improved facilities and rehabilitation programs for those requiring hospitalization.

In the 1830s there were established what were known as insane asylums to house mentally ill patients away from the criminals with whom they had been incarcerated in penal institutions. With this recognition of the nature of mental illness, recreational activities began to be included in the program for the less mentally ill patients. During the last half of the nineteenth century, institutions specifically for the care and treatment of deaf, "feebleminded" * (mentally retarded), epileptic, and "crippled" * (orthopedically disabled) individuals were developed; and in all of these, over time, recreational programs were established.

Recent Years in the United States

With the beginning of the twentieth century, recreational activities for the ill and the disabled became a reality in many of our country's institutions that cared for such persons. The first programs were limited to dancing, table games, and passive entertainment. With the return of many disabled men from military service in World War I, concern grew for providing more complete recreational services, particularly in veterans' hospitals.

Federal legislation and funding helped to strengthen directly programs of rehabilitation, including recreational activities, in the hospitals for veterans and, indirectly, in other types of hospitals. As pointed out earlier, it was in federal legislation that the term *therapeutic recreation* was first

---

*These terms were used during the 1880s. Today the terms mentally retarded and orthopedically disabled, being more descriptive of the actual conditions, are the terms applied.

used; in 1938 the act creating the Works Progress Administration (WPA) used the term to describe all recreational activities intended to serve "disabled, maladjusted, or other institutionalized persons."

The entry of the United States into World War II and subsequent increases in the number of injured and disabled military personnel requiring rehabilitative care and treatment caused a dramatic expansion in therapeutic recreational services. All forms of recreational activities were sponsored with special emphasis given to sports.

In the years following the war, the growth in utilization of sport and other motor activities in recreational programs for disabled clients paralleled the rapid expansion in the use of physical therapy. The early efforts to offer sports and games were for purposes of therapy: the activities were viewed as a natural form of remedial exercises that complemented the conventional methods of physical therapy. However, in recent years sports, particularly competitive sports, for disabled players have come to be viewed as recreational rather than entirely rehabilitative.

At the same time that therapeutic recreational programs were emerging, programs of adapted recreational activities were being initiated. In many instances, they preceded the former because they were the first efforts in hospitals to provide appropriate recreational activities; to enable patients with physical or mental limitations to participate, recreationists modified the activities. With the eventual but inevitable recognition of the importance of recreational activities in the total rehabilitative effort, therapeutic recreational programs became an established service. Recreationists received from the medical doctors prescriptions for certain types of activities and then selected and presented specific activities, adapting them as required. Thus the adapted aspect of recreational services for hospitalized, ill and disabled clients gained professional recognition.

Adapted recreational services also took root in community programs as the efforts to serve all who wished to participate increased. Legislation passed in recent years made it easier for disabled persons to demand and receive all types of public services, including recreational services. In response, community recreational service personnel expanded the recreational opportunities for these individuals through adapting their program offerings as required by the needs of the clients.

In conjunction with the efforts by hospitals and communities to increase their recreational services for ill and disabled clients, interested recreational services personnel and people from the communities have formed several organizations whose objective is to promote such programs. One of the first of these groups was Hospital Recreation, a section of the existing American Recreation Society. Others that have developed more recently are the Recreation Therapy Section of the American Alliance for Health, Physical Education, Recreation and Dance and the National Association of Recreation Therapists (NART). The latter has in more recent years been incorporated into the National Recreation and Parks Association and is known as the National Therapeutic Recreation Society (NTRS). The purpose and work of these groups are discussed more fully in Chapter 2.

RECENT FEDERAL LEGISLATION

The legislative and judicial processes of the United States have affirmed that "handicapped" persons may not be denied equal access to services under any program that receives federal financial assistance. The Rehabilitation Act of 1973 and Public Law 94-112 (popularly known as the Civil Rights Act for the Handicapped) are broad, encompassing all aspects of the handicapped person's life, including the right to participate in recreational activities. The major thrust of the law may be summarized by stating that individuals may not be discriminated against because they are disabled.

In 1975 Congress approved passage of Public Law 94-142, the Education of the Handicapped Act, which establishes the right of all handicapped children to education in the "least restrictive environment." * This law includes several provisions that are designed to ensure that handicapped students receive a free appropriate public education. Each school must write an "Individualized Education Program (IEP)" for each student with a disability. The team responsible for developing the IEP must be composed of parents, the child's teacher, a representative of the school, and when appropriate, the child and other personnel as needed. The IEP team can require the provision of "related services" such as adapted or therapeutic recreation, physical therapy, and occupational therapy, if it is felt that such services are needed to ensure the total education of the child. When recreational service is required, schools must make it available to the child at school or arrange for time for participation in recreational programs outside the school.

OTHER THERAPEUTIC AND EDUCATIONAL MODALITIES

The recreationist working with ill and disabled clients in treatment centers is generally a member of a team of medical personnel and specialists in related therapies who combine their efforts to achieve the objective of recuperation or rehabilitation of the client. In institutions with educational programs for school age clients, the recreationist may be a member of an education team that seeks to help the client achieve optimum educational and social development. The same may be the case in the community where the recreationist may be invited to participate on the educational team for a child who has been diagnosed as needing partic-

---

* This refers to the provision of an educational environment that is *best* for the handicapped child whether the child is mainstreamed (integrated) in the regular class or is placed in a special class.

ipation in recreational activities available in the community but not in the school.

The therapies with which the recreationist is most likely to be involved in treatment centers are physical therapy, occupational therapy, and corrective therapy. Although these therapies are also sometimes found in the school setting, the person with whom the recreationist most often works closely in the school is the adapted or special physical educator. In both settings the team may include representatives of one or more of the activity therapies, among which includes art therapy, dance therapy, equestrian therapy, bibliotherapy, music therapy, industrial therapy, and horticulture therapy.[16]

These are newer, less established therapies that have in most cases developed from recreational activities in the therapeutic recreational program. Usually the activity therapies are not therapeutic in the sense that they are prescribed by medical personnel, but they are nevertheless activities from which ill and disabled clients can benefit. The art form activities like dance and art may be prescribed to promote nonverbal communication and individual expression; they are also frequently used by psychiatrists and psychologists for evaluation and diagnostic purposes.

Because of the interaction between personnel and the overlapping of some activities, the recreationist needs to be informed about the nature and objectives of those fields which are most commonly represented on the therapeutic or educational team.

Corrective Therapy

Corrective therapy is the treatment of ill and disabled individuals by medically prescribed activities designed to develop strength and endurance and to prevent muscular atrophy and general deconditioning (conditions resulting from lack of activity), both physically and psychologically, as the result of lengthy convalescence or inactivity due to illness or injury. The corrective therapy program offers specific exercises (including postural exercises), sports and games, socially oriented activities, and self-care activities. Orientation activities for those who are blind and motivational activities for the aged and infirmed are also included where appropriate.

Physical Therapy

Physical therapy is a therapeutic process to aid patients in their recovery from injury and disease. The primary concern is with impairment related to the neuromusculoskeletal, pulmonary, and cardiovascular systems. The work of the physical therapist includes evaluating the functions of these systems by means of various tests; selecting appropriate therapeutic procedures to maintain, improve, or restore the efficiency of the affected system; and then applying the selected procedures. Among the therapeutic procedures are exercises to increase muscular strength, endurance, coordination, and flexibility; promoting participation in the activities of daily living; increasing mobility; developing the ability to use assistive devices; and relieving pain. In addition, the physical therapist utilizes such modalities as heat, hydrotherapy, diathermy, ultrasound, ultraviolet, and electrical stimulation in the treatment.

Occupational Therapy

Occupational therapy is the art and science of directing an individual's response to selected activities to promote total well being of those who are ill and disabled. The therapeutic process utilizes a "program of normal activity" to promote physical restoration, to assist recovery from mental illness, to aid in training for independent living, and to contribute to psychosocial development. Additionally, in the case of an ill or disabled child, the therapy seeks to stimulate normal development; and in the case of an adult, it is directed toward assisting in vocational rehabilitation.

Adapted or Special Physical Education

The adapted or special physical education program * provides modified individualized or group developmental activities to handicapped students. Generally these activities are offered within the school, although they may be offered in community recreational facilities when these permit experiences needed by the student but not available in the school setting. The basic intent of the program is the development of the student's total well-being with specific emphasis on the improvement of motor skills and physical fitness through selected motor activities. Enhancement of leisure skills is not a primary objective as it is in the program of the school recreationist. Hence, the two programs supplement rather than duplicate each other.

REFERENCES

1. Jay S. Shivers, *Leisure and Recreation Concepts: A Critical Analysis,* (Boston: Allyn and Bacon, Inc., 1981) p. 210.
2. David E. Gray and Seymore Greben, "Future Perspective", (Arlington, Virginia: *Parks and Recreation,* July 1974) p. 43.
3. Office of Education, U.S.A., *Federal Register,* (Washington, D.C.: February, 1975) p. 42478.
4. American Association for Health, Physical Education and Recreation, *Guidelines for Professional Preparation for Personnel Involved in Physical Education and Recreation for the Handicapped,* (Washington, D.C.: American Association for Health, Physical Education and Recreation, 1973) p. 3.
5. Richard Kraus, *Therapeutic Recreation Service Principles and Practices,* 3rd ed., (Philadelphia: Saunders College Publishing, 1983) p. 26.

---

*Adapted physical education indicates a program consisting chiefly of modified activities, while special physical education is an umbrella term that includes all programs of physical education that serve the handicapped, such as adapted, developmental, and individualized. For a complete discussion, see the reference by Fait and Dunn at the end of the chapter.

6. Peter A. Witt, "Therapeutic Recreation: An Out-Moded Model", (Arlington, Virginia: *Therapeutic Recreation Journal,* 2nd quarter, 1977) pp. 31-41.
7. Gerald S. O'Morrow, *Therapeutic Recreation: A Helping Profession,* (Reston, Virginia: Reston Publishing Co., Inc., 1976) pp. 123-124.
8. Philosophical Statement Committee, *Committee Report on the NTRS Philosophical Statements,* University of Illinois, 1982, p. 1.
9. Hollis F. Fait and John M. Dunn, *Special Physical Education: Adapted, Individualized, Developmental,* 5th ed., (Philadelphia: Saunders College Publishing, 1984) p. 452.
10. Ibid, p. 452.
11. Herbert DeVires, *Physiology of Exercise,* 2nd ed., (Dubuque, Iowa: William C. Brown, Co., Publishers, 1971) pp. 278-281.
12. Richard Kraus, *op. cit.,* pp. 44-84.
13. William C. Menninger, "Recreation and Mental Health", (New York: *Recreation,* November, 1948) p. 340.
Alexander R. Martin, "Professional Attitudes and Practices", (Washington, D.C.: *Recreation for the Mentally Ill,* Conference Report American Association for Health, Physical Education and Recreation as reported by Richard Kraus, *op. cit.*) p. 45.
14. David R. Austin, *Therapeutic Recreation Processes and Techniques,* (New York: John Wiley and Sons, 1982) pp. 158-159.
15. Elliot M. Avedon, *Therapeutic Recreation Service: An Adapted Behavioral Science Approach,* (Englewood Cliffs, New Jersey: Prentice-Hall, Inc., 1974) p. 6.
Richard Kraus, *op. cit.,* pp. 19-20.
16. O'Morrow, Gerald, editor, Administration of Activity Therapy Service (Springfield: Charles C Thomas, 1966) passim.

SELECTED REFERENCES

Austin, David, *Therapeutic Recreation Process and Techniques* (New York: John Wiley and Sons, 1982).
Avedon, Elliott M., *Therapeutic Recreation Service: An Applied Behavioral Science Approach* (Englewood Cliffs, New Jersey: Prentice Hall, 1974).
Kraus, Richard G., *Therapeutic Recreation Service,* 3rd ed., (Philadelphia: Saunders College Publishing, 1983).
O'Morrow, Gerald S., *Therapeutic Recreation: A Helping Profession,* 2nd. ed., (Reston, Virginia: Reston Publishing Company, 1980).
Reille, Mary, ed., *Play As Exploratory Learning: Studies of Curiosity Behavior* (Beverly Hills, California: Sage Publications, 1974).

Chapter 2

Professional Development and Responsibilities

The roles, or types of positions, recreationists fill in treatment centers working under the direction of medical personnel or in community recreational centers providing adapted recreational activities entail the performance of specific responsibilities. The effectiveness with which these responsibilities are carried out determines the quality of recreational service that clients receive. A program is only as good as the people who operate it, so it follows that recreationists must not only be fully aware of the nature of their responsibilities, but also have the training necessary to execute them with competence. Certain personal attributes are also important to the effective performance of the obligations inherent in the roles; if these qualities are not already among the attributes the recreationist possesses, effort must be made to develop them. A high level of professional competencies and outstanding personal attributes, however, cannot produce special recreational service of the highest order without there being also strict adherence to standards of ethical conduct.

Even the best recreationists need to expand their knowledge and skills and revitalize their personal commitment. Professional development must continue throughout the career of the recreationist. Many opportunities for doing so are available, ranging from continuing education courses to membership in professional organizations. While they must be concerned with self-improvement, recreationists must also concern themselves with improving the public image of their profession through effective public relations focusing on promoting public awareness and support.

ROLES AND RESPONSIBILITIES

Recreationists who are trained to offer special services to ill and disabled clients fill such professional roles as administrators or supervisors in therapeutic or adapted recreational service programs or as organizers and conductors of the activities offered in these programs.

The chief responsibilities of those in administrative and supervisory roles fall into these broad categories: staffing, long-range planning, personnel problems, finances and budget, maintenance, and public relations. In order to carry out the many activities that comprise each category, administrators and supervisors need to have a good understanding of and a certain proficiency in the skills and abilities associated with organizing and conducting the program activities. In some situations, e.g., in a small community center with limited staff, supervisors or administrators may be directly involved in the responsibilities of recreational participation and leisure education.

Those recreationists who organize and conduct the adapted recreational activities are responsible for the effective daily operation of the program. Their special responsibilities may be categorized as: selection of appropriate activities, scheduling, making equipment and supplies available, instruction of clients in adapted recreational skills, offering guidance and support to clients, and participation as needed in the business and public relations matters of the recreational center.

In community centers, recreationists are involved with the community as a whole. Not only do they organize and conduct adapted recreational activities at the center for clients with special needs, but they actively seek to make all recreational resources in the community available and accessible to ill and disabled community residents. In carrying out this responsibility recreationists become advocates or consultants for the development of community recreational service. Responsibility for leisure education often becomes as integral part of the conduct of the program.

Recreationists may also be employed by private agencies that have programs in which recreational activities have a prominent role and who are, consequently, interested in extending participation to handicapped people in the community. In providing special recreational programs in these agencies, recreational directors and supervisors must make the same considerations in selecting and conducting the activities for ill and disabled clients as those made by adapted recreationists in community centers.

Also, recreationists with training in special recreational services are being increasingly called upon to assist community schools in providing leisure evaluations and leisure education for handicapped students. The need for such services has been given emphasis by the mandate of Public Law 94-142 (requirements of the law are discussed in Chapter 6).

The therapeutic recreationists have slightly different responsibilities due to the usual practice in treatment centers of including them on the rehabilitation team. As members of the team, they participate in setting goals for the clients and identify recreational activities that will assist in reaching the goals; after which, the therapeutic recreationists develop a plan of specific activities for each client, based on prescription or recommendations. Therapeutic recreationists also take on the functions of a leisure educator and share in the responsibility of preparing the client to return to the community and become integrated into the recreational activities offered there.

COMPETENCIES

To fill the important responsibilities of their roles effectively, recreationists must have certain competencies, that is, abilities based on knowledge and skill. The necessary competencies have been identified by the National Council for Therapeutic Recreation [1] and by directors of college and university "competency based programs"* preparing personnel in therapeutic and adapted recreational service. The competencies listed below are representative of those generally included in the competency based programs. They are grouped under four general functions or tasks that need to be performed by recreationists offering special recreational service.

Function 1. Acquiring Accurate Knowledge

Perhaps the most essential function that a recreationist in any role must perform is that of acquiring accurate knowledge for application to the development and improvement of the special recreational service. This is so important because it is fundamental to all other functions. Accurate knowledge is obtained by locating reliable sources of information, which are usually printed materials but can also be examination of reputable programs and discussion with experienced practitioners. Data and pertinent information from these sources are then analyzed and interpreted to assess reliability and determine applicability to the particular situation. Only then can the information be considered worthy of incorporation into the planning, procedures, and practices of the program. The list that follows identifies the specific competencies needed for effective performance of the function.**

- Ability to locate printed and non-printed instructional and theoretical materials from various sources and to utilize these resources, including information retrieval centers, libraries, and other special instructional materials centers.

- Proficiency in interpreting and evaluating research.

- Knowledge of the historic evolution of therapeutic and adapted recreational services; utilization of history in the consideration of contemporary problems.

---

*A competency based program is one in which the competencies (general and specific) have been identified and prepared in written form, and all instructional and evaluation procedures are directed toward competencies achievement through continuous assessment. Programs of this kind whose competencies were reviewed for possible inclusion in this presentation are those of the University of Connecticut, Temple University, and the University of North Carolina at Chapel Hill.

**Competencies are presented in a form known as "program objective." Many educational institutions interpret these competencies as behavioral objectives, i.e., specific outcomes that can be measured quantitatively. The nature and purpose of the types of objectives are discussed in Chapter 6.

- Knowledge of federal and state laws with respect to equal protection and non-discrimination provisions for the handicapped.

- Understanding the responsibility of schools in providing leisure evaluation of handicapped students and leisure education when necessary, as required by Public Law 94-142.

- Familiarity with the state, national, and international agencies and organizations established to serve and promote therapeutic recreational service and establish standards (including certification and registration) for the profession.

- Ability to analyze and evaluate various educational theories of learning particularly as they influence leisure education.

- Knowledge of how recreational skills are learned, utilized, and retained.

- Understanding the process of providing a continuum of therapeutic recreational service to clients.

- Ability to gather input from the client and his or her family in developing a viable recreational program for the client.

- Understanding the need to act in accordance with the highest standards of practice in therapeutic and adapted recreational services, i.e., professional ethics.

Function 2. Utilization of Information

A second important function is the utilization of information and recommendations from various sources to develop an appropriate therapeutic or adapted recreational service program. This involves identifying the social, emotional, and physical needs of the ill and disabled clients as the basis for program development. Accurate observation is essential to the function as is the utilization of appropriate assessment and evaluation tools. The competencies required to perform this function effectively are given below.

- Ability to comprehend basic medical terminology including psychiatric terminology and to communicate with medical personnel concerning therapeutic recreational needs of the ill and disabled.

- Ability to determine whether an individual's performance in social, emotional, and physical settings is appropriate.

- Awareness of the physical, social, and emotional developmental patterns of people.

- Knowledge of anatomy and physiology with particular regard to the development of physical fitness and normal movement.

- Understanding of the adjustment problems created by illness and disability.

- Ability to recognize situations that will negatively affect the self-concept of the ill or disabled person.

- Ability to select the most appropriate environment to ensure effective learning of physical, social, cultural, and other skills.

- Ability to provide leisure counseling and education to families of the client as well as to the client.

- Ability to determine basic facility and equipment needs for the development of recreational activities for ill and disabled clients and to modify and design/construct equipment to be utilized in an adapted program of recreational experiences.

- Ability to work with various agencies, organizations, and institutions, including schools, to develop the most appropriate recreational program for ill and disabled individuals.

Function 3. Organizing and Conducting

The function of organizing and conducting appropriate recreational activities is the core of the program around which all else revolves. The execution of the function requires the performance of a multitude of tasks whose nature can be described as being either the utilization of information about the needs of the clients; the provision of recreational activities that satisfy these needs; or the evaluation of how well the needs have been met. The list of competencies below indicates the breadth of scope in the function of organizing and conducting recreational activities.

- Ability to determine effective learning progression for teaching a variety of recreational activities to each individual.

- Ability to determine objectives and design programs for clients with special needs in recreational service and to recommend recreational objectives for handicapped school children, as provided by federal law.

- Ability to interpret medical prescriptions for individual clients and to select appropriate recreational activities for specific atypical conditions and levels of ability.

- Ability to modify and adapt activities to enable the ill and disabled individual to participate.

- Ability to integrate recreational activities with other social, cultural, educational, and physical programs to meet the needs of the ill and disabled clients.

- Ability to interpret recommendations from clinical reports and the prescriptions from medical personnel as well as from the observations and analyses of the condition and nature of the disabled person by specialists involved.

- Ability to utilize appropriate behavior modification techniques and to recognize their uses and abuses.

- Ability to identify activity tolerance levels for participation in various recreational activities and to apply knowledge of precautionary measures necessary when providing activities for those with various disabilities.

- Knowledge of various assistive devices and techniques to aid clients in ambulation, transfer, and communication.

- Ability to provide necessary safety measures and emergency health care in such cases as incontinence, seizures, and reactions to medication.

- Ability to recognize the reactions to the use of specific drugs administered in the treatment of convulsive and emotional disorders.

- Knowledge of the nature of competition and its use and misuse in adapted recreational service.

- Knowledge of the nature of creativity and the ways it may be stifled or encouraged in recreational activities.

- Ability to work with ill and disabled people from different ethnic and racial backgrounds.

- Ability to develop a plan and procedures for the leisure education of clients, including the development of recreational skills for independent living by severely disabled persons.

- Ability to observe any clients' capabilities and to develop a record of their social, physical, and intellectual performance.

- Ability to develop an evaluation schema to determine the degree of success in accomplishing the objectives of the therapeutic recreational program.

- Ability to assist the client in making the transition from the treatment center to the community when the client is discharged.

- Ability to recommend recreational activities for bedside / homebound clients.

- Ability to organize and prepare routine reports required by the employing agency.

Function 4. Administering and Supervising

The function of administering and supervising therapeutic and adapted recreational service is essential to success in meeting the needs of the clients. The nature of the function can be described as the development of an environment in which the therapeutic or adapted program can function to its optimum in providing a beneficial recreational experience to clients in the program. The competencies required to perform the various tasks associated with producing this desirable environment are presented below. It should be recognized that in small programs there may be no administrative staff in therapeutic recreational service and the practitioner will need to perform some of these functions.

- Ability to formulate a philosophy of recreation for serving ill and disabled clients and to develop policies and procedures consistent with the philosophy.

- Ability to secure adequate staff and other necessary personnel.

- Ability to develop an appropriate budget with clearly presented justifications.

- Ability to conduct or participate effectively in staff and administration meetings.

- Ability to identify funding sources and develop grant applications for additional revenue.

- Ability to prepare a good public relations program.

- Ability to supervise employed personnel, volunteers, and students serving internships.

- Ability to assist staff members to identify and overcome weaknesses and to encourage them to keep abreast of new information and developments.

- Knowledge of current laws that protect and provide services to special populations.

PROFESSIONAL PREPARATION

Although not all professional training programs are competency based, they do all have specific objectives or outcomes that are to be achieved by the students so that they may enter the profession equipped with the knowledge and skills to perform their responsibilities capably and participate in the general community as effective citizens. Toward this end, the curricula of the training programs in therapeutic recreational service are designed to give students exposure to courses of a general educational nature as well as to courses of specialized knowledge. Hence, the first two years of baccalaureate work usually comprise courses in the humanities, physical and biological sciences (anatomy and physiology), social studies (sociology and gerontology), psychology, and the fine arts.

With these courses, students receive the foundation to assimilate more advanced study in the field of specialization during the final two undergraduate years. The specialized courses are directed toward providing information and skill development in each of the basic aspects of well constructed and efficiently operated recreational service for ill and disabled clients. Courses are offered in these general areas: philosophy of recreation, therapeutic recreational service, therapeutic application of the performing arts, recreational skill courses dealing with specific pathologies, community institutions and organizations, administration and supervision, communication arts—public relations, psychology, rehabilitation, psychology of the handicapped, special education, evaluation, and practical experience. The course offering practical experience is usually called the practicum, field experience, or internship; but regardless of the specific course title, the purpose is to provide actual on-the-job participation in a program of special recreational service under the close supervision of professional personnel.

Students who are majoring in recreational service, rather than therapeutic recreational service, need to be prepared to plan programs and offer activities adapted to the needs of those clients who cannot participate in the regular program of the community center because of limitations imposed by illness or disability. To provide the necessary instruction in adapted recreational service, the training program may require an introductory course, like the one for which this book is intended, and offer elective choices from among the therapeutic recreational service courses. The objective is to give the students sufficient knowledge about the etiology and pathology of common illnesses and disabilities to be able to make appropriate adaptations of activities and to understand the medical terminology applied to the conditions thoroughly enough to communicate about the clients with medical personnel and to put their recommendations for recreational activity into effect.

A number of two-year community colleges offer a training program in recreational service with concentration in therapeutic recreational service. The usual curricula of these programs provide courses in both general background and specialized knowledge, although both aspects are necessarily somewhat restricted.

The associate arts degree, which is awarded upon completion of the two-year college preparation, provides the graduate with sufficient skills and knowledge to gain employment in a variety of treatment centers or institutions. Such positions are characterized by direct or face-to-face instruction or programming for patients or clients. For the most part, the two-year degree permits entry level employment. Community college graduates generally have a number of alternatives from which to choose. They may seek additional education by transferring to four-year colleges, or they may gain immediate employment on a full-time basis in the field. The possibility of some combination of work and continued study is also available.

ATTRIBUTES

Perhaps the single most important attribute that recreationists working with ill and disabled clients can possess is emotional maturity. Emotional maturity is the ability to solve problems and adjust to circumstances without undue emotional involvement. Recreationists must be a stabilizing influence, must represent to the clients the ultimate in successful adjustment. Recreationists who are unable to resolve their own psychologic problems are not likely to be able to assist clients in solving their problems. Particularly immature behavior may even contribute to the maladjustment of clients rather than help them make satisfactory adjustments to their illness or disability.

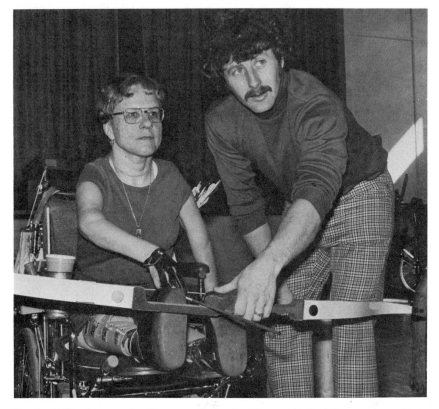

Fig. 2-1 Enthusiasm and patience on the part of the recreationist encourage clients to meet the challenge of acquiring adapted recreational skills. (Greater Hartford Cerebral Palsy Center).

Patience and a sense of humor are indispensable qualities in any good recreationist. Those who work with the ill and disabled need to be endowed with a generous portion of each, for progress is more often than not very, very slow. When the results of long hours of work do manifest themselves, however, they are extremely rewarding to the client and to the recreationist.

A good imagination is yet another desirable attribute in those who work with ill and disabled clients, for it may be necessary to improvise equipment as well as techniques for performing recreational skills. When facilities and equipment for the adapted activities are limited, imaginative recreationists adjust and modify the available facilities and equipment to fit the requirements of the program. They meet the challenge of an unusual handicap by devising suitable adaptations of the activities to meet the needs of the particular individual.

Also important among the attributes that those providing special recreational services should possess is the quality of leadership. An effective leader is more important than good equipment, fine facilities, or any other single contributing factor. Strong recreational leadership springs from great enthusiasm for involving everyone in appropriate activities, regardless of capabilities. Good leaders are convinced of the contributions they can make to the lives of the ill and the disabled and have developed numerous methods and techniques to implement the program. They recognize potential sources of failure and are willing and able to make adjustments that will ensure a successful outcome. Moreover, they have the ability to communicate their enthusiasm and insights to others.

PROFESSIONAL ETHICS

Some long established professions have set standards of conduct for their members, like the Hippocratic oath of the medical profession; others, among them the special recreational services, have no formal statement defining professional ethics. In such instances, individuals must be guided in their professional conduct by personal principles.

All those worthy of being called therapeutic or adapted recreationists are motivated by a desire to enhance the lives of others by enabling them to experience the benefits of recreational service. Service is the heart of their chosen profession and to give the best possible service is a commitment, a guiding principle. Hence, action that benefits the recreationist rather than the client violates the principles of service. Actions that are undertaken for monetary rewards or personal aggrandizement are unprincipled in the extreme. When circumstances require a decision between personal interests and those of clients, principled recreationists put the interest of the client unequivocally before their own.

Because they serve the welfare of people whose lives have limitations imposed by illness or disability, those in the profession regard as a principle the right of all to equal opportunities. Accordingly, recreationists work to ensure that no clients are denied participation in any recreational activity of the program that is not contraindicated by their condition. It would be unthinkable in the context of this principle to allow considerations of color, creed, religion, ethnic origin, sex, or age to enter into a program decision. Equally unprincipled are other actions or comments reflecting personal biases or prejudices against clients or fellow workers.

The need to seek the truth and espouse it is so essential to providing good special recreational services that it serves as a principle to guide ethical conduct. In adherence to the principle, recreationists attempt to discover and analyze all the facts before drawing conclusions. They refuse to bend to social pressure or popular opinion or to yield to expediency when making decisions. They do not attempt to mislead or deliberately falsify information even to benefit the program, nor do they violate the rights and privacy of clients. Ignorance and misconceptions are challenged respectfully but firmly; to do less is to compromise truth.

The democratic ideals that are the basis of government in our country are also good principles for professional conduct in relationships between administration and staff, between staff members, and between staff and clients. Conduct that ignores the democratic process in decision making, that denies presentation of minority or unpopular viewpoints, or that denigrates the worth of the individual is unethical in the most definitive sense of the word.

CERTIFICATION AND LICENSING

Certification refers to the act of attesting to the qualifications of someone or something. Licensing is the act of giving formal permission by a constituted authority to do something. The certification to practice a profession is usually provided by an organization or a college or university, while licensing is the legal right to practice given by a governing body, usually a state, county, or city.

In the case of therapeutic recreational service, certification is granted by the National Council for Therapeutic Recreation Certification,[2] an independent administrative body of the National Recreation and Park Association. The Council has established national standards of training and performance for two levels of certification: (1) Professional: Therapeutic Recreation Specialist and (2) Para-Professional: Therapeutic Recreation Assistant. A complete description of the requirements of each level is found in Appendix I.

Some state recreation and park associations, in addition, although they have not developed certification plans, do have a "registration" program that sets up standards which an applicant must meet before becoming registered as a therapeutic recreationist in the state. The difference between registration and certification has not been clearly established in the states that have chosen to register therapeutic recreationists.

At present, only one state, Utah, has passed legislation for licensing of therapeutic recreationists. The law establishes requirements for various levels of therapeutic recreational service for the issuance of the license and also makes provisions for suspension or revocation of the license.

CONTINUING EDUCATION

The professional in any field must continually keep abreast of new information and developments to maintain the highest possible quality in performance of responsibilities and rendering of service. The means by which this continuing education is achieved are varied according to the profession. For recreational therapists, one way is taking courses or enrolling in a master's degree program at a nearby college or university. Those who develop a special interest as the result of the advanced course work continue to pursue that specialization in work toward a doctoral degree.

Other means of keeping well informed and up-to-date, which are perhaps more readily available to most recreational service personnel, are reading the professional literature and attending workshops, conferences, and institutes. Current issues of books, periodicals, and other publications and audiovisual materials on a wide range of related subjects are available at college and university libraries. Local public libraries generally do not subscribe to professional literature, but they can usually supply a list of publishing companies and their addresses to which requests can be made for catalogs with descriptions of books that may be useful to the practitioner. National professional organizations often publish a variety of materials, as well as scholarly journals, that are available to or may be ordered by the membership, but which can often be purchased by non-members.

Participation in workshops, conferences, and institutes provides unequalled opportunities for continuing education. Many colleges and universities and state agencies conduct workshops and institutes for professionals who live within the service area of the sponsoring institution. National, and also many state, organizations and societies hold annual conferences for professional personnel with the distinct purpose of distributing information about new trends, research findings, methods and techniques, and other relevant developments. While the meetings are open only to members, the information is sometimes available in the form of pamphlets, etc. to non-members at small cost.

PROFESSIONAL ORGANIZATIONS

A number of professional organizations have developed in response to the need those in the field have for assistance and support from authoritative bodies. The help the organizations offer in addition to their continuing education resources, may be in the form of: directly applicable advice, information and materials; sponsoring conferences, workshops, and institutes; creation of public awareness of the values and benefits of the profession; support for research and other scholarly endeavors that add to professional knowledge and improve practices and procedures; establishing standards for professional training, performance on the job, and ethical conduct; and promotion of professional preparation programs.

As might be expected of groups that are organized to serve the profession, changes occur in the organizations in response to significant shifts in emphasis and direction of the profession. In the last decade or so, a considerable number of such changes have been effected among the organizations: Some of the organizations have amalgamated, some have taken new names, and others have discontinued. It is expected that as the nature of therapeutic and adapted recreational service continues to alter, the professional organizations will change as they have done in the past to meet new challenges. At present there are three major organizations on the national level: the National Therapeutic Recreation Society; the American Alliance for Health, Physical Education, Recreation and Dance; and the National Consortium on Physical Education and Recreation for the Handicapped.

National Therapeutic Recreation Society

The National Therapeutic Recreation Society (NTRS) was established as a branch of the National Recreation and Park Association when it was formed in 1965 through the merging of several separate organizations that had developed over the years to represent different aspects of recreational service. All of those groups in the merger that were involved with recreational service for ill and disabled clients became part of the NTRS. In addition to providing the types of services described above, the NTRS publishes a quarterly periodical, *Therapeutic Recreation Journal.* The society's "Philosophical Position Statement" is given in Appendix II. Membership is open to students as well as professionals in therapeutic recreational service.

American Alliance for Health, Physical Education, Recreation and Dance

The American Alliance for Health, Physical Education, Recreation and Dance (AAHPERD), which is an alliance of various groups with related interests, includes two associations that have units within their organization concerned with recreational services for special populations. The two groups are the Association for Leisure and Recreation (ALR) and the Association for Research, Administration, Professional Counseling and Societies (ARAPCS). The units of the two associations provide assistance and support to professionals in special recreational service by means of the activities identified above. Student memberships are invited.

National Consortium on Physical Education and Recreation for the Handicapped

Established in 1973, the National Consortium of Physical Education and Recreation for the Handicapped (NCPERH) was originally called the National Advisory Council on Physical Education and Recreation for Handicapped Children and Youth. It is an organization of individuals with expertise and extensive work in the fields of adapted physical education and therapeutic recreational service. Its purpose is to promote professional preparation programs and research in physical education and recreational service for special populations. In addition to conducting an annual meeting, NCPERH publishes a quarterly newsletter and is active in supporting legislative efforts to improve conditions for those who are handicapped.

PROMOTION OF THE PROFESSION AND PUBLIC RELATIONS

Members of a profession have a responsibility to enhance and promote the profession. The easiest and most obvious way of doing this is joining one or more professional organizations like the National Therapeutic Recreation Society, and then becoming an active participant by attending meetings, serving on committees, and filling offices. The support of many members enables an organization to provide better service to those in the field and to conduct more effective public relations to make the public aware of the value of the profession in meeting society's needs.

On another level, promotion of the profession is accomplished through the sharing of experiences either in the form of informal lectures or scientific papers or as published materials in magazines, scholarly journals, and books. Useful ideas for practical application are developed continuously by practitioners in response to specific program needs, and new information is constantly being discovered by researchers and investigators in the profession. The communication of these innovative practices and newly discovered knowledge is essential to the vitality of the profession; and everyone has a responsibility to participate in it.

Promotion of the profession must occur also at the local level in the community or general service area of the program. In addition to building understanding and respect for the service being provided by therapeutic and adapted recreationists, public relations efforts at this level serve several other important purposes:

- To inform ill and disabled individuals of the recreational opportunities available to them and encourage their participation.

- To stimulate financial support by the municipal government and local philanthropic and service organizations and by individual donors.

- To encourage schools to provide leisure evaluation of handicapped students and education in leisure skills when necessary as required by federal law.

- To interest people in volunteering their assistance.

Specific ways of reaching the public include news stories and feature articles in newspapers and on radio and television. Also, opportunities can be created to attract people into the recreational facility such as an open house, special program, or guided tour. Attractively printed flyers and brochures that can be handed out to the visitors and also distributed at local stores, library, and other places where people go frequently represent another effective public relations endeavor.

REFERENCES

1. National Council for Therapeutic Recreation Certification, "Current Revision," February, 1983, p. 4.
2. Ibid, p. 2.

SELECTED REFERENCES

Carter, Marcia and James, Ann, "Continuous Professional Development Programs for Therapeutic Recreation," *Therapeutic Recreation Journal,* 3rd Quarter, (1979), p. 13.

Goldstein, Judith E., *Consultation: Enhancing Leisure Service Delivery to Handicapped Children and Youth* (Arlington, Virginia: National Recreation and Park Association, 1977).

Navar, Nancy and Dunn, Julia, eds., *Quality Assurance—Concern for Therapeutic Recreation* (Champaign–Urbana: University of Illinois Department of Leisure Studies, 1981).

Van Andel, Glen E., "Professional Standards: Improving the Quality of Service," *Therapeutic Recreation Journal,* 2nd Quarter, (1981), pp. 23-26.

Witt, Peter A., "Professionalism / Certification / Accreditation: What's At Stake?" *Leisure Commentary and Practice* (Denton, Texas: North Texas State University, Division of Recreation and Leisure Studies, March, 1982).

Chapter 3

Theories, Processes, and Instruments

All effective programs for special populations involve theories, processes, and instruments to accomplish their objectives. Theories, which are particular concepts or views of the way in which something should function, form the foundation and point the direction for the special recreational service program. The processes or systematic actions and procedures and the specific instruments, i.e., the tools, devices, and activities, are sanctioned by the theories that guide the program.

In the discussion that follows, theories from several fields of study are presented to develop an understanding of the source of specific processes and instruments that are used in therapeutic and adapted recreational service. It should be remembered while studying the various theories, processes, and instruments, that no one of them is always effective with clients. Because this is true, knowledge of many ways to reach and help the client is extremely important.

THE REHABILITATIVE PROCESS

Rehabilitation is the provision of a variety of specific services to effect restoration of the patient to the highest possible level of health and capacity to function socially and economically when these have been impaired by disabling illness or injury.* From a purely medical view, rehabilitation can be said to be the utilization by medical personnel of all measures in the realm of medicine that hasten the patient's recovery. In the broader sense, which is the interpretation applicable to this discussion, rehabilitation includes various services that are supplemental to the medical treatment and continue beyond the time that medical treatment is

---

*The rehabilitative process for criminal offenders and juvenile delinquents has a different focus from that of rehabilitation of ill and disabled clients and will, therefore, be discussed in chapter 11.

the preemptive service. Rehabilitation begins when the patient is sufficiently recovered for medication to be discontinued and/or has regained full, or is able to utilize residual, physical function; it ends when the patient is restored as fully as possible to normal social and economic functioning. A succinct description of the rehabilitative process is offered by Krusen:

> Rehabilitation is a creative procedure which includes the cooperative efforts of various medical specialists and their associates in other health fields to improve the physical, mental, social, and vocational aptitudes of persons who are handicapped, with the objective of preserving their ability to live happily and productively on the same level and with the same opportunities as their neighbors.[1]

Rehabilitation—Multidisciplinary Practices

Rehabilitation is a multidisciplinary practice in which a variety of medical and therapeutic specialists combine their expertise in evaluating, treating, and optimizing the social, emotional, physical, and occupational capabilities of the client. The team approach enables concentration of collective effort on enhancing the residual functions to effect the fullest possible recovery of the individual being treated. Included on the team are medical doctors, therapists, and other specialists from the four basic areas of rehabilitation: biophysical, psychologic, social, and occupational. The therapeutic recreationist is one of the team members.

After an initial appraisal is made of the client's abilities and needs by members of the team, a group conference is held for the purpose of reaching an understanding about the kind of individualized treatment plan that can be developed to enable the client to be restored to the fullest degree of independence possible. Each specialist contributes suggestions based on assessment and/or observations made of the client to help establish general objectives for the rehabilitation program. When these have been established, the specialists make specific recommendations and choices of activities that each will offer to effect achievement of the objectives. The members of the team conceive the purpose of their program as being not just the repair or restoration of the individual but preparation for the complete integration of the client into the community with all of the prerogatives and skills necessary to ensure self-respect, personal fulfillment, and social acceptance.

HOMEOSTASIS

The theory of homeostasis helps to explain why therapeutic recreational service contributes so significantly to the rehabilitation of those who are ill and disabled. The theory advances the idea that the life process is homeostatic, i.e., it has a tendency to maintain internal stability;[2] therefore, a balance between tension and relaxation is essential to human beings. The human body has a need for both physiologic recovery and for psychologic recuperation after intensive work performance. As people deplete physical and psychic energy during the survival or work phase of their lives, they must recover their equilibrium during the recreational and rest phase. The accommodation between survival expenditure and recreation for recovery is vital for a balanced life and the maintenance of the healthy organism.

Deviation from the typical patterns of health—illness, trauma, or permanent crippling—is capable of interrupting the cycle of the homeostatic process. In these circumstances it becomes difficult, because of increased emotional stress and physical pain, to achieve the necessary counterbalancing effects of relaxation and recreation. Rehabilitation assists the restoration of the desired balance. Therapeutic recreational service plays a vital role in the rehabilitative process and thereby contributes to homeostasis. The adapted recreational service program continues the contribution to the development and maintenance of the homeostatic process upon the client's return to the community.

MOTIVATION

According to Wloodkowski the word motivation applies to processes that can (a) arouse and instigate behavior; (2) give direction or purpose to behavior; (3) continue to allow behavior to persist; (4) lead to choosing or performing a particular behavior.[3] Consideration of the ways in which the process can be utilized to achieve desirable behavior has produced several theories on motivation. Two of the most popular of these theories are humanism and behaviorism.

Humanism

Humanism regards the use of the reasoning process as the most important factor in behavior. If individuals utilize reasoning in arriving at decision about their actions, according to this theory they will behave in ways that are best for themselves as individuals and for the society in which they live.[4] Thus desirable behavior is motivated by the reward of knowing that an action or response was the best possible one in the situation.

Extrinsic rewards are not utilized to influence the outcome of the reasoning process. Basing behavior on the receipt of an extrinsic reward tends to make the reward become the goal and not the behavior. This view is supported by evidence to the effect that intrinsic rewards are much more effective in altering behavior of a permanent nature than are extrinsic rewards.

The humanistic approach may be utilized by recreationists to help clients alter behavior to their advantage. These clients need to assess past experiences to identify what happened and why it happened. Analyzing former experiences and their results develops insight into the relationship between thought and action. This leads to examination of how the results in a former experience would have been changed had a logical choice of action been made through the process of reasoning. Encouragement and support are given as the client applies the reasoning process in new situations.

It should be noted that the humanistic approach to motivating behavior cannot be applied in every situation. Fait and Dunn have observed that, "Experience with learners of various levels of intelligence confirms the development of a reasoning process that enables a person to make a decision with respect to most desirable behavior is dependent upon the capacity to reason and possess an adequate degree of emotional stability." [5] Consequently, the humanistic method is most effective when there is no intellectual limitation and no emotional problems are involved.

Behaviorism

Behaviorism is a theory that regards the observation of the behavior of an individual as the basis of understanding the psychology of that person's behavior. This is in contrast to theories that have developed on the premise that hidden unconscious forces underlie the behavior of an individual. Behaviorism emphasizes that behavior is controlled by its consequences. In general, behaviors that are rewarded will continue, those that are not or have negative outcomes will not. This concept is the basis for a method of motivation to change behavior known as behavior modification.

Behavior Modification. Behavior modification or operant conditioning is defined as a systematic use of selected reinforcers (rewards or punishments) to weaken, maintain, or strengthen behavior. There are several techniques and the degree of success that can be had with each depends upon the nature of the intellectual or emotional problems of the individual with whom the technique is being used.

With mentally retarded individuals, for example, positive reinforcement and modeling are used. Positive reinforcement refers to providing a reward, usually extrinsic, for the performance of a desirable behavior. Modeling is a technique whereby an action or a skill that is to be learned is demonstrated for the learner.

The two techniques can be used in combination, so that success in performing the action that was modeled is a reward. With severely retarded individuals it is sometimes necessary to provide the reinforcer for their having allowed a part of the body to be moved in simulation of the desired movement or for their responding to a demonstration by turning the head or eyes.

Types of Reinforcers. Several types of reinforcers may be used. These include favorite food items, toys or trinkets, and auditory or visual stimuli such as showing pictures or films or playing records. Verbal praise and attention are often effective reinforcers and ones that are easily administered. Selection of the optimum reinforcer depends upon the likes and dislikes of the client and the ability of the client to understand. For a large majority of the mentally retarded clients, praise or acknowledgment of the success of their attempt is the most effective reinforcer. It is also an excellent reinforcer in many cases for the emotionally disturbed. For severely retarded clients a reinforcer of food is more effective in inducing the desired results.

Regardless of the type of reinforcer used, the time between when the desired reaction or movement is made and when the reinforcer is given should be as short as possible to increase the probability that the client will recognize a relationship between the reward and the action. It is obvious that the reward should be given consistently and only for the desired performance.

Other techniques of behavior modification that are frequently used are negative reinforcement and extension. While these are appropriate under specific circumstances for the mentally retarded, they are generally used for those with behavior problems. However, positive reinforcement and modeling are also used effectively with clients who have behavior problems and also with those who are emotionally disturbed.

Negative Reinforcement and Punishment. Negative reinforcement, sometimes referred to as adverse control, is the use of punishment as the reinforcer. It is used to reduce or eliminate the use of a specific behavior. Punishment as defined in behavioral terms is an event that follows an undesirable behavior by the client which because it is distasteful to the individual decreases the occurrence of the behavior in the future.[6]

In selecting the punishment to be used as a reinforcer, the reason for the undesirable behavior must be determined and consideration given to the kind of punishment most likely to decrease the behavior. The preponderance of evidence indicates that corporal punishment is not an effective reinforcer and should not be considered. Laws in all states prohibit the use of corporal punishment for adults and in a large number of states its use is illegal for children as well. Regardless of the matter of legality, much more productive forms of punishment are available.

Research has shown that the most effective punishment is denial to the individual of something that the person wants or desires. One form of negative reinforcement that is popularly used because of its great effectiveness with children who have severe behavior problems is a technique known as "time-out." Time-out refers to the removal of the individual from the situation in which the undesirable behavior occurred if the situation is one in which the individual would prefer to remain. Often an individual responds in an unacceptable way to get attention. If that person is then simply removed from the environment with no fanfare and placed in an area where there is no one to respond to the misbehavior, the motivation that prompted the undesirable behavior disappears.

Extension. Extension refers to the disappearance of a behavior because the reinforcers for that specific behavior have been limited. Bandura explains that, "In naturally occurring situations response patterns sustained by positive reinforcement are frequently eliminated simply by discontinuing the rewards that ordinarily produce the behavior." [7] The simplest form of extension, and the one most frequently used, is the ignoring of the unacceptable behavior; if the behavior fails to elicit attention from those present, which is often the case, the individual will not persist in the bad behavior.

PSYCHOANALYSIS

Psychoanalysis is a systematic structure of theories concerning the relation of the conscious and subconscious. This structure is the basis of a method for investigating unconscious mental processes and for treating psychoneurosis. Psychoanalysis is not a procedure that therapeutic recreationists will make direct application of in their work with clients. However, some programs for treating psychiatric patients are based on psychoanalysis and it is, therefore, useful for the therapeutic recreationist to have a basic understanding of its nature.

Sigmund Freud, the father of psychoanalysis, contended that within each person there is a tendency to gratify the inherent instincts—self-preservation, sexual desire, and aggression—in the face of the demands of society to act otherwise. Psychologic problems arise from the conflict between satisfying instinctual desires and fitting into the molds of society. Then individuals often cope unconsciously with the problems by erecting the protective shield of a defense mechanism.

A defensive mechanism can be said to be a means of subconscious avoidance of the psychic pain of the problem by focusing on a substitute for the real cause of the problem. This description can be better understood by examining several commonly employed mechanisms:

- Sublimation—the replacement of a desire or impulse that cannot be satisfied with one that can be fulfilled.

- Compensation—an attempt to offset some shortcoming or limitation by developing some special talent or ability.

- Identification—the conscious or unconscious assuming of the attitudes, manners, and so forth, of another admired individual or group.

- Projection—placing the blame on others for one's own shortcomings.

- Escape—an attempt to avoid reality by escaping from it in daydreams or fantasy.

- Rationalization—the substitution of reasons other than the real ones for a certain act.

- Displacement—the release of emotions by expressing them toward another individual or object rather than the one which provoked the emotion.

All individuals make use of such mechanisms to some degree in achieving personal adjustment. Serious psychologic problems are created when the mechanisms are used excessively; then professional help is often required. The therapy offered by psychoanalysis is directed toward self-discovery of the reasons for one's behavior and, based on this under-standing, developing more appropriate mechanisms of adjustment.

Play Therapy

Play therapy is a procedure based upon principles of psychoanalysis. In play therapy children are encouraged to portray in a play situation the unsatisfactory experiences they have had. It is postulated that in this way the child brings real life problems to the play situations and is more able to deal with them there because it is just "play." The therapist, utilizing psychoanalytic techniques, helps the child to understand the meaning of these play activities and to develop ways of adjusting to the problems.

PSYCHOTHERAPY

Psychotherapy is a form of treatment for disturbances of a psychologic or emotional nature whereby a professionally prepared individual inten-tionally establishes a clinical relationship with a patient or client. The primary purpose of such a professional relationship is to delete, change, or diminish existing symptoms. In conjunction with the reduction or re-moval of disturbed behavioral patterns, encouragement is offered to achieve positive personality growth and development.

Psychotherapy emphasizes the humanistic approach through the spe-cial interpersonal relationship between the patient or client and the ther-apist. The reasoning process is utilized to achieve an understanding of the reasons for certain behaviors so that they can be replaced with more appropriate responses and actions. The process of assisting clients to examine their behavior and to make decisions about future conduct is sometimes termed values clarification.[8]

GROUP THERAPY

Group therapy is, as its name suggests, the involvement of a group of clients in a therapeutic process—the process being that of interacting with one another to examine their problems and their reactions to them. In the dynamics of such a situation, clients tend to reveal the attitudes and habits of thought and behavior that have contributed to the devel-opment of their maladjustment and interpersonal problems. Because members of the group can, by virtue of their own experiences, relate to the problems of one of their number, mutual support is generated for that person as he or she strives for self-acceptance and understanding. In the environment of the group, free from the strictures of the usual social environment, the client feels more secure about attempting a replacement of former negative and destructive patterns with more constructive atti-tudes and behavior. At the same time, the client becomes more capable of seeing the point-of-view of others and acquires skill in developing satisfactory interpersonal relationships.

Group therapy has certain advantages that can be explicitly stated. Among them are:

- Self-knowledge is developed in an environment that is analogous to the real world.

- Because adjustment to a variety of personalities is essential, a range of inter-personal skills is achieved for flexible response as conditions change.

- With the group serving as a protected situation, experimentation with new attitudes and behaviors is possible without the recriminations or rejection that might accompany behavioral lapses in the real world.

- Knowledge that feelings and anxieties are shared by other members of the group permits the rebuilding of self-respect and self-confidence.

- Elimination of artificially contrived defensive interpersonal barriers enables relationships to be formed without fear and awkwardness.

- Acceptance of criticism and the dropping of pathologic interpersonal defenses fosters a more realistic self appraisal of social capacities as well as inhibitions.

- Simultaneously with the advent of increased precision of insight greater accuracy in the observation of others is attained which permits the gradual reduction of previous tendencies toward warped perceptions of interpersonal responses.

- With the development of respect for the feelings of others, shared perspective and mutual resolution of problems become possible.

Despite these apparent advantages, critics of group therapy indicate that many of the sources of disruptive behavior are typically by-passed and remain unsolved. The fluidity of group dynamics and the swiftness of group interaction may not provide sufficient time for the inquiry necessary to bring to light and gain insight into the origins of the problems. This is especially true of shy, withdrawn, or hesitant clients. Indeed, group contact can be so rapid that some clients can be hurt in terms of undermined personal security, terminating in withdrawal from treatment before these traumas are subdued.

Types of Groups

Among the various kinds of groups that are formed for therapy are activity groups, discussion groups, analytical groups, role-playing groups, and family groups, Each of these groups attacks a behavioral or attitudinal problem from a different tack. Activity groups pursue a common set of experiences of a reacreational nature. Discussion groups participate either in therapist-directed or unstructured discussions which can focus on specific topics or be entirely free-wheeling. Analytical groups take their point of departure from intrapsychic theory wherein an attempt is made to expose unconscious attitudes, defenses, ventilation of repressed emotions, and the reconstruction of childhood-based pathologic behaviors. Role-playing groups use psychodrama which simulates people who are significant in their lives. Family groups are composed of family members who share certain behaviors, attitudes, and deep-seated emotional problems that are made more complex because of the intra-family relationships. Family group therapy is directed toward intervention by family members in counter-productive and pathologic behaviors of one of the family and also toward intervention to break a cycle of poor responses to negative behavior that produces poor responses.

THERAPEUTIC MILIEU AND MILIEU THERAPY

Therapeutic milieu is a term used in reference to the treatment of mental disturbance. It may be defined as a propitious environment within the treatment center in which prescribed treatments can be carried on effectively. Environmental factors include the physical situation: the living and recreational facilities, the attitudes of the staff, and the general social atmosphere.

Milieu therapy is a different term which refers to a form of treatment. The treatment consists of attempting to change behavior by altering the environment, or milieu, in which the individual lives, or by placing the patient in systematically and progressively different environments. The patient's reactions to the specific environment are carefully monitored and changes in the environment are made as needed to elicit the desired behavior.

The significance of the social elements of the environment are highly regarded and individually developed for each patient. Socializing activities for a regressed patient may be elementary while for another individual the social activities may be highly "reality-oriented" to challenge the capacity of the patient.[9] The social environment is changed as the patient improves or regresses.

PRESCRIPTION

Prescription, as noted in the first chapter, is the element that transforms the recreational experience into a therapeutic modality. Specifically, prescription is a medical term that refers to an order usually written, although it may be oral, by a doctor to designate a course of action in the treatment of a patient. In the circumstance of the doctor designating recreational activities for therapeutic purposes, the prescription may be directed to different personnel depending upon the nature of the treatment center and the specialists who are on the staff.

Where there is a rehabilitation team working with physically disabled clients or with psychiatric patients, all the members offer input to the development of the prescription by the doctor. In some general hospitals, the only therapeutic specialists may be the physical therapist and the recreational therapist; then the physical therapist generally receives the prescription from the doctor, and the recreational therapist works closely with the physical therapist to provide a program of complementary activities.

Considerable variation occurs in the way the prescription for recreational activities is developed, if it is used at all, in institutions or group homes for mentally retarded persons. In some instances there is a rehabilitation team (with the client's doctor as a member) who develops prescriptions, designating the type and purpose of recreational activities that are to be presented. More often, the recreational specialist on the staff of the facility is responsible for developing the total recreational program based on the established recreational objectives, which frequently have been prepared by the recreationist. In this instance, the designation of appropriate activities is not a prescription.

In correctional institutions the recreational program is usually left entirely to the recreational service staff. Even though very limited, there has been some effort made by criminologists to involve recreational services directly in the rehabilitation program through coordination of the recreational program with whatever rehabilitation services are offered.

Contents of the Prescription

The prescription for the therapeutic recreational program generally includes besides name, age, sex, and other vital statistics, a diagnosis of the disorder, aims of the treatment, precautions, limitations, and potentialities. In unusual circumstances the specific types of activity to be presented are designated as well as the attitude the recreationist should assume in working with the client. However, in the majority of cases only the needs of the client that the therapeutic recreational program should work to meet are indicated.

The needs to be met through prescriptive programming fall into several broad categories. Several examples of these general categories of need are offered here to indicate the nature of the prescription:

1. Physical activity
   a. general conditioning
   b. strengthen muscles and develop tonus
   c. increase flexibility
   d. increase cardio-respiratory endurance
2. Social interaction
   a. large and small groups
   b. other individuals
3. Better self-image
   a. mental
   b. physical
4. Emotional support
   a. groups
   b. individuals
5. Working out problems
   a. art forms
   b. psychodrama
   c. discussion
6. Success
   a. motor performance
   b. mental
   c. appearance

7. Increased attention span
    a. work
    b. play
    c. listening
8. Cooperation
    a. play
    b. planning with others
    c. work
9. Skill building
    a. mental
    b. gross motor
    c. fine motor
10. Understanding positive use of leisure
    a. passive
    b. active
    c. individual
    d. group

Irrespective of the type of information and amount of detail which is provided in the prescription, the recreationist must try to discover as much as possible about the client. There is an absolute necessity to know the client's potentialities and limitations and those activities that are contraindicated. Additional information concerning the client's likes and dislikes, general attitude, and specific idiosyncracies are helpful in developing a recreational program appealing to that person.

SENSORY OR PERCEPTUAL TRAINING

Sensory or perceptual training is a process utilizing various activities to improve the perception of those with disabilities in perceiving and interpreting stimuli. It is a neurologic and psychologic process, not necessarily involved with the physical loss of hearing or sight or any other of the senses.

In the early 1900s it was felt that perception was not learned but was instead a factor of maturation. However, today there is sufficient evidence available to support the concept that the process of perceiving can be improved through the use of specific activities and educational procedures.

One of the first uses of sensory training was with geriatric patients in whom there had been a decline in receiving and interpreting stimuli. Other special populations with whom sensory training has been effective are the mentally retarded and learning disabled.*

---

* Learning disabled is an educational term that refers to children who have severe learning problems usually in language and mathematics, but who are not mentally retarded or emotionally disturbed. It is thought that the basis of the disorder is the inability to perceive accurately.

Remotivation, Resocialization, and Reality Orientation

Remotivation, resocialization, and reality orientation are terms, most commonly used in geriatric settings, for the processes that are directed toward helping the disoriented and the confused aging client. All three methods are personalized, i.e., attention is provided to each client personally.

Resocialization emphasizes increasing the personal awareness of other people.[10] The client is helped to form relationships with others, make friends, and explore new social interests. Remotivation is concerned with social relations but also promotes renewed interests in the environment. The process consists of group meetings where features of everyday life are discussed. The meetings are kept as lively and friendly as possible, avoiding discussion of personal, emotional, or health problems. Reality orientation attempts to combat confusion and apathy by continually involving the client in the repeating of basic facts and constant orientation to time, place, familiar names and items, and events of the day. All staff members in contact with clients contribute to the continuous drill of the client on such things as the names of people in the room, the food eaten at lunch, the time of day, the items in the client's immediate environment, etc.

RELAXATION

Achievement of a relaxed state is important to the promotion of the well-being of ill and disabled persons. Relaxation is the abatement of tension, tension being a stretched or strained condition. Tension can be used to describe a psychologic state of strain or anxiety, but relaxation is used more frequently to refer to the releasing of tension in muscles of the body. It has been established that a relationship exists between psychologic tension and physiologic tension, i.e., muscles in a state of tension. As muscular tension is reduced, in many cases a parallel reduction in psychologic tension occurs and vice versa.

The positive effects of relaxation on physiologic functions have been well established. Blood, which is impeded in its flow by the constriction of the blood vessels in tense muscles, circulates more freely so the work of the heart and the stress on the blood vessels are reduced. Because relaxation conserves energy, it prevents undue fatigue. The removal of waste products, which are increased when muscular tension is present, is facilitated by increased blood circulation in the relaxed state. Fatigue can often be alleviated by relaxation exercises and they are often used for those who are chronically fatigued and have trouble falling asleep.

Another beneficial effect of relaxation on physiologic functions is that breathing often becomes easier after relaxation exercises. Lung capacity is smaller when the chest muscles are tense, but when they relax the capacity is increased and the rate of breathing is decreased. A relaxation program designed to develop slower or more relaxed breathing is frequently of benefit to those with breathing problems.

Relaxation Programs

Relaxation programs may be based on several different procedures or may be a combination of several. The ones most commonly used are described below.

Progressive Relaxation. The most popular method used in therapy is progressive relaxation or Jacobson's method of relaxation.[11] The basis of the method is awareness of the difference between a relaxed muscle and a tensed one. This is achieved by having the client alternately tense and relax one set of muscles. After the difference has been well established in the client's mind, practice follows on relaxing each of the major muscle groups of the body one at a time until all the groups are relaxed. When relaxation of each new group has been attempted, attention is focused on relaxation of all groups simultaneously.

Yoga and Tai Chi. Both Yoga and Tai Chi originated in early Eastern cultures. Hatha Yoga is a form of Yoga which is particularly effective in learning to relax. There are many different techniques; the most widely used is called asana, which is performed by moving the body slowly into a prescribed position, stretching each segment of the body that is brought into the movement as far as it can be comfortably stretched.

Tai Chi Chan is an ancient Chinese exercise or dance which comprises various movement patterns called forms. The exercise concentrates on specific movement forms, linking one form with others in continuous movement. No form is held even momentarily, rather each flows gently into the next.

Imagery. This method may be used effectively separately or together with other methods in inducing relaxation. Imagery is the formation of mental pictures evoked either internally or externally. Individuals who do not have an active imagination may be stimulated by the spoken word or a musical mood.

The theoretic basis for the use of imagery is the help individuals receive from matching movements to concepts that strongly suggest relaxation. Evidence indicates that concepts and feelings have a strong influence on the tension of a muscle. To imagine a tight muscle is to produce one. The converse is also true. Suggestive phrases such as "make your body feel like a rag doll" or "fall slowly to the floor like a balloon that is floating to the ground" usually produce a relaxed state of the muscles.

EXERCISE AND PHYSICAL FITNESS

A large segment of most recreational programs is devoted to physical activity: sports, games, physical conditioning exercises, etc. Consequently, it is essential to understand the effects of exercise on the body in order to plan appropriate programs, particularly for clients with disabilities.

There appears to be no universally accepted definition of physical fitness. However, it is common among exercise physiologists to define physical fitness by identifying its components, components being those physical qualities that are influenced by progressive overloading.* They are muscular strength, muscular endurance, cardiorespiratory endurance, and flexibility. Although body fat or body composition is not a true component of physical fitness, it is often included with physical fitness since it has a close relationship to cardiovascular fitness, a true component of physical fitness.

Concepts of Fitness Development

Improvements in the physical fitness components is accomplished as a result of the body's responses to the stress of exercise (reaction to progressive overload). The components of physical fitness are separate entities and must be developed with separate procedures.

Physical fitness programs for the ill and disabled should be individually tailored for each client and all activities for those who are ill or physically disabled should be approved by a physician. Most physically disabled individuals can participate in physical fitness activities.

Stress Reduction and Physical Activity

Casual evidence that individuals feel better after exercise abounds. When asked why they exercise, people often respond "I feel better," "I am more relaxed," "Relieves my anxiety." Joggers in particular find their type of activity reduces stress and fosters positive psychologic effects.[12] It should be noted that exercise appears to reduce anxiety only when direct competition is held to minimal level. Competitive sports tend to cause anxiety not only temporarily but over longer periods of time, especially in those who lose in the competition.

Aggression

It is a commonly held belief that certain types of recreational activities provide an opportunity for the release of feelings of aggression in a socially acceptable manner. Participation in sports, especially those with body contact, is frequently cited as an example of an activity in which violent action occurs with social sanction, thereby enabling aggressive feelings to be released without experiencing guilt. The assumption is made that this is entirely beneficial to the individual and to society.

---

* Progressive overload refers to the continual increase of the work load of the body over a given period of time to produce an increase in the efficiency of the organ or muscle receiving the overload.

However, evidence is accumulating that release of aggressive feelings in violent activity is harmful rather than wholesome. In 1954 Fait pointed out that empirical evidence did not support the contention that students became less aggressive after participating in or viewing contact sports. He observed that there was a positive relationship between aggressive and violent behavior on university campuses following football games and the hostility and violence expressed by spectators during the games.[13] Quanty in a review of evidence on aggression cartharsis found that viewing or participating in aggressive activities does not decrease aggression in the participants but actually increases it.[14] Austin makes a similar observation: "Aggression when rewarded, or at least condoned, simply brings about further aggression."[15]

ACTIVITY ANALYSIS

Activity analysis is a procedure to determine the essential features of an activity. This has value in therapeutic and adapted recreational service because the analysis gives insight into the nature of the activity; then, if the limitations and needs of the client are known, the possible effects participation in the activity may have on a client can be determined.

There are various activity-analysis models, some of which are limited to one behavioral area, usually the psychomotor, and therefore have limited value for the recreationist. Behavioral areas other than the psychomotor or physical are the cognitive or intellectual, affective or emotional, and social.[16] The recreationist needs to take all of these areas into consideration when analyzing an activity, since the needs of a client will likely involve all areas.

The four areas of behavior and the items in each area that will provide information about the activity are given below:

Physical Demands
1. Types of perception necessary. (Example: sight, sound, touch, proprioceptor reaction)
2. Types of motor movement required. (Example: catching, throwing, running, batting, grasping)
2. Amount of strength and muscular endurance needed and parts of the body where needed. (Example: maximum or minimum amount in fingers, arms, legs)
4. Amount of speed of movement necessary and parts of the body where needed. (Example: maximum or minimum in arms, fingers, legs)
5. Specific coordination required. (Example: threading a needle, bouncing a ball, sawing a board)
6. Amount of flexibility needed and movement where required. (Example: maximum in reaching up with arms; minimum in bending over)
7. Amount of cardiorespiratory endurance required. (Example: maximum to minimum)
8. Amount of stress to the joints and parts of the body where stress occurs. (Example: maximum to knees because of need to dodge)

9. Degree of possibility of injury and nature of the danger. (Example: medium danger of finger injury in catching a ball)

Cognitive or Intellectual Demands

1. Degree of complexity of the rules. (Example: very complex and requires much memory retention)
2. Degree of complexity of strategy development. (Example: various, depending upon the level of individuals involved)
3. Communication skills required. (Example: limited to high level of word recognition)
4. Complexity of scoring. (Example: complex but easily kept by the recreationist)
5. Leisure educational value. (Example: considerable carry-over value)
6. Steps involved in performing the skill and their complexity. (Example: one-strand braiding = three steps with last step repeated over and over, moderately simple)

Affective or Emotional Demands

1. Level of competition. (Example: can be kept to a minimum by de-emphasizing winning)
2. Possibilities of the activity producing emotional responses and the likely responses. (Example: maximum possibility; joy, frustration, guilt)

Social Demands

1. Degree of communication required between participants. (Example: minimal)
2. Number of people interacting with one another and the degree. (Example: 10 people; intimate to distant)
4. Tendency of the activity to include or exclude participants. (Example: very inclusive—interaction throughout activity)
5. Opportunities for participants to share in the limelight. (Example: at least one chance—each participant has chance to score)
5. Intrinsic or extrinsic rewards. (Example: extrinsic—praise and cheers from other participants)

In utilizing the results of activity analysis, concern must be given to the limitations and needs of the client. If the prescription does not provide sufficient information or there is no prescription, as in the case of community programs, additional information about the client will need to be obtained, e.g., residual weakness, attitude toward such factors as competition and cooperation, ability to communicate, socialization level, and intellectual capacity.

KINETIC OR SKILL ANALYSIS

Kinetics or skill analysis refers to determining the movements that are required to perform a specific skill. In doing this, the skill needs to be broken down to its movement components.

The components of the skill that is to be performed can be identified by careful examination of movements in the three phases of the performance: preparatory, executionary, and recovery. To illustrate using the example of the underhand toss of a small ball, the skill is divided into phases and the movement components in each are identified. The first phase, preparatory, comprises the grasping of the ball with the four fingers spread and in opposition to the thumb. This is followed by swinging the dominant arm from the shoulder backwards, and stepping forward on the opposite foot. (The distance the arm is brought back depends upon how far the ball is to be thrown.) In the executionary movement phase, the components consist of swinging the ball forward in an arc, shifting the weight of the body over the forward foot, and releasing the ball (when the release is made is dependent on the distance the ball is to be thrown.) In the recovery movement, the only component is the follow-through of the arm, which continues the arc until the momentum begun by the execution is dissipated.

The utilization of the results of the kinetic analysis in selecting and adapting the skills appropriate for any given client is a process similar to that of activity analysis. The movements that are required for performance of the skill are compared with the movements that are possible for the client to make and then, if necessary, modifications in movements are made to enable the skill to be performed. For example, if the client cannot grasp the ball but is able to make a cup with the fingers, the swing of the arc can be modified so that the ball remains cupped in the hand. This may require bending the elbow so the ball will stay in the "cup" and also stopping the forward movement abruptly without a follow-through to allow the ball to be thrown forward from the cupped hand.

LEISURE COUNSELING AND LEISURE EDUCATION

Considerable difference of opinion exists among those in the field of therapeutic recreational service about the nature and function of the processes of leisure counseling and leisure education. There are those who feel that in actual practice the processes are so overlapping that there is no need to recognize a difference between them. Others see a definite distinction between leisure counseling and leisure education. They regard the function of leisure counseling as being the development of clients' awareness of the nature of leisure and the instilling of positive leisure attitudes and values, as well as expanding the ability of clients to make appropriate decisions about participation in leisure. In their view, the function of leisure education is to impart knowledge to clients about leisure resources and to develop their skills in order to perform activities well enough to find pleasure and satisfaction in them, alone or in groups.

Leisure Counseling

Leisure counseling, when first used in psychiatric hospitals, was directed toward providing clients with the information and skills needed to identify, locate, and use recreational resources in the community to which they return after treatment. Today leisure counseling is not necessarily limited to the goal of preparing clients for easier re-entry into community recreational activities but may be an integral part of the psychiatric treatment program. In this case, one of the primary concerns is to modify the client's attitudes, concepts, and values with respect to the use of leisure.

Hence, it is possible to identify at least three major functions of modern day leisure counseling:

- developing clients' recreational skills, including social skills;
- providing clients with information about recreational resources;
- promoting attitudes, values, and concepts that lead clients to appropriate use of leisure.

The first two of these functions are educational and so are also functions of leisure education, and it is here that the two processes overlap. However, the third function is complex in nature and requires the recreationist to have the specialized knowledge and skills of the art of psychologic counseling. Recreationists who wish to make leisure counseling the major emphasis of their work need to take special training in counseling.

Leisure Education

Leisure education, identified as one of three major elements in therapeutic recreational service by the National Therapeutic Recreation Society in its "Philosophical Statement,"[17] is an educational process that endeavors to impart knowledge to clients about leisure resources and to develop skills to enable satisfying performance of leisure activities. Leisure education utilizes a wide variety of educational techniques such as discussion, demonstration, and behavior modification to accomplish its goal. Originally used mainly with school children to promote worthy use of leisure in after school hours, leisure education is today an integral element of the recreational service provided to those who are ill and disabled.

NORMALIZATION AND MAINSTREAMING

Normalization and mainstreaming are terms that are sometimes regarded as synonymous; however, the concept of mainstreaming is actually an offspring of normalization. Normalization is a process of human management applied to those whose behavior deviates from the norm to the detriment of the self or society. "One of the basic principles of normalization is that behavior deviancy can be reduced by minimizing the degree to which persons are treated differently from 'normal' persons. Conversely, deviancy is enhanced by treating persons as if they are deviant".[18]

Mainstreaming refers to the concept of providing appropriate service to handicapped individuals in a regular setting. For recreational service, the program in the community center is a regular setting. Mainstreaming has come to be associated with the concept of integration but it is actually much more than that. It involves not only placing the individual in a regular setting for a specific service, but also providing supportive services to ensure successful participation in the regular setting. Not all handicapped individuals can be successful in a regular program even when the optimum supportive services are provided because of limitations that cannot be satisfactorily compensated for. An example is that of mainstreaming a non-verbal mentally retarded individual into a discussion group on world politics.

REFERENCES

1. Frank Krusen, *et al.,* (eds.) *Handbook of Physical Medicine and Rehabilitation* (Philadelphia: W. B. Saunders Co., 1966) p. 1.
2. Walter Cannon, *The Wisdom of the Body* (New York: W. W. Norton and Company, 1963) p. 24.
3. Raymond Wloodkowski, *Motivation,* Washington, D.C.: National Education Association, 1977, p. 6.
4. Albert Ellis, "Rational-emotive Therapy" in *Current Psychotherapies,* by Raymond Corsini, *et al.* editors, 1976, *passim.*
5. Hollis Fait and John Dunn, *Special Physical Education: Adapted, Individualized, Developmental* (Philadelphia: Saunders College Publishing Company, 1984) p. 99.
6. Robert Presbile and Paul Brown, *Behavior Modification,* (Washington, D.C.: National Education Association, 1976) p. 12.
7. Albert Bandura, *Principles of Behavior Modification* (New York: Holt, Rinehart and Winston, Inc.) p. 355.
8. Sidney B. Simon, *et al, Values Clarification* (New York: Hart Publishing Company, Inc., 1972) *passim.*
9. E. Mansell Paterson, "The Relationship of the Adjunctive and Therapeutic Recreation Services to Community Mental Health Programs" *Therapeutic Recreation Journal,* (1st Quarter, 1969) p. 19.
10. Eleanor Barns, *et al,* "Guidelines to Treatment Approaches," *The Gerontologist* 13, 1973, p. 313.
11. Edmond Jackson, *Progressive Relaxation,* 2nd ed. (Chicago: The University of Chicago Press, 1938) p. 40.
12. A. Ismail and L. Tractman, "Jogging the Imagination," *Psychology Today* Vol. 6, No. 10, 1973, p. 78.
13. Hollis Fait, "Lecture Notes, Principles of Physical Education," (Storrs, Connecticut: University of Connecticut, 1954-1964).
14. Michael Quanty, "Aggressive Catharsis: Experimental Investigations and Implications" in *Perspectives on Aggression* edited by Russel Green and Edgar O'Neal, (New York: Academic Press, 1976) p. 99.
15. David Austin, *Therapeutic Recreation Processes and Techniques,* (New York: John Wiley and Sons, 1982), p. 14.
16. Carol Peterson and Scout Gunn, *Therapeutic Recreation Program Design—Principles and Procedures,* 2nd. ed., (Englewood Cliffs: New Jersey, Prentice-Hall, Inc., 1984) p. 276.
17. Philosophical Statement Committee, "Committee Report on the NTRS Philosophical Statement," (Washington, D.C.: National Therapeutic Recreation Society, 1982) p. 1.
18. Wolf Wolfensberger, *The Principles of Normalization in Human Service,* (Toronto: Leonard Crainford, 1972) p. 28.

SELECTED REFERENCES

Baker, M., *et al. Developing Strategies for Biofeedback Applications in Neurologically Handicapped Persons* (Washington, D.C.: American Physical Therapy Association, 1977).
Basmajian, J. V. and Kirby, R. L., *Radical Rehabilitation—A Student's Textbook* (Baltimore: Williams and Wilkins Co., 1983).
Berryman, D. L. and Lefebvre, C. B., *Recreation Behavior Inventory* (Denton, Texas: Leisure Learning Systems, 1981).
Braun, S. J. and Lasfer, M., *Are You Ready to Mainstream: Helping Preschoolers with Learning and Behavior Problems* (Columbus, Ohio: Charles E. Merrill Publishing Co., 1978).

Goldenson, Robert M., Ed., *Disability and Rehabilitation Handbook* (New York: McGraw-Hill Book Company, 1978).

Grief, E. and Matarazzo, R., *Behavioral Approaches to Rehabilitation: Coping With Change* (New York: Springer Publishing Company, Inc., 1982).

Loring, J. and Beum, G., eds., *Integration of Handicapped Children in Society* (Boston: Routledge & Kegan Paul, Ltd., 1975).

Mundy, J. and Odum, L., *Leisure Education: Theory and Practice* (New York: John Wiley and Sons, 1979).

Pattison, E. Mansell, "The Relationship of the Adjunctive and Therapeutic Recreational Services to Community Health Programs," *Therapeutic Recreation Journal,* 1st quarter, 1969, pp. 19-20.

Robertson, E., *Rehabilitation of Arm Amputees and Limb Deficient Children* (Philadelphia: W. B. Saunders Co., 1979).

Wehman, Paul and Schlein, S. J., *Leisure Programs for Handicapped Persons* (Baltimore: University Park Press, 1981).

Wright, G. W., *Total Rehabilitation* (Boston: Little, Brown & Co., 1980).

Chapter 4

Special Recreational Service in Treatment Centers and Community Settings

Therapeutic recreational service in treatment centers and adapted recreational service in community programs have much in common but there are significant differences. The contradistinctions are produced by the nature of the settings in which the programs function. In treatment centers most of the clients are much more ill or disabled than participants in community adapted recreational programs. Consequently, the program emphasis in therapeutic recreational service is rehabilitative in nature, and the recreationist usually follows a prescription from the doctor, psychiatrist, or rehabilitation team in developing the program. The people whom the therapeutic recreationist serves are residing in the treatment center or come to it as out-patients so that, unlike the adapted recreationist, there is no need to plan transportation services for disabled clients, take recreational services to homebound clients, and coordinate services with the adapted programs of other local agencies and organizations.

The dissimilar natures of the settings which influence differences in programs also require different administrative structures. Treatment centers, which provide a variety of care and treatment services, are organized to enable efficient coordination of these services by different disciplines. Adapted recreational service is usually a function of the community recreational department, which is one of several governmental agencies; the administrative structure in this case is organized to respond effectively to community needs within the limitations of the financial support provided by the residents.

THERAPEUTIC RECREATIONAL SERVICE IN TREATMENT CENTERS

The treatment center is any agency of society that provides some sort of health care on a residential or out-patient basis. Broadly, a treatment center may be said to include all of those agencies that supply needed care, treatment, and remedial assistance to children and adults with any of the physical or mental conditions that prevent individuals from living and performing optimally. Agencies most frequently characterized as treatment centers are hospitals, nursing homes, clinics, and institutions and specialized schools for the handicapped. Of these, the clinic is the one place where treatment is offered only to non-residential patients.

Treatment centers may be classified by (1) sponsorship or control, (2) type, or (3) term.

The first classification includes governmentally operated and privately owned treatment centers. In the former instance the hospital is supported through tax funds as well as by fees or charges for services based on the patient's ability to pay. In the latter case, private corporations, physicians, or groups own the treatment center; usually it is operated on a nonprofit basis, although there are private treatment centers that have a profit motive. When the center is operated not for profit, but for altruistic purposes, it is more likely to be sponsored by a philanthropic foundation, private corporation, church group, fraternal or benevolent order or protective society, or voluntary community (but nonpublic or nongovernmental) institution. Those treatment centers which are controlled by governmental agencies may be at any level—local, county, state, or federal.

Classification of treatment centers by type involves identification of the special kind of illness or disability for which the center provides treatment and care. There are general medical hospitals in which all types of diseases and injuries are treated. As medicine has become more highly specialized, however, some clinical departments which once functioned within the general hospital have separated themselves and become organized as specialized hospitals. For example, there are hospitals for: joint diseases; eye, ear, nose, and throat infirmities; cancer; maternity care; children's chronic diseases; convalescence; orthopedic conditions; neuropsychiatric problems; and rehabilitation. Also, some clinics are specialized; the most common of these are cancer, mental illness, diagnostic, and eye, ear, nose, and throat. Specialized schools include those for blind, deaf, mentally retarded, orthopedically handicapped, and emotionally disturbed children. Nursing homes, because they have a predominantly elderly clientele, specialize to a certain degree in geriatrics.

Treatment centers may also be classified by term or length of the patient's stay. Hospitals or other treatment centers that treat emergency situations and acute illnesses or provide intensive care may be categorized as short-term or acute; those that handle chronic diseases, rehabilitation procedures, or convalescence cases are termed long-term or custodial institutions.

Nature of Therapeutic Recreational Service

Recreational experiences are necessary to all people in whatever situation they may find themselves. In the normal routine of living they expect to find time for recreational activity. The disruption of routine which accompanies confinement in a treatment center can be mitigated somewhat by the inclusion of at least some activities which recall participation in routine events. Recreational service may be just that bridge which can link the patient to his / or her community existence thereby sustaining an important psychologic association which preserves identity and courage. If recreational experiences are a part of a person's life, they should not be curtailed because he or she moves into a treatment center. If anything, such experience should be reinforced as it encourages attention to ideas, objects, or performances which are associated with meaningful, satisfying, and enjoyable impressions.

Types. Patients enter treatment centers for different reasons, and the nature of the recreational program is determined by the reason for the patient being there. For example, there are those who arrive for observation only. They will have no medical treatment other than diagnostic tests which, while time-consuming, are seldom painful, and do not leave the recipient impaired in any way. For these individuals, confined to the hospital but not undergoing treatment, time may hang heavy. Recreational activities of a diversional nature are needed to fill the hours in a pleasant and satisfying way. A full range of recreational activities may be planned and organized, insofar as space limitations permit, to meet the needs of such a patient. Activities will not be therapeutic, although, to the extent that they support morale and reduce stress, they might be considered as such.

Some patients enter the treatment center in emergencies. They are victims of more or less serious injuries resulting from accidents, or they are sufferers of a sudden onset of illness so severe that it forces immediate hospitalization. Under these circumstances there can be no thought of anything but swift medical attention and therapy. There will be a time lapse, short or long depending upon the nature of the malady, until the patient has recuperated sufficiently to be aware of his or her surroundings. Once the initial debilitation has receded or the pain and acute discomfort have diminished, a regimen of therapeutic recreational activities may be begun. However, some kinds of recreational activities will be contraindicated for certain patients. For example, activities that involve exercise cannot be offered to those with acute cardiac problems or rheumatic fever and those who are in shock, under sedation, and with high temperatures. Exercise activity is not given to patients with acute respiratory infection when that activity will cause overwork of the lungs. When an area of the body is immobilized, as in a fractured leg in traction, excessive movement is not permitted in that area in any activity.

The length of time between admission to the treatment center and desire to be involved in something other than medical and nursing routine varies with the nature of infirmity or ailment. The time may be as short as 36 hours after initial surgery has been performed, e.g., for hernia, joint derangement, hip fracture, or appendicitis; or it may be much longer due to the degree of complication or involvement. Whenever the patient is sufficiently recovered from the initial trauma to be bored is the right moment for the inception of therapeutic recreational services. This rule-of-thumb does not apply to mentally ill patients. Depending on the state of the patient's condition, rehabilitation may begin immediately after hospitalization or sometime thereafter. Therapeutic recreational service is initiated when the rehabilitation process begins.

In acute or short-term physical illness, the patient may be in and out of the treatment center within days of admission. This should not impede the development of recreational services which can be of value to that patient. Even in short periods there may be much which the patient can learn that will have carry-over value long after the disease or injury incident has been forgotten.

By law, some treatment centers are required to offer therapeutic recreational service before they can be registered and licensed by the state. Typical are nursing homes or institutions which deal with geriatric conditions. For the most part, such agencies are looked upon as long-term custodial centers and rightly need to provide a recreational outlet for their clients. In such an institution, therapeutic recreational service might be subordinated to diversional recreational activity. However, if there are clients under treatment for psychiatric problems or involved in a rehabilitation program, these individuals may have a prescribed recreational regimen.

Organizational Structure

All treatment centers, large or small, specialized or general, have governing or policy making bodies. These may variously be called boards of directors, trustees, or some other suitable designation, based upon ownership, sponsorship, and / or operational control. The primary responsibility of the governing body is to ensure that the center is rendering appropriate health care to the center's clientele and to the community at large in the most economic and efficient manner possible. It carries out this function by setting policy by which the institution is guided in its efforts. The governing board invariably delegates the authority and responsibility for daily operation of the center to an appointed administrator.

Duties and Responsibilities. Among the duties and responsibilities of those who serve as administrators are preparation of all financial statements as well as the annual budget, assessing the physical plant needs of the center, maintaining records on all operational departments, and direction of personnel management. The final authority on employment and discharge of personnel and, within the restrictions of available funds, control of all salaries of the institution are administrative functions as are the planning and designing, or evaluating designs, for the physical plant.

The administrator of a treatment center that has a large number of clients usually has assistants to enable full coverage of administrative duties, day or night. Additionally, there are heads of various departments and other suitable personnel to carry out the functions for which the treatment center is established. The departments, comprising in-patient and out-patient services, are subdivisions of two major divisions into which the functions of the treatment center are separated: a division of business management and a division concerned with patient care and treatment.

The division dealing with patient care and treatment further subdivides into four groups, the major responsibility of which is patient health and rehabilitation. These four are: (a) admitting, records, social service; (b) diagnostic and therapeutic departments or medical services; (c) nursing services; and (d) dietary service. The division of business management includes all of those functions dealing with accounting, auditing, personnel management, physical plant maintenance, housekeeping, public relations, and non-medical record keeping. In smaller institutions, departmental functions may be combined and integrated into fewer groups. Responsibility for the care of patients, insofar as diagnosis and treatment are concerned, is the function of the professional medical staff which works in close relation to the center's administrator. Record keeping related to patient care is a function of medical personnel.

Typical Organization. In Figure 4-1 the relationships of those charged with direct supervision and responsibility for specific functions are identified for a typical, large treatment center, such as a hospital that offers general health care services. The flow of authority and responsibility for the care and treatment of patients as well as for the management of the entire hospital administration may be seen from the diagram.

In such a structure, the therapeutic recreational service section reports to the Director of Special Services, who coordinates the work of the subdivisions. In this situation, the therapeutic recreational service staff is

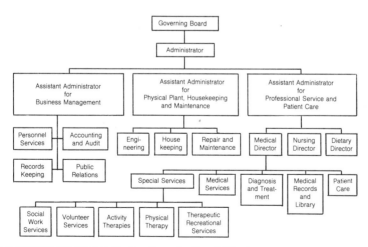

Fig. 4-1 Typical Treatment Center Organizational Chart

responsible to the Assistant Administrator for Professional Service and Patient Care and works under the auspices of the Medical Director. The operation of recreational service in this arrangement may be either therapeutic or diversional or, possibly both, depending on the commitment of the medical director to incorporation of the therapeutic recreational program into an ongoing team orientation, where each medical or paramedical discipline is responsible for a segment of the total treatment and / or rehabilitation regimen.

Alternate Organization: Under One Department. A different but not unusual organizational scheme coordinates all recreational services in the treatment center under one department which is directly responsible to the top level administration (Figure 4-2). This effectively ends duplication of effort, enhances the effectiveness of the overall program, and reduces expenditures. Perhaps the single most important advantage is that the director of therapeutic recreational service and the professional staff are in a better position to benefit from medical supervision.

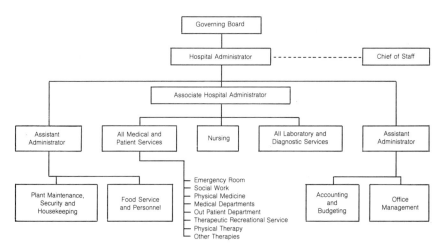

Fig. 4-2 Alternate Organization

In this organizational structure, the staff of recreationists is given the status and discretionary responsibility to affect directly the rehabilitation of the patient and to coordinate efforts with other members of the rehabilitation team. A member of the therapeutic recreational service staff is present at every patient evaluation. Such conferences are held regularly to determine patient progress. At such meetings medical and paramedical personnel present their observations and analysis of the patient's behavior and progress. Reports of certain behavioral patterns, attitudes, interests, characteristics, needs, and abilities may be evaluated, and corroborated by others on the team to offer a complete picture of the patient's care and treatment needs.

With a supportive administrator at the head of this type of organizational structure, the therapeutic recreational service department and its program are increasingly called upon to carry out specific prescriptions for recreational activities which physicians feel are beneficial to the patient, while hospital aides conduct some of the diversional recreational activities. Such practices improve the atmosphere for the patients, lessen demands upon the time and effort of the professional personnel, and tend to encourage patients' interests in matters other than their own illness or impairments.

Alternate Organization: Along Medical Lines. In some treatment centers, therapeutic recreational services are organized along medical service lines. This means that, if there is an office or bureau providing recreational activities, it is administratively the direct responsibility of the physician in charge of a medical specialty. Thus, it is not infrequent that therapeutic recreational services are situated in departments of physical medicine and rehabilitation. When this is the situation, recreational service is recognized for its value to patients in terms of therapeutic impact, rather than as diversion, and the recreationist is welcomed as an integral part of the rehabilitation team, as in the Veterans' Administration system (Fig. 4-3). The recreationist functions at the same level and with equal status to the occupational therapist, physical therapist, vocational guidance counselor, and psychologist. In fact, all members of the rehabilitation team are peers and each has an important role in enabling the patient to reach a level of emotional and physical fitness for optimum performance.

In the treatment centers that are organized along medical service lines, there may be several departments in which recreationists are situated. Each section or office operates as a separate entity, answering only to the medical director of that particular service. Thus, the orthopedic, geriatric, psychiatric, pediatric, or general section may each have its own

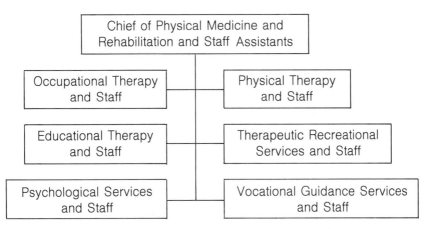

Fig. 4-3 Typical Veterans Administration Hospital Departmental Structure.

therapeutic recreational service. In other institutions, only one service in the entire treatment center may have a therapeutic recreational service attached to it. Typically this has been the pediatric or psychiatric service, or services dealing with chronic diseases. The recreational service offered is generally diversional rather than therapeutic because the need to keep these kinds of patients happily occupied in recreational activities takes precedence over the treatment benefits of therapeutic recreational service.

Alternate Organization: Under Division of Special Services. A third variation of hospital organization occurs when a division of special services is created and a department of therapeutic recreational service is housed in this division. The recreationist then reports to the director of special services who is responsible to either the medical director or to an assistant administrator. In the former, the relationship between the therapeutic recreational service staff and the patients is such that the service can be therapeutic in nature. However, in the latter situation, the program is very likely to be merely diversional, for when the recreationist moves out of the sphere of responsibility covered by medical services, there is a great likelihood that the program will become one of entertainment and diversion rather than one of therapeutic intent and scope.

Alternate Organization: Under Department of Activity Therapies. A fourth variant occurs when therapeutic recreational services are administered from a department known as Activity or Adjunctive Therapies (Fig. 4-4). In such a situation, sections within this department are organized along activity lines for patients and there may be established such programs as: (a) manual arts therapy which employs industrial arts and crafts, e.g., metalworking, woodworking, electrical wiring, graphic and applied arts, and agricultural activities; (b) educational therapy which employs instructional activities like those of the school curriculum; (c) occupational therapy which employs arts and crafts activities; (d) music therapy; and (e) therapeutic recreational service. There is some overlapping and duplication of services through such a particularized program.

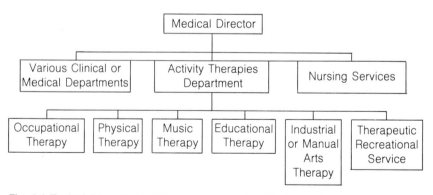

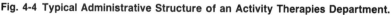

Fig. 4-4 Typical Administrative Structure of an Activity Therapies Department.

With so many clinicians and therapists operating around the same patients, confusion rather than resolution of the patient's problems can occur. However, if the treatment center has a rehabilitation team to make recommendations and provide prescription for clients the duplication is less likely to be detrimental.

Alternate Organization: Function of Hospital Auxiliary. In at least one other variant, the recreational service function is instituted and grows out of the hospital auxiliary, an organization of supporters allied to the hospital. Under such circumstances, there is little direct connection between the recreationist-in-charge and hospital administration; from the time of its establishment, the recreational service functions as the creature of the auxiliary. This is so particularly because no financial aid needs to be diverted to this program. Under such conditions, the onus is upon the recreationist to provide the services to patients almost without sanction of the hospital administrator. Depending upon the strength of the auxiliary and its influence on the hospital administration, the recreational service either suffers from anonymity or flourishes as an informal entity within the structure of the institution.

Other Organizational Schemes. Obviously there are other organizational schemes depending upon the size, type, specialization, and sponsorship of the treatment center. When the treatment center is a nursing, convalescent, or geriatric institution, the department of therapeutic recreational service is often responsible directly to the chief executive of the agency. To a lesser extent this is also true for centers which specialize in children's diseases or impairments, although it is not unusual to find that therapeutic recreational service, when it is considered to have significant value, has direct responsibility to the director of all medical services.

In institutions which lay emphasis on the re-education and re-socialization of individuals committed to its responsibility, therapeutic recreational service is administered as a section within a division or department of the institution. Some penal institutions, for example, house recreational services within a department of education or social services, with the director of the program reporting to an intermediate administrator and not to the executive of the institution. In such an organizational hierarchy, therapeutic recreational service does not function in any way except as a diversionary experience, which fills time and provides enjoyment.

Another ramification of organizational control exists in institutions for the mentally retarded, where the therapeutic recreational service is responsible directly to the administrator of the institution. The director, then, serves as a senior staff adviser to the administrator and is, in this way, enabled to offer therapeutic recreational service in close coordination with other departments in the institution.

Recreational service may also, in institutions for mentally retarded clients, be placed under the jurisdiction of the school department, where the physical education unit of the school program generally combines with recreational service in developing a suitable program of recreational activities. The program is largely diversionary in nature, but there is usually a strong element of leisure education.

Client-Centered Organization. Gunn and Peterson point out that organizational flow charts like those that have been described emphasize upward responsibility, that is, people at the lower levels are responsible to those at higher levels of the structure. This, they feel, is both an undemocratic process and one which inhibits the highest quality service being given the client. To overcome these weaknesses, the pair advocates the client-centered organization flow chart shown in Figure 4-5, which "illustrates the necessary commitment of all staff members to meet the needs of the client."[1] In such an organizational structure, the team member who has the best rapport and is the most effective with the individual or group of clients assumes the leadership role in providing therapeutic recreational service.

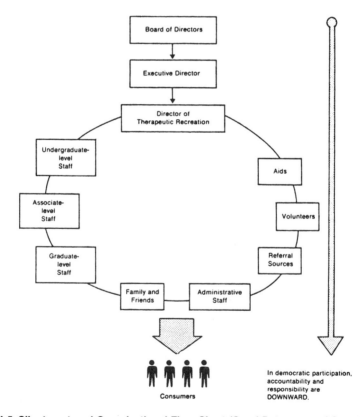

Fig. 4-5 Client-centered Organizational Flow Chart (Carol Peterson and Scout Gunn, *Therapeutic Recreation Program Design-Principles and Procedures,* 2nd ed. Englewood Cliffs, New Jersey, Prentice-Hall, Inc., 1984.)

Therapeutic Recreational Service in Schools. Finally, therapeutic recreational service may in rare instances be a subordinate section within a public or private school structure where the principal of the school has a staff of therapists including a recreational therapist. Unless the principal has a good understanding of the values of therapeutic recreational service, and medical personnel is available to provide prescriptions, the program is limited to activities of diversion and entertainment. However, when handicapped children in the school need to acquire appropriate leisure skills, PL 94-142 mandates that such instruction be provided by the school.[2] The recreational department, if there is one, will have this responsibility; otherwise, arrangements must be made by the school for such children to receive recreational services as out-patients of a treatment center or participate at a specified time in the community recreational service program.

ADAPTED RECREATIONAL SERVICE IN COMMUNITY SETTINGS

In every community there are numerous ill and disabled persons of every age group who are not so severely handicapped as to require confinement in treatment centers. These people obviously have special recreational needs, yet they do not require therapeutic recreational services. It is for such individuals that the adapted community recreational service program has been developed. Adapted here refers to the adjustment or modification of the activities, the facilities, and/or the programming of the community recreational services in any way necessary to enable the handicapped person to participate successfully.

Adapted recreational service programs are offered in a variety of community settings, but the most common is the publicly funded community recreational service department of the local government. Other settings include public schools and special centers and private and public organizations, societies, and agencies.

Nature of Adapted Recreational Service

As stated many times before, recreational activity is as important to the health and well-being of people as physiologic sustenance and social equilibrium. The sick or otherwise handicapped individual requires recreational activity to the same extent, if not more greatly, than one who is not handicapped. Adapted recreational service meets the needs of ill and disabled persons within the community setting in two significant ways. First, the adaptation of recreational experiences enables clients to engage in a much wider range of active recreational pursuits than is otherwise possible; the modification of recreational activities reduces the restrictive effects of the disability, promoting compensation for the handicap while stimulating residual capacity. Second, adaptation supports the individual psychologically and encourages participation in activities that build confidence in the ability to perform what was previously thought impossible; this alone often improves morale and builds self-esteem.

Obligation to Provide Community Adapted Recreational Service. Aside from the importance of community adapted recreational service to the handicapped individual, there is an indisputable reason for provision of this special service: It is the responsibility of community recreationists to offer their professional services to their entire community. Handicapped individuals residing in a community that has a public recreational service department are entitled to the same opportunities and choices as their non-handicapped compatriots. Recreationists owe their professional service to all; they cannot decide that one shall receive and another not on the basis of incapacity or any other contrived reasons.

This ethic of recreational service is reinforced by the mandate of federal law. Section 504 of the Rehabilitation Act of 1973 forbids discrimination in providing recreational service to anyone because of a disability.[3] The legislation reflects society's judgment that recreational service for all is, indeed, a societal benefit and should be provided for the good of the public welfare. Whatever adaptation is necessary to include the ill and disabled in the program of recreational activities and experiences must be undertaken.

Number in the Special Populations to Be Served

Unlike treatment center recreational programs, the community recreational program, because it serves all individuals in the community, must be prepared to offer programs for clients with many types of physical, mental, and emotional illness and disabilities in varying degrees of incapacitation. The kinds of handicapping conditions to be served are the kinds that are found in the community. Their number and variety depends on the size of the community in which the recreational program is located.

It has been estimated that 10% of the total population of this country have serious handicapping conditions.[4] To provide an idea of the number and kinds of handicaps that may generally be expected in a community, the chart in Table 4-1 presents the estimated percentages of various prevalent types of handicapping conditions.[5] By multiplying the population of a given community by the percentage of people with a certain handicap, the number of individuals with that specific disability living in the locality may be determined. The figure will, of course, be only an estimation since it is based on imprecise national data. The reliability of the figure as an indication of the number of community residents with the specific disability is less if the size of the community is small.

Obtaining precise data concerning the number of individuals in any classification is difficult for several reasons: many persons are multi-handicapped and so fall into more than one category; there is often no standardized criterion for indicating the presence of the disorder; and the methods of reporting handicaps are inadequate and inconsistent. Hence,

TABLE 4-1. ESTIMATED PERCENTAGE OF HANDICAPPED PERSONS WHO MAY NEED ADAPTED RECREATIONAL SERVICE

Visual handicaps		3%
Auditory handicaps		1%
Cardiopathic conditions		1%
Endocrine disorders	Less than	1%
Blood disorders	Less than	1%
Respiratory disorders		3%
Neurologic disorders		1%
Mental retardation		1%
Orthopedic disabilities	Less than	1%
Other	Less than	1%

the figures presented in the chart are at best rough estimates. They are useful, however, in giving recreationists an idea of the number of potential clients in special populations to whom adapted recreational services should be extended, especially in large cities where enumeration is usually impractical. In small communities enumeration is often possible and yields more accurate information on the number and types of handicapped persons to be served than the calculation of percentages based on the national data.

Other Information Needed About Clients. As important as knowing the number of handicapped people for whom adapted recreational services must be provided is information about the severity of their conditions. Such information is much more difficult to obtain and may not be available except from the persons themselves or the medical records they provide. The kind of initial information that is helpful to obtain includes degree of self-care skills, level of mobility, intelligence level, presence of emotional problems, availability of transportation.

Extent of Recreational Experience of Clients. Handicapped residents in the community who become clients in adapted recreational service bring to the program assorted backgrounds of recreational experience. Some have participated extensively in therapeutic recreational programs in treatment centers and have developed good recreational skills; others have limited experience and a few skills; and still others have led such isolated and restricted lives that their recreational experiences are nil. Recreationists must begin with the clients at whatever point of recreational development they are.

Those clients who have had no previous or limited opportunities to engage in recreational programs require a thorough orientation to the recreational services that are available. They need to have programs of progressive recreational skills development tailored to their needs and capabilities. Integration with other clients is effected as often as feasible to stimulate social interaction and motivate participation. Considerable time may be spent in developing adaptations.

For those rehabilitated clients who are re-entering the community, opportunities are provided to utilize and expand the skills and abilities that have been developed in the therapeutic recreational program of the treatment center. Communication between the treatment center and community recreational personnel alerts the latter about clients who are returning to their homes and supplies information about the abilities, interests, and special needs of the individual clients. In many cases, the client is able to participate in community programs with no special accommodation, but in other cases adaptations need to be made. In general, these will be the same as or similar to modifications made by the therapeutic recreationist in the treatment center.

There are always some clients whose stay in the treatment center was so short that they had little exposure to the therapeutic recreational services. Their integration into the community recreational program requires a different approach from that used with clients who enter after extended hospitalization in treatment centers. These clients need to receive more extensive introduction to the community recreational services and more individualized attention in adapting and developing recreational skills. Also, a larger portion of time is devoted to leisure education.

Departmental Organization for Community Adapted Recreational Service

Generally, public recreational service departments have a special office, bureau, or section solely responsible for programs for the ill and disabled residents of the community. Ideally, these programs are organized so that handicapped clients are integrated or mainstreamed into the regular program of recreational activities. This may require elimination of artificial barriers that prevent access of disabled clients to playgrounds, centers, parks, swimming pools, bleachers, etc. In those instances where the handicap is so severe that integration is not possible, sequestered or special programs are offered to these clients at specifically designated locations. For those whose disabilities are extreme or profound and who are, therefore, homebound, a series of activities is planned and conducted in the home to serve their particular needs.

Provision of all these special recreational services requires an effective organizational structure of the agency or department offering the services. Figure 4-6 shows an organization flow chart that might be utilized in a medium to large department. Small departments or one-person operations do not need an organization plan of this magnitude.

In this chart of organization, the overhead administrative staff is composed of the chief executive and administrative assistants. The program

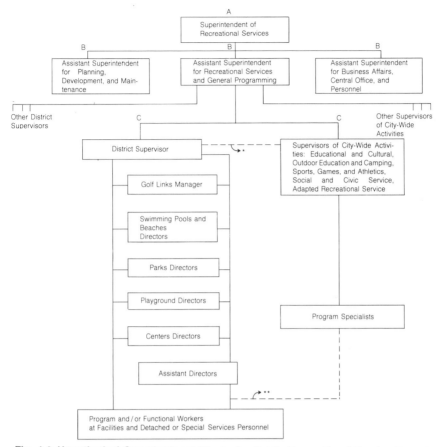

Fig. 4-6 Hypothetical Organizational Chart of a Public Recreational Service Department that Offers Adapted Activities.

A —Chief executive officer
B —Administrative assistants at divisional level
C —Middle managers
* —Liaison or coordinationg relationship
** —Coordination for instruction and programming

division is ramified in this schematic to indicate line and staff relationships as well as specialties. This chart can best be understood as the organization diagram of a large metropolitan or county recreational service department which serves a hypothetical community that is divided into a number of districts. Supervisors (C) of the districts are responsible to the assistant superintendents (B). These supervisors control all facilities and personnel within their respective districts. Each district contains not less than four neighborhoods in which local playgrounds, centers, parks, and other recreational facilities are situated.

All programming is administered through the Assistant Superintendant for recreational services and general programming and is, in turn, coordinated at the district supervisory level. City-wide events are developed at the supervisory level, whose specialists are charged with whatever special services, projects, or in-service education is necessary for program level recreationists within the department. Close liaison is maintained with district supervisors as indicated by the broken line in diagram. The city-wide supervisors may be looked upon as staff personnel as are the program specialists. Supervisors of city-wide activities schedule classes conducted by activity specialists at the various recreational facilities by arrangement with district supervisors who clear program calendars with managers or directors of facilities. City-wide events and special projects are cleared in the same way.

The adapted recreational service specialist is considered as a city-wide supervisor and is responsible for the development of all those special services which are geared to enabling the aging, ill, homebound, or handicapped to participate in some capacity in recreational experiences. If there are special facilities for the handicapped, the adapted recreationist would also maintain direct supervision over the personnel and programs originating in such facilities. Naturally, there would have to be some arrangement made with any supervisor in whose district the special facilities were situated. If the community has the financial capacity, it may employ several activity specialists who work with ill and disabled clients in their homes. Few communities now do this, however, preferring to have the clients, who can be, transported to central facilities particularly adapted to meet their needs.

The ultimate responsibility for utilization of specialists lies with the executive in charge of recreational programming for the system. The line of authority in the employment of staff specialist enables the program executive to channel staff personnel into the operation at a point which is convenient for accomplishing the aims of city-wide activities, providing instructional services both to staff and clients, and arranging for schedules.

The organizational form indicated here is neither the only method by which line and staff arrangements may be developed, nor the most appropriate for all agencies. It is offered as a possible model for medium and large metropolitan communities and counties. Its utility comes in the provision of direct recreational services to various clients and the administrative effectiveness of the delivery of service. It also specifically indicates the responsibility of each staff member for presentation of recreational opportunities that exist.

Clients in Other Programs

In many communities, children and adults with illnesses and disabilities are receiving supportive and/or educational service from various agencies. Examples are special service centers for the handicapped, senior citizen centers, group homes, and public schools. Recreational activities are an important element in the programs of the sponsoring agencies, and when the size warrants it, a recreationist with training in therapeutic or adapted recreational service is employed as the director. Otherwise, the director of the center or of the overall program has responsibility for the recreational activities. In both cases, those who are in charge usually work closely with the community recreational service department and use its special services when appropriate.

Recreational Centers for Handicapped Individuals. Because mainstreaming of handicapped people into the regular recreational program does not provide recreational opportunities to all those who are disabled, some communities have established recreational centers for handicapped participants. All community activities offered for those who are incapacitated originate in the center. The director of the center is usually directly responsible to the chief executive of the community recreational service department. In urban areas where the center is large in size and scope of activity, its program may be departmentalized by types of activities, e.g., music department, crafts department, sport department.

Senior Centers. With the increasing population of elderly citizens, special centers to serve the needs and interests common to older age groups have become popular. Generally the centers are supported by public funds, but some are sponsored by churches or private agencies and organizations. Programs at the centers are largely recreational service although educational and health care activities are often included. The director of the center or the recreational service director, if the center is large enough to employ one, usually with the assistance of volunteer senior citizens, plans the recreational activities. The program is customarily coordinated with the community recreational service department to enable the widest possible range of services, particularly adapted recreational activities.

Group Homes. A group home is a house or apartment in which several adults or juveniles with a common disability live together as much like a family-situation as possible. Group homes are presently established for mentally retarded individuals, addicts, delinquents, and those with psychiatric problems. In most states, group homes are administered by a department within the state government.

Directing the activities of the home are an adult woman and man, usually a married couple, with training in helping residents cope with the problems they encounter as the result of their disability and also those they confront as responsible members of a group living together. Some of the residents may be employed at jobs in the community, but others are incapable of outside work and remain at the home to care for it and to assist any residents who have difficulty with self-care.

Recreational Activities in Group Homes. Recreational activities in the home are patterned as closely as possible on those that constitute the leisure choices of the families of the group home residents. This helps to reinforce the concept of being a part of a family. However, there is also an effort to introduce new recreational pursuits that will expand interests and spur latent talents and abilities so that the lives of the residents may be enriched.

Use of recreational resources outside the home is a definite part of the planned recreational service. There may be trips to local movies, play productions, concerts, and exhibits, to name a few possibilities. Participation at local commercial recreational facilities like the bowling alley, golf driving range, and swimming pool, are also arranged; often these establishments are willing to reduce the fees for group attendance. The interaction with the community outside the group home and the opportunity to practice social skills is of great importance to the residents. So, in addition to the initiation of activities utilizing community resources, there is a coordinated effort to mainstream the residents into the program at the local community recreational center.

Adapted Recreational Service for School Children. In a few isolated cases, as pointed out earlier, large school systems may employ a recreationist who can provide activities for students with handicapping conditions. Most schools, however, when required to comply with the legal mandate to offer a program of recreational activities to meet the specific needs of students make arrangements with the community recreational center or with a treatment center with a therapeutic recreational department to offer the needed services.

Individualized Education Program. The Individualized Education Program (IEP), required by Public Law 94-142, is a plan of study designed for a particular handicapped student. The law states that for each handicapped school age child, there must be developed an IEP, indicating short-term objectives and yearly goals based on needs determined by evaluation (see Chapter 6 for discussion of assessment and evaluation procedures). Members of the IEP team must by law comprise the child's teacher, an administrator of the school, parent(s), and the child when appropriate. If one of the objectives determined by the team necessitates the child's receiving recreational service, the school is required to provide activities to meet the need. Under these circumstances, the school is permitted the option of electing a community recreational program to provide the activities the student needs.

Community Groups. In nearly every community there are various kinds of privately supported groups developing opportunities for handicapped residents to engage in recreational activities. Civic and social groups often sponsor social events, like parties, dances, and holiday celebrations, especially for those who are handicapped. These events occur only occasionally and are usually conducted by volunteer members of the host organization. Other groups offer year-round programs of recreational activities, open to handicapped people of all ages and degrees of disability.

Prominent among these organizations are the Boy Scouts of America, the Girl Scouts of America, the Young Men's Christian Association, the Young Women's Christian Association, the Catholic Youth Organization, the Young Men's Hebrew Association, the Young Women's Hebrew Association, the Boy's Club of America, and the Girl's Club of America. There is much effort made in the programs of these groups to mainstream handicapped participants in the regular recreational activities. The recreational leadership in the organizations of this kind is usually professionally trained, but much use is made of volunteers.

Other than these groups, there are some that have organized for the purpose of serving single groups of handicapped individuals. The Association for Mentally Retarded Citizens, the United Cerebral Palsy Association, and the National Easter Seal Society are examples. These organizations conduct recreational events for special populations in the community and in treatment centers. Many of them have focused on sports and sponsor competitive events at all levels from local to international; some offer special coaching clinics to ensure application of the national rules and regulations adapted for the specific handicapping condition. Campaigns are conducted to recruit vast numbers of volunteer helpers at the sport events.

All types of groups may need to borrow facilities and equipment from other groups or from the local recreational service department in order to carry out planned activities on a hoped-for scale. Staff assistance may also be requested. Often the arrangements for such use, especially in small communities, are informal. However, it is always a good idea to have developed written statements on policies and procedures to avoid misunderstandings that often produce poor community relationships.

Transportation Services

Transporting participants is a major problem in the organization of recreational services for handicapped clients in the community recreational program. Often there are many adults who are without personal transportation and who cannot utilize public transportation because of their personal limitations or because of the inadequacies of the public vehicles. To enable participation in the recreational program by these people, the recreational department needs to devise transportation services.

Communities have solved the problem in various ways. Volunteer and private vehicles are used in some instances with drivers recruited from among parents, relatives, and volunteer agencies. The arrangement is not entirely satisfactory, however, because of problems of insurance coverage and also the difficulty of ordinary vehicles carrying wheelchairs. Sometimes community service organizations like the Rotary or Lions Club purchase a van with a loading ramp for wheelchairs and donate it, along with the services of a driver and the maintenance of the vehicle, to the

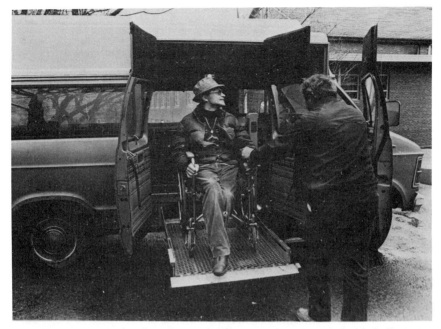

Fig. 4-7 A van with a loading ramp facilitates transportation of disabled clients to recreational activities.

recreational service department for its use in transporting disabled clients. Or such a van may be purchased by the department itself if funds are adequate. Procedures must then be established for insuring the vehicle and occupants and employment standards set for the driver.

Facilities and Equipment

Programming is determined to a considerable extent by the facilities and equipment available. A community that has even a moderately good recreational program will probably have adequate facilities and equipment to accommodate handicapped clients. The chief problem is generally an architectural one—the presence of stairs that make entrance to the facility difficult or impossible for those with lower limb involvement. Possible solutions range from carrying the clients up the stairs to installing ramps and elevators.

Some of the older treatment centers, built before the recognition of the importance of recreational service in the hospital setting, have little in the way of facilities planned specifically for recreational use; consequently, recreational space is available only through conversion of visiting rooms, porches, corridors, and other unused space. Treatment centers of more recent vintage usually have areas specifically planned for recreational use, although where conditions are crowded, the space is often utilized for beds or other hospital needs. If facilities are inadequate, the recreationist must exercise his or her ingenuity to make the most productive use of the space available. The selection of activities must be appropriate for facilities that are provided and consistent with the idea that these facilities must be used in the most effective way possible.

Most of the recreational equipment that is used in the regular recreational program can in most instances be used effectively in the adapted program. However, at times the equipment will need to be modified to meet the specific needs of a handicapped individual, or a piece of equipment must be used in a way that is different from its standard usage. An example of the former is the modification of a softball bat by sawing several inches off the end so that it can be more easily swung by a child with one arm; an example of equipment used in a different way to accommodate a disability is the space ball net substituted for a table tennis paddle by a blind player.

In addition to modifications that can be made by the recreationists, there are various pieces of equipment on the market that have been especially designed for use by handicapped participants. These range from outsized scissors to be used in cutting by those with problems in gripping to devices for guiding the bowling ball down the alley for those with limited mobility.

Still another way of providing equipment for recreational activities for handicapped clients is the use of items not normally associated with recreational use. Possibilities include scarves, rolls of twine, balloons, and boxes of various sizes and shapes. They can be endlessly fascinating to groups of all ages. Ideas for their use and other suggestions of items and adapted equipment are found in the chapters of section 3.

Scheduling in Treatment Centers

Scheduling recreational activities will depend upon the routine of the treatment center. Recreational time should be scheduled so that it does not interfere with the medical treatment and care of the patients. However, therapeutic recreational activity should have an important place in the day's schedule and should not be subject to cancellation in order to accommodate other activities. Schedules should be flexible enough to be adapted readily if emergencies arise and yet provide consistent daily opportunities for the patient to engage in recreational pursuits. A certain flexibility also allows the recreationist to take advantage of unique opportunities for programming that may arise, such as a visit to the treatment center by a well-known personality who may give an impromptu program of entertainment.

As a general rule with respect to scheduling, it is best to schedule activities that are more strenuous in the morning or after the rest period in the afternoon; quiet games, movies, musical programs, etc. are more appropriate in the evening hours. Of course, it is also necessary to consider the attitudes and interests of a specific patient, as well as his or her physical condition, in scheduling activities. The amount of time to be allocated to recreational participation by any one patient varies with the patient's condition. Some patients are able to participate even in quiet activities for only brief periods while others with the same illness or disability may be able to engage in recreational activity for an extended period without undue fatigue.

Scheduling in Community Settings

The schedule of recreational activities for special populations in community settings should parallel that of the regular program. There are some exceptions, however. If there are sheltered workshops in the community, a check to determine the hours of their workday will indicate if scheduling specific activities at times other than when they are regularly scheduled is desirable to ensure opportunities for the workers to participate. Checking their schedule of activities with the directors of group homes is useful for the same reason.

Offering activities for special populations at the same time that the regular clients participate in these activities has the advantage of dual scheduling. The dual system enables special clients to move between the program designed for them and the regular program as their abilities and needs indicate. For example, if mentally retarded clients are scheduled for table tennis at the same time the activity is being offered to regular clients, it is possible to move a mentally retarded client with exceptional skill in the game into the regular group where the challenge is greater and the opportunity to develop social skills is greater.

Regardless of other factors involved in scheduling, a continuous canvassing of clients should be made to determine the best day and times for offering special events for handicapped clients.

Participant Planning

Involvement of clients and patients in the program is still another phase of the process of organizing special recreational services. The term applied to this phase of the operation is participant planning and it refers to the utilization of clients in community recreational settings and patients in treatment centers in advisory capacities with regard to the planning and conduct of the activities of the program. Participation by clients and patients may be informal in structure; but, particularly in treatment centers, formally organized advisory committees and councils are favored.

Community Setting Participant Planning. At the most informal level participation by clients in the community setting occurs in interviews and discussions with clients to learn about their interests and attitudes. This less formal participation can be advanced to client membership on committees to assist with program planning and to provide advisory services. The recreationist benefits from the reactions and recommendations from the "consumers" of the program, while they acquire greater self-realization, mastery of the skills of social interaction, and personal satisfaction.

Treatment Center Participant Planning. In the treatment center, the prescription for the patient's activities is merely the first step in the initiation of therapeutic recreational services. When patients can be influenced to be actively concerned about the setting up of their own activities, it is more likely that they will experience gratification and immediate satisfaction. If clients do not have the ability to spontaneously select or reveal activity choices, then the recreationist must offer several attractive alternative activities that have been suggested in a previously conducted interview. Gaining the client's confidence, reinforcing correct behavioral patterns with positive rewards, and gradually leading the individual into an expression of likes and dislikes can be instrumental in meeting the prescribed treatment goals.

By the recreationist's working closely with the client at every step of the way and literally forcing decisions, the activities selected will have greater meaning for the client and have a more intense effect in rehabilitation. Obviously, one cannot force another to enjoy an activity or impose an activity against the person's will or interests. Only by gaining the client's interest through his or her own apparent selection of activities will the recreationist have a chance to make the recreational experience beneficial. Participant planning may be one important method for motivating the client.

Advisory Committee. Whenever treatment centers have wards or units, i.e., those divisions of hospital space into which predetermined numbers of patients are placed for residence and therapy, recreationists may find it beneficial both to patients and program to form committees of patients in each unit. Membership on the committee may be by election or appointment.

The committee can be most effective in generating patients' interests in participation and activity. When patients feel that their ideas, suggestions, and advice are taken into serious consideration in the development of the program, there is greater likelihood they will personally identify with the program and support the planned activities. The importance of the committee is that it permits patients to function in a responsible role to make a contribution to their own situation, and to have some say about how their body and mind will be employed.

In the heady pursuits of suggestions, plans, and selection of activities patients tend to forget the prescription which literally forces them to participate. The consequences may be wonderfully therapeutic and stimulate further involvement. It is this additional involvement, now grown beyond the point of involuntary participation, which provides the essential satisfactions and brings to fruition the effects for which the therapeutic recreational service is striving.

Councils. Self-governance by patients and the benefits that derive from it can be further developed through an all-institution client council, functioning in much the same manner as do unit committees. Interested representatives may be elected from the unit committees to participate in a variety of planning and decision-making functions. Among these may be the setting of behavioral codes and expected levels of conduct, determining visitation privileges and hours, planning community trips, and other relevant activities that have normally been the purview of hospital administration. Naturally, patients need to be in sufficient contact with reality and have the necessary emotional maturity to serve on such a council.

Use of Volunteers

The utilization of volunteers in the recreational program of both treatment centers and community settings offers an unparalleled opportunity for extending recreational services to clients who might otherwise not receive the guidance or help they need to benefit fully from an activity. For this reason, use of volunteers is considered part of program organization.

Volunteers may be lay people in the community or clients who are capable of helping other clients. Almost anyone who has the time and some interest, talent, or skill to share is a potential volunteer. However, some screening is necessary to eliminate individuals who are motivated by abnormal personal needs rather than by a genuine desire to help others. After the screening, volunteers need to receive orientation to the therapeutic recreational department of the treatment center or in the community setting, to the recreational facilities and program.

The orientation is essentially the same in both settings. Volunteers are made aware of the philosophy, policies, and objectives of the program. They are informed about the activities of the program, the kinds of clients being served, and the ways in which they as volunteers will be used. As much information about individual clients as possible for the volunteers to know without violating the client's rights of privacy is provided to promote understanding and appreciation.

The primary purpose of orientation is to give the volunteers the necessary information to develop insight into the behavioral and adjustment problems and physical limitations that patients have in order to better understand what they can do to help. Secondly, orientation suggests ways that volunteers may be useful in the overall program operation. Finally, orientation establishes the importance of communication about the clients so that staff and volunteers may learn more about those whom they are serving through the exchange of observations about clients' behavior and ideas for enhancing their recreational experiences.

Volunteer activities range from helping with office routines to assisting in the conduct of the program. Volunteers with training or expertise in any of the activity areas of the program can provide valuable teaching or supervisory assistance to a group or in working personally with an individual client. Volunteers with no special skills can contribute in a multitude of other ways, to name a few: take messages, run errands, keep records, transport clients, decorate for parties and special events, make and serve refreshments, read to or simply chat with clients. A particularly valuable service by volunteers is assisting with the program for homebound clients to whom they give the personal contact needed to motivate continued participation in recreational activities.

REFERENCES

1. Carol Peterson and Scout Gunn, *Therapeutic Recreation Program Design—Principles and Procedures,* 2nd. ed., (Englewood Cliffs: New Jersey, Prentice-Hall, Inc., 1984) p. 276.
2. Federal Register, "Education of Handicapped Children, Part II, Implementation of Part B of the Education of the Handicapped Act (Department of Health, Education, and Welfare, Office of Education, Aug. 23, 1977) p. 42478.
3. Federal Register, "Handicapped Persons, Part V. Section 504 of the Rehabilitation Act of 1973" Department of Health, Education, and Welfare, Office of Education, May 17, 1976) p. 20309.
4. John Nesbitt, "The 1980's Recreation a Reality for All" in *Education Unlimited* (Boothwyn, Pennsylvania, Educational Resources Center, June 1979) p. 2.
5. Hollis Fait, "Random Survey of State Departments of Education to Ascertain Numbers of Handicapping Conditions," *Professional Preparation of Personnel in Physical Education for the Handicapped* (Storrs, Connecticut, University of Connecticut, 1981) p. 5.

SELECTED REFERENCES

Case, Maurice, *Recreation for Blind Adults: Organized Programs in Special Settings* (Springfield: Charles Thomas, Publishers, 1965).
Edginton, R. E., Compton, D. M. and Hanson, C. J., *Recreation and Leisure Programming: A Guide for the Professional* (Philadelphia: W. B. Saunders, 1980).
Farrell P. and Lundegren, H. M., *Recreation Programming: Theory and Technique,* 2nd. ed., (New York: John Wiley and Sons, 1983).
Levine, Susan P., *Recreational Experiences for the Severely Impaired or Nonambulatory Child* (Springfield: Charles C Thomas, 1983).
Peterson, Carol and Gunn, Scout, *Therapeutic Recreation Program Design—Principles and Procedures,* 2nd. ed., (Englewood Cliffs, New Jersey: Prentice-Hall, Inc., 1984).
Witt, Jody, Campbell, Marilyn, and Witt, Peter, *A Manual of Therapeutic Group Activities for Leisure Education* (Ottawa, Canada: Leisurability, 1975).

Chapter 5

Understanding Problems of Adjustment Caused by Illness and Disability

Normality of appearance and behavior is a distinct concept on which certain social attitudes and practices are formed. The way others view an individual, as well as an individual's own view, produces specific responses. Based upon particular cultural preconceptions, people react in ways that are influenced by conditioning factors of their environment. In the same way, individuals observing unusual physical characteristics or extraordinary behavior will respond in accordance to their personal appraisal of these characteristics. The success of the therapeutic recreationist in working with those whose appearance and behavior is affected by physical disabilities or mental deficiencies is to a large extent dependent upon an understanding of the behavioral responses of general society and the influence this has on the adjustment of those who differ from society's concept of "normal."

ATTITUDES TOWARD DISABILITY

All biases are learned. No one is born with preconceived attitudes about anything or anyone. The specific ignorances and prejudices which people manifest in the normal course of daily routine are conditioned from earliest remembrances of what was said and how such expressions were delivered and received in the home environment. Thus biased remarks are learned and accepted as factual information and repeated as such. From earliest childhood on, individuals are influenced by the attitudes of family, peers, and associates in countless ways. Consequently, those whose appearance is not considered normal, due to disabling illness or injury, encounter negative reactions fostered by society's prejudices and ignorance about physical disabilities.

Individuals with mental deficiencies are even more subject to negative responses for they are likely to deviate from the accepted norms in both appearance and behavior. The cause or agent of their mental impairment often produces physical disability as well. Even when no physical problems are apparent, mental incapacity may influence development of characteristics that are perceived as being unattractive, e.g., the gaping mouth, awkward posture, and nervous ticks or extraneous movements. To the extent that mentally retarded individuals are capable of responding to their social environment, the attitudes of others toward them affect their adjustment, just as in the case of those who are physically ill and disabled.

Early Home Environment

The impairment, as such, does not typically result in personality distortion, but the treatment that impaired individuals receive from earliest childhood often produces maladjustments. Parents who are generally the most constant element in the child's environment often either cannot or do not accept the condition of the child and so compound the problem by the manner of their response.

Parental reactions directed toward the disabled child, particularly when there is severe physical impairment or mental incapacitation, are sufficiently typical to be identified by categories. These are:

- Overprotection: The child is in effect wrapped in a cocoon of parental protection to avoid exposure to the negative reactions of others or to prevent possible injuries due to movement limitations. Overindulgence of the child's behavior and the satisfying of every want are common.

- Overt rejection: Association, even communication, with the child is avoided because the parents are so greatly affected by the disfigurement or incapacity that normal parental acceptance and love are not possible. Neglect and even cruel and inhuman treatment of the child occur in extreme cases.

- Vacillation between affectionate care and animosity: Because they alternate between feelings of love and hate for their impaired child, parents express their emotions either with lavish attention or hostile reactions. An environment of insecurity results as a consequence of the vacillation.

Desirable parental attitudes are those based on acceptance of the child's deformity or illness, rather than on irrational explanations, e.g., punishment by God, or guilt about some fantasized or suspected taint in the family. The parental behavior most beneficial to satisfactory adjustment is that which is accepting, loving, and security-providing, which recognizes the child's limited capacity but does not smother the child with overprotection. Realistic acceptance of the problem should preclude emotional dependency by the child on the parents.

Group Attitudes

A whole range of prejudicial attitudes is revealed whenever a sampling is taken of the general population's views of mentally retarded, disabled, or chronically ill individuals.[1] Most people hold stereotyped concepts of mentally and physically handicapped persons and are frequently afraid to associate with them. The usual reactions are either overt or covert cringing. It is also possible that the unafflicted individual is subconsciously

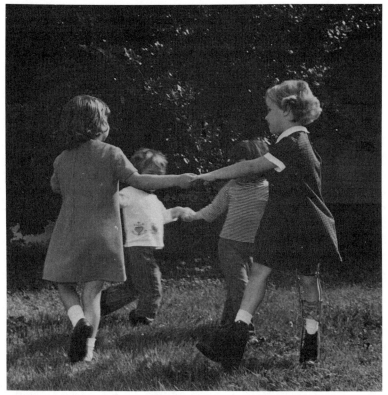

Fig. 5-1 Satisfying experiences contribute to positive attitudes about the self. (March of Dimes)

breathing a sigh of relief and saying, "There, but for the grace of God, go I." In this very act of thankfulness, the person may also be experiencing a twinge of guilt.

ATTITUDES TOWARD SELF

Physically disabled individuals may accept their permanent disability, but frequently also feel fear, isolation, and sensitivity about the handicap. Optimal development of good interpersonal relations between disabled and nondisabled persons necessitates communication about the disability. However, those who are disabled often reject any sign of interest by an acquaintance. Initially, they may believe that such curiosity represents a negative reaction toward them as persons. Secondly, mere discussion of the disability may activate remembrances of earlier unsatisfactory experiences with others and thus becomes anxiety-provoking. Finally, disabled individuals can have completely negative feelings toward themselves insofar as the disability is concerned, viewing it as a shameful stigma, as a mark of inferiority, and something to be kept from view.

Disabled people often feel that they are not really accepted as members of social groups in terms of their ability to become actively engaged in group activities. This may occur because they believe their abilities are underestimated and that for this reason they are excluded from group activities. Feelings of being left out hamper the disabled persons' ability to communicate about themselves thereby intensifying the feelings of exclusion; and so a vicious cycle of negativism is perpetuated.

In diseases that affect the body, the perception of the body commonly undergoes modification as the body changes. However, in certain situations changes in the body structure may take place without associated changes in the body image. This happens most frequently in imperceptibly developing chronic diseases that slowly alter the body structure. When physical deformity takes place, frustration of the social, occupational, and normal sexual behaviors suitable to the body image occurs because the behaviors cannot be actualized by the ruined physique. This discrepancy, in turn, leads to emotionality, fantasy, friction, and delusional processes.

In instances where psychotic reactions are not present, individuals tend to deny their disability through a repression mechanism that obliterates any conscious recognition of their disability. Furthermore, such individuals will not admit to their incapacity to perform. While the latter may be a desirable adjustment pattern, it is probable that the discrepancy between the actually disabled body and the hoped-for-normal body will become so great that the individual loses contact with reality. Under such circumstances maladjustment results, and in severe cases delusional overtones with regression to psychotic reaction can develop.

PSYCHOLOGY OF ACUTE ILLNESS

With the realization of their illness, individuals' range of vision is suddenly reduced. Almost all situations which once assumed paramount importance lose their immediacy and importance. Such conditioners of behavior as business matters or professional obligations, family affairs, studies, and other forms of social interactions are important when individuals are well; in illness, such factors cause only self-centered behavior. One of the supreme examples of this type of behavior is related by the Nobel prize winner Solzhenitsyn in his novel *The Cancer Ward*. A patient with a tumor is admitted to the hospital specializing in the treatment of cancer. He is a respected functionary within the current political administration. After his physical examination and confrontation with the physician who diagnoses and will treat him, the following is recorded:

> But in a few days this whole close-knit, ideal Rusanov family—with two older and two younger children, with their completely well-ordered life, and their spotless apartment, unstintingly furnished—had receded until it had vanished on *the other side* of the tumor. No matter what happened to the father, they were alive and would go on living. No matter how they might worry, exhibit concern, or weep now, the tumor had divided him from them like a wall, and he remained alone on this side of it.[2]

The author here brilliantly captures the psychology of the sick person: The letting go of everything that, up to the time of diagnosis, had assumed importance in the individual's life. The central focus of the individual's attention is his or her own pain, deformity, or affliction. The things that tend to influence the obvious behavior of an individual become restricted to the requirements of a select circle of people—physicians, nurses, aides, specialist technicians; a select group of physical conditions—noise, light and darkness, heat and coldness, physical comfort; and the incessant demands of a few personal needs—absence of pain, nourishment, rest, and shutting out thoughts of distressing symptoms and prognosis. The sick person's world becomes so reduced in content, scope, and meaning that it closely resembles that of an infant, and the behavior resulting from these factors is often infantile also.

Egocentricity

Infantilism can be the product of illness at any time, but it is seen most dramatically when illness is acute and severe. The person who is ill becomes the center of a universe designed especially to cater to his or her needs. Situations are appropriately adjusted to the demands of the sick person to a greater extent than to the needs of the healthy. An ill individual's behavior, like that of a child, is less restrained by previous experience and the knowledge that others exist. In such a restricted universe the individual's needs, desires, and perceptions are the chief determinants of all behavior and intellectualization and social response are therefore much more egocentric as a result.

As the world closes about the sick person and the strength of external behavior conditioners is weakened, internal agents of behavior become more significant. The healthy person is nearly oblivious of physiologic processes, but the sick person frequently agonizes over them and in the process suffers pain and torment. The importance of minor bodily variations such as temperature, pulse rate, digestion, elimination, and breathing is exaggerated and these receive concentrated attention. Again, the observers may recognize the similarity to the world of the infant whose behavior is almost always determined by proprioceptive and interoceptive stimuli, i.e., stimulation from the ligaments, muscles, and organs.

Regression

Because the ill adult's situation is like an infant's in terms of narrow scope, egocentricity, and the influence of internal rather than external determiners of behavior, it follows that regressed or infantile behavior should also be a part of the sick person's reaction. Among the kinds of behavior that accompany sickness or impairment are:

- The number of interests will decrease. Fewer stimuli will arouse the individual, since the range of interests in the physical and social world is reduced and the power of several internal stimuli, e.g., hormone production or other chemical changes, decreases. The ill person becomes relatively parochial in comparison to a former broadly oriented viewpoint. Regressive behavior is characteristic and not unusual.

- Sick persons tend to become autocratic, partial, and self-indulgent. Since they inhabit a narrowly restricted environment, they are incapable of understanding the needs of others; their behavior is determined by their own selfish interests to the exclusion of all others. There have been countless narratives of experiences where invalids literally took over the lives of those devoted to them, by playing upon their sympathy and / or affection.

- At particular periods during the illness, individuals become indifferent to the world around them. Such reactions are encouraged by the tight circle of sympathizers and attendants who make no demands upon the sick person. The reduced scope of the patient's world does not require adjustment to the varied and frequently contrary realities of life.

- The more sudden the onset of severe illnesses or the longer the duration of illness, the more frightened, susceptible to insecurity, and dependent sick individuals become. They may feel ambivalence; they have enormous influence on the lives of those who are caring for them, and yet they are absolutely dependent upon these people. This situation is similar to that of children who love their parents yet are fearful about losing them since they are absolutely dependent on the parents for survival. Adult patients may develop a similar love-hate relationship because of the conditions of helplessness and dominance which coexist.

- Hypochondriacal behavior is very likely during any prolonged period of illness. The stimuli which tend to motivate the behavior of sick persons are almost always going to be those internal and physical manifestations of which they are most aware. In this case, they typically become the center of their universe and direct unceasing attention on themselves. Every thought and communication focuses on how they feel, look, or sound. They become preoccupied with their own symptoms. Overconcern with personal physiology is another indication of regressive behavior.

PSYCHOLOGY OF PHYSICAL DISABILITY

Even moderate degrees of functional deficiency may insidiously, yet definitely, intervene with daily living. Obviously impairments in structure and function frustrate self-fulfillment. If the frustration is not to become psychologically debilitating, the individual must accept the disability or impairment for what it is and must renegotiate an appropriate system of values. A personal acceptance of the self is concomitant with the acceptance of a disability. However, the individual is not necessarily resigned to the inevitability of impairment nor to liking the condition. Instead there is acceptance of the self as a human being with certain structural deficiencies, recognizing that these do not devaluate the individual as a person. The disability still restricts, but effort continues to improve the capacity to perform. There are no feelings of shame or guilt—nor should there be—about the disability.

Broad Values

No one can say that it is not of major importance for individuals to have the full use of their neural apparatus and anatomic structure. However, where impairment results, either as a congenital defect or as a result of accident or injury, personal values may tend to compensate for and offer support in the face of loss. Thus, life itself and skills or talents already acquired, plus social acceptance, intellectual acuity, or other current and potential strengths provide a base of support. An individual with a disability is emotional over his or her loss in terms of personal and social achievements and rewards that might now be closed. The loss of range of motion and function permeates the thoughts of the disabled individual at least at first. For example, at the onset of blindness following accident:

> The shock consists of depersonalization followed by depression. The depersonalization usually lasts 2 to 7 days. The patient is immobile, or almost so, facial expression is blank, there is a generalized hypoesthesia or anesthesia, and mutism, or speech is meager, slow, muted. Superficially, the condition may resemble catatonia. But the patient does not utter the delusional or dissociated remarks of a schizophrenic: rather he is likely during the acute stage, or more often later, to say that he has no feeling or that he feels as if he were unreal or the world were unreal . . . The depression which follows may be an acute reactive depression or an agitated depression . . . And it is a state of mourning for the loss of the eyes.[3]

This form of depressive reaction is not unusual, nor is it the only type of behavioral pattern observed in individuals who experience a sensory of motor function loss. Combat casualties, although depressed by wounds suffered, have manifested reactions that can only be termed happy in comparison with what might have been expected. While depressed at the loss of limb or sight, the depression occupies a secondary place in the hierarchy of emotions. The fact that the soldier is alive rather than dead provides the rationale for feelings of relief. In order to adjust and compensate for the state of loss, the individual must concentrate on the possibilities remaining and the satisfactions that can be achieved despite the loss. When disabled individuals recognize that they still have the potential to engage in many activities, although perhaps not as wide-ranged as formerly, and that they can make their own way, then the process of reappraisal has begun in earnest and the scope of values enlarges.

As the range of values broadens, the importance of physique may diminish. If physique becomes less dominant, then its effects become of less concern. The reverse also holds: reducing the attention given to physique downgrades its place in the hierarchy of values. It is not difficult to appreciate the fact that persons who widen their value horizons by subordinating the importance of physique and perceiving it as a lesser value, will achieve improved self-acceptance.

Model of Response to Crisis

The responses by so many to the personal crisis of an illness or disability that is progressive or permanent in nature have such similarity that a typical pattern has been identified. A model of the pattern of a crisis developed by Fink has four phases in the response pattern: shock or stress, defensive retreat (blocking out or denying), acknowledgement, and adaptation and change. The model given in Table 5-1 also provides information about the typical nature of the patient's perception, the emotional reaction, and the reasoning process as well as the status of the disability at each stage of the pattern.

The patient passes through the various stages more or less slowly depending on the way the circumstances are perceived. Movement back and forth between phases can be expected during the initial period of entry into a new stage. Some individuals regress after having passed one or more stages, or they may be unable to go beyond a certain phase.

SOCIAL PROBLEMS OF DISABLEMENT

Rarely do individuals who are not themselves disabled understand and appreciate the problems encountered by those who are disabled. That most of these problems result from the attitudes and values of society rather than the disease, deformity, or sensory loss, is difficult for the healthy person to recognize. While it is easy to see that a disabled person does not have the full use of his or her body and to appreciate the restrictions of the condition because of a previous experience of one's own with a fractured bone or muscle strain, comprehension of a disability arising from a birth defect or accidental loss is quite another matter. The able-bodied have never had to face the great frustrations encountered in satisfying the daily activities of living nor have they needed to abandon objectives toward which they strived as a result of impairment. It is hard to comprehend, for example, how the problems of traveling by oneself threaten the blind and why the great difficulty in communicating is such a thwarting social obstruction for the deaf.

The problems which confront those who have been physically disabled as a result of accident or war injury are somewhat different from those who are congenitally disabled. Individuals who are blinded or deafened in later years have had past experience with vision and sound. They know what color is and can remember the nuances of language and sound. This definitely affects their rehabilitation, although their sense of loss and frustration at having to give up occupational goals they may have had and worked toward should not be minimized. They will, most certainly, make the devastating comparison between what has been and what remains.

The degree to which those who are disabled can achieve satisfaction in their lives will be immeasurably increased if popular myths, negative attitudes, cosmetic aversion, and hypocrisy can be replaced by frankness, disinterested acceptance, and truth on the part of society. It is probable that the often negative attitude toward the disabled, rather than the im-

TABLE 5-1. PSYCHOLOGIC PHASES OF CRISIS*

Phase	Self-Experience	Reality Perceptions	Emotional Experience	Cognitive Structure	Physical Disability
Shock (Stress)	Threat to existing structures	Perceived as overwhelming	Panic; anxiety; helplessness	Disorganization; inability to plan or to reason or to understand situation	Acute somatic damage requiring full medical care
Defensive retreat	Attempt to maintain old structures	Avoidance of reality; "wishful thinking"; denial; repression	Indifference or euphoria (except when challenged, in which case anger); (low anxiety)	Defensive reorganization; resistance to change	Physical recovery from acute phase; functional return to maximum possible level
Acknowledgement (renewed stress)	Giving up existing structure; self depreciation	Facing reality; facts "impose" themselves	Depression with apathy or agitation; bitterness; mourning; high anxiety; if overwhelming, suicide	Defensive breakdown; (1) disorganization; (2) reorganization in terms of altered reality perceptions	Physical plateau gradual slowing of improvement until no change is experienced
Adaptation and change	Establishing new structure; sense of worth	New reality testing	Gradual increase in satisfying experiences; (gradual lowering of anxiety)	Reorganization in terms of present resources and abilities	No change in physical disability status

* Joan Luckman and Karen Sorensen, *Medical-Surgical Nursing: A Psychophysiologic Approach*, 2nd ed. (Philadelphia, W. B. Saunders Co., 1980).

pairment itself, promotes serious problems of adjustment and encourages a great degree of frustration. Undoubtedly, maladjustment among disabled persons is more often a result of an inability to break through the customary rebuffs and thwartings of society than of failure to accommodate successfully to the physical condition itself.

PERSONALITY CHARACTERISTICS OF THE IMPAIRED

It is often stated that specific disabilities—in particular, blindness, deafness and epilepsy—have characteristic personality patterns associated with them. However, a common behavior pattern evidenced by a group of individuals with the same impairment is a reaction to the obstacles and common misconceptions and attitudes of a negative society. The impairment is not in and of itself the cause of a characteristic pattern of behavior.

Some conditions of disability, particularly those which accrue from head injuries, involve damage to the brain and thus changes in behavior are not unexpected; but generally, any personality characteristics that appear after the onset of some accident or injury can be explained in terms of the type of personality that had been developed prior to the disability. The individual and the environment in which he or she was nurtured have the greatest influence on a person's reaction to impairment—and not the disability itself.

REFERENCES

1. John M. Dunn and A. Marie Boarman, "A Need: Better Understanding of People With Special Need," *Campfire Leadership,* Winter: Vol. 6 (1979) p. 6.
2. Aleksandr I. Solzhenitsyn, *The Cancer Ward* (New York: Dell Publishing Co., Inc., 1968) p. 18.
3. H. R. Blank, "Psychoanalysis and Blindness," *Psychoanalytic Quarterly,* Vol. 26 (1957) pp. 1-24.

SELECTED REFERENCES

American Medical Association, *Guides to the Evaluation of Permanent Impairment* (Chicago: AMA, 1983).
Biklen, D. and Bailey, L., eds., *Rudely Stamp'd: Imaginal Disability and Prejudice* (Lanham, Maryland: University Press of America, 1982).
Darling, R. B., *Families Against Society: A Study of Reactions to Children with Birth Defects* (Beverly Hills, California: Sage Publications, Inc., 1979).
Kessler, H. H., *Disability: Determination and Evaluation* (Philadelphia: Lea & Febiger, 1970).
Wright, Beatrice, *Physical Disability: A Psychological Approach* (New York: Harper & Row, 1960).

Chapter 6

Determining Status and Progress: Assessment and Evaluation

No program in therapeutic or adapted recreational service can be fully successful in serving clients without an accurate basis of information for setting goals and for clear determination of the progress being made in achieving the goals. Therefore, some systematic assessment and evaluation procedures must be established to comprehend fully the characteristics of the client, to understand the nature of the special services required, to identify the procedures and techniques that are most effective with the client, and to facilitate monitoring the client's progress.

Programs of recreational service for ill and disabled clients also require periodic review and evaluation. Only in this way can it be known if the program is truly operating efficiently and effectively in agreement with the basic philosophy of special recreational service. Evaluation of the program provides information to judge the adequacy of equipment and facilities and the quality of performance of personnel. Program evaluation is, however, an administrative function and beyond the scope of this book. Therefore, the discussion in this chapter is concerned only with assessment and evaluation as it relates to serving clients.

Because the terms assessment and evaluation are used in different ways by writers in the field of recreational service, there is a need to define their meaning. Some authorities use the terms as synonymous, making no distinction between them. Others regard assessment as a process used only with individuals (clients) while applying evaluation to those determinations made of the status of programs, facilities, regimens, etc. The majority of writers in therapeutic recreational service, however, use the term assessment to indicate a procedure for gathering information to enable objectives and goals to be set and evaluation to indicate the process of determining the degree of achievement of those objectives and goals. It is in this light that the terms are used in this chapter.

EVALUATION AND LEGAL REQUIREMENTS OF PL 94-142

Although the provisions of the Education of the Handicapped Act, PL

90

94-142, focus on handicapped children in a school setting, consideration is also given to the development of recreational skills in the total education of the handicapped student. For this reason, the basic concepts of the law and the way the law relates to recreational services are of interest to recreationists in schools and in community adapted recreational programs who may be involved in directing recreational skill development of handicapped students.

Screening and Identification. The first procedure in the provision of the services to handicapped children required by the law is the screening of the general school population to locate those with handicapping conditions and, then, identification of those who need special assistance and the kind of assistance required. The screening and identification are usually carried out by the state's department of education in conjunction with local school districts or regions. Students with handicapping conditions that restrict their opportunities to engage in recreational activities are identified as are children whose recreational development deviates so significantly from the norm as to constitute a handicap. In the evaluation of these students, observations by teachers and recreationists are important, particularly if they have developed skill in using observation as an assessment tool. (A discussion of observation in assessment appears in a section later in the chapter.)

Due Process

Due process in PL 94-142 refers to the guaranteed procedural safeguards provided handicapped children and their parents. Parents and children must be informed of their rights; special emphasis is given their right to challenge educational decisions that they consider inadequate or unfair. This includes decisions concerning recreational services.

In situations requiring tests to be given to determine whether a child requires special educational services, written permission must be secured from the parents before the evaluation can be conducted. A letter to the parents must include a reason for the evaluation and a statement indicating the nature of the test(s). Public Law 94-142 establishes that "assessment of leisure function" may be a part of the evaluation to determine the need for special education procedures to be used. A sample form for requesting parental approval for evaluation of their child, which recognizes the need to evaluate leisure functions, is shown in Figure 6-1.

The letter must, if necessary, be in the native language of the parents. In addition a copy of the parents' rights must be included. Most states have a form developed for this purpose, but the notice includes information about due process, right of privacy, right to outside evaluation, right to qualified testers, right to know of results, and the right to a hearing (see discussion that follows).

The results of all evaluations must be given to the parents of the child and if necessary the results interpreted for them. In addition the parents

CONSENT FOR ASSESSMENT

Dear _____ :

Your child _____ is being referred for assessment to assist in the development of his/her educational program. To secure information that will enable teachers to give your child the best possible instruction for his/her needs, the tests in the following list that have been checked will be given to your child with your approval.

1. Academic achievement—level of basic academic skills, i.e., reading, writing, mathematics, and other appropriate areas
2. Behavior—emotional and social development or adapted behavior
3. Oral communication—ability to communicate the spoken word
4. Hearing and sight—level of ability to hear and see
5. Cognitivity development—degree of verbal and non-verbal intellectual functioning
6. Physical—ability to perform basic motor skills
7. Leisure function—skill and ability to take part in recreational activities

Enclosed please find a copy of explanation about your rights concerning the education of your child. Since the law requires that written permission be given for the testing, if you agree to the assessment procedure, please sign below, and return to this office.

_____

I, the undersigned, agree to have the above described testing be given to my child. I understand that the granting of this consent is voluntary and that I may request discontinuance of the testing at any time. I have received a copy of my rights with this letter.

Signed _____

Parent or Guardian

Date _____

Fig. 6-1 Parental consent form.

must be informed if the testing indicates a handicapping condition sufficiently severe to require special educational procedures. If the parents are dissatisfied with the test results (this includes leisure function assessment), the parents may ask for an independent evaluation of their child. Only if the findings are the same as the original evaluation do the parents have to pay for the evaluation.

If they do not agree with the school authorities, the parents have a right to a hearing by an impartial officer selected by the state department of education. The decision of this hearing officer is final unless appeal is filed. All test results and reports, including assessment of leisure functions, are confidential. Only school authorized officials may review the records unless special permission is given to others by the parents.

ADMINISTRATIVE EVALUATION AND ASSESSMENT REQUIREMENTS

Agencies, organizations, and clinical facilities often have various requirements for documenting the effects of treatment or rehabilitation programs on individual clients. In some instances, the requirements are initiated within the agency; but in other cases, like the Veterans Administration Hospitals, standardized policies are established by the federal government and these prescribe the record keeping procedures to be used and the types of evaluation and assessment information to be collected. Also, agencies and organizations that belong to accreditation bodies must meet specific standards of reporting evaluation and assessment results to achieve and maintain their accreditation. Most of such bodies do not dictate how the information is to be gathered, only the kind of information that must be reported.

Administrative evaluation and assessment are required not only for documentation of treatment and rehabilitation of clients, but to assemble information for third party payments. Third party payments are made by outside groups like insurance companies and governmental agencies for services which clients are entitled to receive by contract or law.

BASIC TYPES OF INSTRUMENTS OF ASSESSMENT AND EVALUATION

Two terms are used to indicate the way in which, and the time when, assessment and evaluation are used: summative and formative. Summative refers to the final determination of the quality and quantity of the item being measured and is used primarily for processes that determine if established objectives and goals have been met. Formative is applied to an ongoing evaluative process that measures progress during the formative stages or before the situation is terminated. Any particular test instrument may be summative or formative depending on how and when it is used.

Reliability and Validity

Reliability and validity are terms for defining the worthiness of a test. Reliability refers simply to consistency in the results of a test, that is, a test administered to a client one day and then again on another day produces the same results, if no changes occurred in the quality or quantity of the factor(s) being measured. Validity refers to the accuracy with which a test measures what it purports to measure.

In many situations statistical procedures are used to determine the degree of validity of tests. However, some tests have face validity, i.e., it is self-evident that the test is measuring what it purports to measure. For example, in a test to determine the ability of a client to cut along a line on a piece of paper with a pair of scissors, the result of the client's performance of the task provides evidence that the test produces the intended measurement. Tests created on the spot by recreationists for measuring simple tasks like this one should have face validity to ensure that the result obtained is the one that was sought.

Statistical Validity. There are three commonly utilized statistical procedures for determining validity of more complex tests. These procedures test the content validity, criterion referenced validity, and construct validity.

Content validity is demonstrated by showing how well the chosen test items sample knowledge of the total information (testing universe) presented to the testee. If the recreationist wished to know, for example, if a group of clients had enough information about the rules of bridge to play the game, a test containing sample questions drawn from the rules of the game (testing universe) could be prepared and administered to the clients. If the scores on the test of sample questions compared favorably to complete knowledge of all the rules, the same test would have content validity.

Criterion-referenced validity is demonstrated by comparing the test with a specific criterion. This is commonly done in two ways: comparison of the test results with a test whose validity has been established and comparison of the test results with the results of the opinions of a select group of experts in judging the characteristics being tested. In the first instance, the second test is the criterion and in the second case, the expert opinions become the criterion.

Construct validity is used to estimate validity when a test purports to measure an attribute or quality that is too complex or nebulous to be precisely measured. In other words, a criterion is not available or readily established for comparison purposes. The "construct" is some postulated attribute or quality assumed to be reflected in the test performance; anxiety, friendliness, proneness to violence are examples of constructs. One of the common means of investigating construct validity is factor analysis, a statistical procedure that shows interrelationship between the results of test items.

Correlation Coefficient

The reliability and validity of standardized tests are reported by the use of coefficient correlations. These are computed mathematically and designated by the symbol r. If there is perfect agreement between the test and what it is compared to, the r equals 1. If there is perfect negative agreement, i.e., one score goes up and the other goes down, the r is -1. An r of zero indicates no relationship. Scores ranging between 1 and -1 indicate the degree of agreement.

The type of characteristics being tested influence how the correlation coefficient score is interpreted in determining the degree that can be considered a fairly good relationship. Usually, however, .7 is considered the cut-off point for acceptable tests. Scores of .9 indicate a very high relationship. For the r of .7 the percentage of the test items being valid is 49% (.7 $\times$ .7) and for .9, is 81% (.9 $\times$ .9).

Norm-Referenced Tests

A norm-referenced or standardized test is one in which the results are compared to established criteria. Such tests have been or are commonly used in psychiatric testing; however, they have not, in the past, been widely used by recreationists. As their value in determining status or quality in therapeutic and adapted recreational programs has become increasingly recognized, these tests are being used more frequently by recreational service personnel. This kind of evaluation involves the development and administration of the test to a randomly selected group of people representing the type of individual the test has been designed to evaluate. For example, a test to measure cerebral palsy children must use a random selection from a group of children with cerebral palsy. The results of the testing become the criteria against which other cerebral palsied children can be compared. If the random selection of subjects is from non-handicapped children, the test can be used with handicapped children to determine how far they deviate from the norm and to identify individuals who are in need of special services. In the examiner's manual that accompanies norm-referenced tests, directions about how the test is to be administered are provided as well as how to score and interpret the results when making comparisons with established norms. In addition information is provided about the test's reliability, i.e., the degree to which the test provides the same results each time it is given, and the validity of the test, i.e., the extent to which it measures what it purports to measure.

Criterion-Referenced Test

Another type of referenced test is the criterion-referenced test which because of its versatility is well suited to assessment or evaluation in recreational programs. In the criterion-referenced test, the criterion or level of accomplishment for mastery is established arbitrarily for each item on the test and/or for the complete test. The scores indicate the level of achievement.

Performance and Item Analysis

The performance analysis and item analysis are frequently employed by recreationists. (The activity analysis, described in Chapter 3, is an example of item analysis.) These evaluation procedures are not criterion-referenced. They consist of determining the status at a given time without making comparisons to criteria or objectives; the analysis only provides information on the quality or quantity of performance or item being evaluated. The effectiveness of evaluation by analysis depends entirely on the level of knowledge and degree of objectivity of the individual making the analysis.

Instruments and Testing Procedures

Recreationists may select instruments and procedures for evaluation or assessment from among those that are available from professional publishers, or they may develop their own. In either case, the first consideration is the qualities or elements that are to be measured. Then, if a selection is being made and the test is to be norm-referenced, available tests appropriate to the subject must be examined to choose the most suitable. Factors to be considered in selecting a test are: (1) the ease of giving a test, (2) the kind of subjects used to develop the norm, (3) the cost of the test, (4) the length of the test and the validity and reliability of the test.

Criterion-Referenced. When a test is to be developed for use in a specific situation, the most appropriate type is the criterion-referenced test. In developing a test of this kind, a domain about which the evaluation is concerned is established. A domain is a pattern of behavior (the forms of behavior are psychomotor, affective [emotional] and cognitive [intellectual]). A domain is made up of various components. To illustrate using an example involving chiefly affective behavior: cooperation of children in play is a domain; sharing of toys by children is an important component of that domain (cooperation in children's play), but it is not the domain.

After the domain has been established, the test maker must decide which components of the domain or pattern are to be examined. The selection is based on the importance of the component to the performance of the behavior pattern (domain). For each of these components a criterion is set based on the level of mastery that is desired. In the example above, a possible criterion is: the child gives a toy in his or her possession to a playmate 8 out of 10 times when the playmate asks or reaches for the toy. A numerical score can then be recorded after observing the child's performance in play.

Offering an example relating the criterion-referenced test only to the affective form does not in any way infer that the test is most effective in this particular area. The test is readily developed for assessment or evaluation of psychomotor and cognitive forms as well.

Observation. All assessments and evaluations involve observation of subjects to some degree. However, when observation is formally utilized as a technique to assess or evaluate, there is a greater reliance on systematic procedures in recording of results.

Two procedures are primarily used: total observation and specific behavior observation. In both procedures a given time period is established for the observation of the client's recreational activity. The time may vary from 15 to 30 minutes to several days. The observation may be in the client's regular environment which is termed naturalistic observation.[1] Also, the environment may be contrived in order to observe how the client will react in a given situation.

Total observation may be referred to as watching all actions and responses of a client during a given time. Unless the time is short, observation is best limited to only the unusual or abnormal actions of the client. Care should be taken that expectations of the way an individual reacts do not color the observer's interpretation of what is happening. Constant awareness is required to prevent a preconceived concept of someone's behavior from producing misinterpretation of observations. It is extremely important when using observation as assessment or evaluation procedure that results should be recorded as soon as possible after the observation. Doing so ensures against possible influence by a later observation.

Total observation procedure is more difficult than specific behavior observation and probably less accurate because it requires alertness to all that is happening and because of the difficulty in accurately recording the numerous observations. However, it has the advantage of providing information about the relationship of one behavior to another that may not be evident during the brief specific behavioral observation.

In specific behavior observation an interval is selected, usually a period of an hour or two at a predetermined time of the day. During that period the observer looks for the occurrence of a specific behavior and records the frequency with which it happens. For example, the number of times the client hits, strikes, or takes other physically aggressive action against another person is observed and recorded. To further increase the usefulness of this observation, the apparent reason for the aggressive action can be noted.

Total observation and specific behavior observations may be combined to produce a method of observation more effective in some instances than either alone. The combination is used when knowledge about how a client may react in certain situations is required; an individual in a social situation or a child at play are common situations where observations occur. To guide the observer a list of significant actions or responses is prepared. Takata[2] has developed such a list in question form for guidance in the observation of a child at play. They are:

- With what does the child play?
- How does the child play?
- What type of play is avoided or liked the least?
- With whom does the child play?
- How does the child play with others?
- What body posture does the child use during play?
- How long does the child play?
- Where does the child play?
- When does the child play?

Interviews

Interviews, both casual and structured, are effective in gaining information in all situations where assessment of clients is involved. The casual interview may be no more than a conversation between client and recreationist but the astute recreationist can gain much insight about the client from such an exchange. Asking a simple question about how the client enjoyed a certain activity can produce interesting responses that will be of assistance in serving the client more effectively in other proposed activities. Some of the questions may be preplanned and then altered to fit the situation. It is essential that clients be made to feel they can express their thoughts freely; otherwise useful information will not be obtained.

The structured form of interview requires the selection of an area to be examined, e.g., interest in recreational activities or likes and dislikes of socializing situations in recreational activities. The interview is directed toward the objective of acquiring information about the selected area or subject.

To ensure meeting the objective in the interviews, specific questions are prepared for use prior to the interview. Austin[3] suggests open-end questions, ones that tend to produce further questions. Following are some examples of open-end questions that could be used by the therapeutic recreationist in determining likes and dislikes of a client in recreational participation:

- What do you usually do in your free time?
- Do you have a favorite game? Hobby? Pastime?
- Do you like to do activities with others or by yourself?
- Whom do you prefer to have fun with? Family? Friends?
- When (part of the day or time of the week) do you usually participate in activities for fun?
- Where do you usually participate in these activities?
- Do you have your own equipment for your favorite activities?
- Do you have any equipment that you have never used?
- Would you like to learn to use the equipment?
- Is there any activity that you have always wanted to do but have never had an opportunity?

Preplanned questions are to be regarded only as guidelines, not as items that must be strictly adhered to. Often it becomes necessary to deviate from the prepared questions to follow-up on a client's reply in order to determine the real feelings of the client. Before the interview is held, in addition to planning the questions, other preparations should occur: (1) investigation of the client's background; (2) selection of an environment for the interview in which the client is at ease; and (3) setting of a definite time for the interview.

Care should be taken to establish good rapport between client and recreationist so that the client feels comfortable about divulging accurate information because he or she knows that it will be personally beneficial, rather than detrimental, to do so. In the actual interview, the interviewer should be attentive to discern the necessity to repeat or explain a question. Concern should be given to detection of vague, contradictory, evasive, or deceptive answers; in such instances an alternative or more penetrating question can be asked to elicit an accurate and straightforward answer. Information from the interview should be recorded immediately afterward. Notes may be made during the interview to record significant emotional display or obvious omissions in response to questions. Such notes should be recorded as unobtrusively as possible.

Inventories

The inventories are instruments that attempt to assess one or more acts of a client's behavior. An inventory presents a list of items related to the one being appraised; clients are asked to indicate their preference by checking the appropriate items. Inventories can be used to obtain information on almost any subject but their most frequent use in special recreational service is to determine activity interests.

Recreational interest inventories can be scientifically constructed and norm-referenced or informally developed by the recreationist for local program planning. To be certain that the items listed in the inventory really provide information about total recreational interest, the items must agree highly with some other reliable device for measuring interest in recreational activities. Such comparisons establish the validity of the testing instrument. However, a test constructed for local use without its validity being established still provides accurate information if correct construction of instructions and proper interpretation of the responses by the recreationist occurs. To illustrate why this is so, the following example is offered. An inventory is developed listing all the activities that are feasible to present in a special recreational program. The clients are instructed to check those activities in which they would like to participate. This type of inventory has "face validity"; that is, it asks the respondents only to check those activities they would like to participate in, and their answers provide that information (assuming the clients are being truthful). Interpretations of the clients' total recreational interest are not possible because the inventory's validity as a measurement of total interest has not been established.

Various validated recreational interest inventories can be obtained for use by recreationists. They include self-Leisure Interest Profile, Leisure Activities Blank, Miranda's Leisure Inventory, and Avocational Activities Inventories. These and other inventories are published in professional journals, copies of which are available in most university or college libraries. In selecting an interest inventory consideration should be given to the following:

- Does the inventory measure what it purports to measure (Is it validated by appropriate procedures or are the test items of "face validity")?

- If it is "face validity," does the inventory include activities that could be presented in the program?
- Is the inventory appropriate for the age group to be inventoried?
- Are the items easily understood and checked by the group to be inventoried?

Questionnaire

A questionnaire is a list of questions submitted for replies which can be analyzed for useful information. Although the questionnaire may be used for evaluation, its chief use is assessment of the status quo, or at least that which the respondents regard as the status quo. Use of the questionnaire has limitations in that it is impersonal and, unlike interviews and observations, the assessor is not present during the response period and so cannot make adjustments in questions or observe clients' behavior in the context of the environment that produced the response. Nevertheless, the questionnaire is a useful instrument because it provides a considerable amount of information from large groups in a relatively short period of time. Consequently, it is utilized more often as a research tool than as a program tool. However, it could be used effectively to assess the opinions or beliefs that a given group holds concerning a specific question; for example, ascertaining the general response of the local residents to the community adapted recreational program.

Construction of a questionnaire is relatively complex because more is involved than just posing questions. Writing questions that are readily understood and interpreted in the manner intended by a large group of people is more difficult than it may seem. Those who wish to make use of the questionnaire to gather information are advised to consult textbooks on research that detail questionnaire development (see references listed at the end of the chapter).

Sociometric

Of the various sociometric devices (tools for measuring social interaction), the most functional in therapeutic recreational services is the sociogram. This is a technique for assessing or evaluating peer acceptance and rejections by asking participants in a given activity to write down on paper the names of two individuals whom they like, admire, or respect. (The actual wording will depend upon the age of the individuals involved.)

The results are diagrammed as shown in Figure 6-2. Those whose names were mentioned most frequently are the ones most liked by their peers, and those whose names appeared infrequently or not at all comprise the rejected group. On the basis of this evaluation, then, the therapeutic recreationist may make special efforts to help the rejected clients improve their social interactions with the peer group.

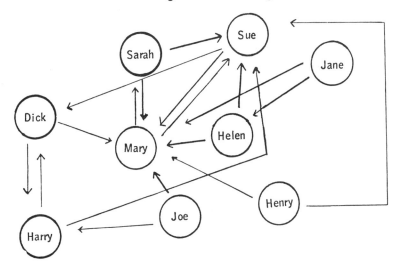

Fig. 6-2 Sociogram and its interpretation.

Sarah: Mentioned only once but probably is accepted by peers to some degree because she shares friendship with most popular child in the class.
Joe: Has no friends; needs help.
Henry: Has no friends; needs help.
Helen: Has someone who likes her but does not share the friendship; perhaps needs some attention.
Jane: Has no friends; needs help.

Motor Performance or Skill Tests

Most of the motor skill tests that have been developed measure gross (large muscle) motor performance rather than fine motor movement of the small muscles of the body, like those of the fingers, which are frequently used in recreational activities. The motor skill tests given in this section exemplify tests that provide valuable information about clients' ability to perform recreational horticulture, games and sports, and other activities requiring large muscle performance. The nature and structure of these tests are such that they can be readily adapted to the construction of informal tests of fine motor skills by the recreationist for assessment of fine motor movement abilities.

Motor performance can be measured by a number of tests. The types that can be most useful are: (1) basic skill tests and (2) screening tests.

Basic skill tests are evaluation or assessment instruments to measure the basic or fundamental skills of motor movement: those motor skills that are used most frequently and are most important in the daily life and recreational functions of an individual.

The Texas or Ness Revision of Fait's Basic Motor Skill Test[4] is an example of a basic skill test for profoundly retarded children and young adults (see Appendix III). The test is designed to evaluate the basic skills commonly utilized by many profoundly mentally retarded individuals. The test has been validated, using the techniques of face or content validity, and has a high test and retest reliability.

In giving this test to profoundly retarded individuals care must be exercised that clients are sufficiently motivated to perform the test items; otherwise, the score will represent the level of motivation rather than basic skill performance level. To ensure motivation, extrinsic rewards are given for appropriate responses. If this fails, an evaluation can be obtained by observing the clients over a long period of time during which they will likely be self-motivated sufficiently to perform the activity of the test item. Performance analysis is applied in making the evaluation of the observed movement.

Basic skills of physically handicapped clients can be evaluated with the Basic Skill Motor Profile (BSMP), which is also used with moderately and mildly retarded individuals. Developed by Fait and colleagues at the University of Connecticut,[5] the test consists of items that measure specific motor skills utilizing the process of task analysis. A skill is analyzed to determine which movements are necessary to perform the skill most effectively. In the analysis consideration is given to the physical maturation level and the motor movement limitations of the client.

Analysis of the performance of a basic skill such as throwing overhand by a mature individual with no physical limitations[6] produces these results:

- Turns dominant shoulder away from direction of throw as hand is brought back behind head and turns dominant shoulder forward as ball is thrown.

- Cocks wrist as it is brought behind head and snaps it forward when ball is released.

- Brings upper arm parallel with ground and points elbow away from body as ball is brought back behind head.

- Changes body weight and steps forward with correct foot.

- Follows through.

- Other.

However, if there are physical limitations that affect how the throw is made, the results of the analysis of movements would be different. For example, a partially paraplegic client, who has no arm movement except flexion and extension of the fingers and wrist, flexion but not extension of the arm, and forward and backward movements of the shoulder, can not make the throw as described above. The throw can, however, be made over the shoulder. In analyzing this skill possibility, the following movement components are produced: (1) grasp of the object to be thrown; (2) arm lowered as far as possible, (3) wrist hyper-extended (bent back), (4) sharp contraction of bicep (muscles of upper arm), (5) sharp flexion of the wrist, (6) release of the object at the proper time so that it is propelled in a straight line. The list of movements produced by the analysis becomes the criteria for judging the test results. In the case of the example, if the test results indicated that the object was not traveling in a straight line after it was released but was instead being directed down-ward, it would be established that the release movement did not meet the criterion of "releasing the object at the proper time so that it is propelled forward."

Basic skill tests of this nature can be used not only to assess or evaluate the skill level in performance of a basic motor skill, but to indicate where corrections are needed to achieve proper performance of the skill.

Screening Tests

Motor performance screening tests are used to determine base line performance, that is, the level of motor skill development of a client before instruction. They are generally norm-referenced tests so that by com-paring an individual's performance score with the norms for a given group, determination can be made of the individual's level of performance and its comparison to the performance of others.

The Bruininks-Oseretsky Test of Motor Proficiency[7] is a popular screen-ing tool. While it does successfully identify poor motor skills, the test is not appropriate for measuring progress, although it and other general motor performance tests are sometimes used for this purpose.

Perceptual-Motor Tests

Because recreationists may be exposed to the use of perceptual-motor tests in school programs, they need to be informed about them. The best known of the perceptual-motor tests used to measure motor skills are the Frostig's Developmental Test of Visual Perception, Kephart's and Roach's Purdue Perceptual Motor Survey, and Ayres's Southern California Motor Tests. These tests, once popular, are not now being used as extensively because of accumulating evidence that brings into question the validity of overall measurement of motor ability that was frequently claimed for the tests.

These tests purport to assess perception as it is involved in movement by measuring certain movement patterns. It had been assumed by their makers that the tests measured an overall ability to perform motor skills because they measured perception which is basic to all movement. How-ever, later investigation has not confirmed this assumption but has found, rather, that the tests offer specific motor skills information, which does not necessarily provide a clue to overall motor performance.

DEVELOPING GOALS AND OBJECTIVES

The function of assessment is gathering pertinent information to be used in establishing goals and objectives. Setting of goals and objectives has been mandated by PL 94-142 for all handicapped school children. Public Law 94-142 requires that a statement of annual goals, including short-term instructional objectives, must be included for all handicapped children in the school system. Also, prescriptions for therapeutic recreational activities for the ill and disabled clients imply, if they do not actually state, objectives. Not as obvious but no less important are objectives for individuals in adapted recreational services.

In determining objectives for an individual two considerations must be made: (1) what the environment demands of an individual and (2) what abilities the individual needs to function effectively in the environment. Determining the environmental demands is largely subjective. For example, one may judge that in a given playground environment a boy in a wheelchair should be able to play "catch and throw." Identifying the abilities needed for this activity is an objective procedure. Analysis of the boy's performance may reveal that he is physically capable of catching and throwing but he doesn't know how. Consequently, learning to catch and throw is an appropriate objective for that boy in the recreational program.

Classification of Objectives

Objectives may be devised for short or long periods. A long-term objective is frequently called a goal and is a generalized statement setting forth overall accomplishments for a long period. For example, a long-term goal for a given client may be to participate in social activities without feelings of anxiety.

A short-term objective is more specific, indicating a more readily accomplished achievement that helps to satisfy the long-term goal. In reaching the goal of socialization, a short-term objective might be to circulate in a given social gathering and converse with at least 25% of the people present.

Objectives are also classified as behavioral and curriculum. The latter are generalized in nature and are used as long-term objectives. The former are specific and short-termed.

Behavioral objectives are widely used in education, especially in developing short-term objectives for the IEP of a handicapped student. Through their work with educators on recreational objectives for the individualized program, recreationists have become aware of the value of behavioral objectives, and the practice of utilizing them has spread to programs in adapted and therapeutic recreational service.

A behavioral objective is stated in terms of behavior, i.e., the desired behavior is described in a way that is observable and measurable, and the kind of performance required is identified. Stated another way, the behavioral objective indicates what is to be performed and the quality and quantity of the performance. This requires that the words in which the behavioral objective is written be precise and that the performance be easily measured. Terms like understand and appreciate used as part of an objective do not lend themselves to easy measurement in the way that list, state, and demonstrate do. An objective that reads: "To develop art appreciation" is far less precise in indicating the quality and quantity to be measured than an objective that states: "To be able to distinguish impressionistic paintings 9 out of 10 times in a pre-selected group of 10 paintings." The first of these objectives is not a behavioral objective according to the definition of such an objective. The second is a behavioral objective because the participant must identify (performance) 9 out of 10 times (quality) in 10 paintings (quantity).

ASSESSMENT AND EVALUATION MODELS AND SYSTEMS

Various models or systems have been developed for use in assessment and evaluation. They offer a definitive procedure for conducting assessments or evaluations based on a specific concept. The three most commonly used are the Discrepancy Evaluation Model and the systems called SOAP, Subjective Data, Objective Data, Assessment and Plan, and CERT, Comprehensive Evaluation in Recreational Therapy.

Discrepancy Evaluation Model

The Discrepancy Evaluation Model[8] utilizes pre- and post-testing as a basis for evaluation. The difference or discrepancy in results on a test administered prior to and after a period of learning provides evidence of progress or lack of progress in the client's achievement. Consequently, the model is useful in establishing the degree to which objectives, criteria, or standards set for the program have been met; it also provides an effective means of monitoring progress.

Subjective Data, Objective Data, Assessment and Plan

Subjective data, objective data, assessment and plan (SOAP) refers to a process of assessment and evaluation, use of the results in developing a rehabilitation plan, and reporting of the data.[9] Subjective data in this process are defined as information verbalized by the client as, for example, "I don't want to go to the party. I want to be left alone." Objective data are that information obtained directly by the recreationist as a result of either observation or testing; personal opinions or conjectures of the recreationist are not objective data.

Assessment in SOAP is not used in the same sense as defined earlier in this chapter; in this case, assessment refers to the interpretation of the subjective and objective data. The assessment can indicate progression, regression, or no change in the client's condition. However, specifics are needed to provide concrete information about the client.

The plan of SOAP presents what is to be done for the client based upon the assessment. For example, for a specific client, one phase of the plan could be "to slowly expose the client to an increasing number of individuals over a 30-day period, with support from the recreationist, to develop ability to communicate with various people."

A sample showing the reporting of SOAP results is given below:

Date	Problem	Client Status

		Subjective Data
5/8/85	Patient lacks recreational skills to participate in community recreational activities	Patient (pt.) states: "I don't participate in recreational activities because I don't know how."

Objective Data

(1) Observations indicate pt. is poorly coordinated in racket games, dancing, running, arts and crafts.

(2) Results of test using Basic Motor Skills Profile indicate inadequate skills in 11 of the 12 items.

(3) Observation of pt. identifies lack of information about how to perform the motor skill to succeed in the activities in item 1.

Assessment

5/13/85   As above.

(1) Pt. has developed adequate basic motor skills but cannot perform effectively in complex activities.

(2) Pt. lacks varied experiences in recreational activities and so has not had opportunity to develop recreational skills.

Plan

5/13/85   As above.

(1) Schedule pt. for 30 minutes per day in performing and practicing skills to develop abilities; build confidence by focusing on skills pt. does well.

(2) Enroll pt. in beginning arts and crafts activities.

(3) Schedule pt. in one gross motor activity for daily 30-minute period.

(4) As motor skills develop, introduce pt. to more complex activities, offered with guidance from the recreationist.

(5) Formal re-evaluation will not be necessary because the nature of the plan will provide daily observations of improvement in skills.

Comprehensive Evaluation in Recreational Therapy

Comprehensive Evaluation Recreational Therapy (CERT) is a behavioral scale developed for use in psychiatric settings.[10] The instrument is designed to monitor different behaviors frequently displayed during participation in recreational activities. The items of behavior, of which there are 25, range from attention span to expressions of hostility to display of sexual role in the group. On a chart listing the behaviors, five levels of responses are indicated for each behavior and space is provided for recording the date on which the patient was observed making the particular level of response. An example of this is shown below for the item Attention Span, which is in the category of Individual Performance on the CERT scale:

Attention Span	Date	Date	Date	Date
	12/1	12/7	12/14	12/21
0—Attends to activity				
1—Occasionally does not attend				
2—Frequently does not attend	✓	✓		✓
3—Rarely attends			✓	
4—Does not attend				

Recreationists may use a specific model if they wish; however, in the majority of circumstances an eclectic approach is more desirable since it can be developed to fit the specific situation. The evaluation or assessment procedure must, however, provide valid information about the client and the program.

As assessment of the client needs to provide base-line data, that is, what the client is like, what the nature of the disorder is, what the strengths and weaknesses of the client are. From this information the goals and objectives can be derived and the foundation established for the client's rehabilitation. The assessment can also offer vital information about the program and its structure. Among the questions that need to be addressed in the assessment are:

- Is there an overall statement of purpose for the recreational program with established guidelines for its conduct?
- Is there an adequate number of staff members with appropriate training to deal with the expected number and kinds of clientele?
- Is there a written plan of operation for the recreational program that provides general information on procedures, e.g., the specific programs to be offered, the roles of the recreationists, and the types of assessment and evaluation procedures to be used?
- Are the supplies, materials, equipment, and facilities sufficient for the program?
- Are the activities adequate and appropriate for the anticipated needs?
- Are the sequences of activities planned to serve the anticipated clients?
- Does it appear that the time allotments for the various activities to be presented are sufficient to achieve ultimate benefit from participation?
- Have appropriate assessment and evaluation procedures been developed?

Evaluation procedures are usually based on objectives sought so that a determination can be made as to whether they have been achieved. By its very nature evaluation indicates continuous observation or testing to ascertain degree of achievement. Therefore, the evaluation instrument must be constructed to provide information about achievement. For example, if a prescription calls for increasing the length of the client's attention span, this becomes an objective; measuring to determine its accomplishments may take the form of actual timing of the length of the span of attention devoted to a certain activity. (This test would have face validity.)

REFERENCES

1. Eveline D. Schulman, *Intervention in Human Services,* 2nd ed., (St. Louis: The C. W. Mosby Co, 1978) p. 42.
2. Nancy Takata, "Play as a Prescription" in *Play as Exploratory Learning: Studies of Curiosity Behavior* by Mary Reilly, ed. (Beverly Hills: Sage Publications, 1974) p. 209.
3. David Austin, *Therapeutic Recreation Processes and Techniques* (New York: John Wiley & Sons, 1982) p. 64.
4. Hollis Fait and John Dunn, *Special Physical Education: Adapted, Individualized, Developmental,* 5th ed. (Philadelphia: Saunders College Publishing, 1984) pp. 129, 131.
5. Ibid, pp. 128-129.
6. Ibid, p. 130.
7. Robert Bruininks, "Bruininks-Oseretsky Test of Motor Proficiency" (Circle Pines, Minnesota: American Guidance Service, 1978), passim.
8. Diane K. Yavorsky, *Discrepancy Evaluation: A Practitioner's Guide* (Charlottesville, VA: University of Virginia, 1976), passim.
9. Lawrence L. Weed, *Documenting Patient Care, Responsibility* (Horsham, Pennsylvania: Intermed Communication, Inc., 1981) p. 30.
10. Robert Parker, *et al.,* "The Comprehensive Evaluation in Recreation Therapy Scale: A Tool for Patient Evaluation," *Therapeutic Recreation Journal,* 9, 4, 1975, p. 143.

SELECTED REFERENCES

Barrows, H. S., *Guide to Neurological Assessment* (Philadelphia: J. B. Lippincott Co., 1980).
Miller, T., *Evaluating Orthopedic Disability* (Oradell, New Jersey: Medical Economics Books, 1979).
Mulliken, R. K. and Buckley, J. J., *Assessment of Multihandicapped and Developmentally Disabled Children* (Rockville, Maryland: Aspen Systems Corporation, 1983).
Murray, J. N., *Developing Assessment Programs for the Multi-Handicapped Child* (Springfield: Charles C Thomas, 1980).
Stimmel, B., eds., *Evaluation of Drug Treatment Programs* (New York: Haworth Press, Inc., 1983).

Section 2

Conditions of Illness, Disability, and Maladjustment

Chapter 7

Physical Disabilities

Physical disabilities are all those pathologic conditions of the body not primarily involved with psychologic aspects of body function. The physical disabilities most commonly found in the general community population are orthopedic, neurologic, cardiac, and pulmonary disorders and visual and auditory impairments.

To provide effective therapeutic and adapted recreational services to the physically disabled client in any of the treatment centers or community settings, the recreationist must have considerable background information about the disability. It is not enough to know that a client's disability falls into a certain category, such as for example, orthopedic disorder; nor is it sufficient to know the particular kind of disorder, for instance, that the orthopedic problem is juvenile arthritis. Some knowledge of the cause of the disease or disability and its treatment is needed so that it is possible to understand and respond appropriately to the special problems the condition imposes on the client. Such problems *may* include restrictions on movement, avoidance of stress and fatigue, and debilitating effects of the drugs used for treatment. With such information, the recreationist can assess the special recreational needs of the individual client, as well as identify limitations and capabilities in performing activities that will satisfy those needs. Knowledge about the disability creates an awareness of the precautions that need to be observed and develops insight into the recreational potential of the client.

Furthermore, for the therapeutic recreationist basic information and familiarity with medical terminology enable effective communication with others on the rehabilitation team concerning the possible effects of the recreational activities. This is particularly important in working with the physical or occupational therapist whose programs the recreationist can so effectively supplement and complement with an appropriate individualized therapeutic recreational program.

It has been suggested that familiarity with the etiology (origin), pathology (nature), and treatment of diseases and disorders tends to compartmentalize the thinking of recreationists so that they are more likely to regard all clients with a certain disability as requiring the same treatment and safety precautions and, therefore, as having identical recreational needs that can be served with the same program. It is our experience that the opposite is true: the more recreationists learn about a disability, the more aware they become of the need to treat each client as an individual with unique problems and needs.

ORTHOPEDIC AND NEUROLOGIC PROBLEMS

Orthopedic and neurologic disorders are two distinct and separate problems although they may cause similar types of limitations. Neurologic disorders involve the central and peripheral nervous systems directly, while orthopedic disorders entail only the bones, joints, and associated ligaments and muscles. Both disorders can, for example, cause movement problems that confines the individual to a wheelchair. In terms of programming recreational activities for clients in wheelchairs, the similarities in limitations of those with orthopedic and those with neurologic disorders makes possible the utilizations of many of the same activities with, of course, modifications for specific differences.

Orthopedic Disabilities

Orthopedic is defined as pertaining to the correction of deformities of the skeletal system, while orthopedics is a surgically oriented branch of medicine that is specifically concerned with the preservation and restoration of the functions of the skeletal system and associated structures. An orthopedic problem refers to a disability that prevents the effective performance of motor movement. Such a disability involves the bones and their articulations (joints) and associated structures (tendons, bursae, muscles, and peripheral blood vessels and nerves).

Treatment. The emphasis in treatment today is placed equally on prevention and correction of deformity and disability, often involving the use of mechanical devices. For example, possible deformity that may follow a disease can be prevented by the use of splints, circular casts, braces, traction devices, and straps. These devices may also be used to correct a disability. Correction is also effected through surgical procedures. Surgery is performed on both hard tissue—such as bone—and soft tissue—such as tendons and muscles.

Etiology and Pathology. In this section, the nature, origin, and cause of a number of different types of orthopedic problems are briefly discussed. It is recognized that not all the problems that the therapeutic or adapted recreationist will encounter are included—due to space limitations only the most common problems can be presented. It is hoped that this background information will motivate students to expand their knowledge of the etiology, pathology, and treatment of a wider range of orthopedic problems, in addition to performing the primary function of enabling them to enter the profession better equipped to serve disabled clients.

Trauma. Trauma is an injury caused by an external force, often resulting from surgery or accident, and occurring in any part of the body. Examples range from a bone that has been fractured to a nerve that has been severed or damaged in some way.

Trauma is an increasingly frequent cause of amputation, which may occur as the result of accident or surgery. Surgical amputation is performed when the patient's welfare will be improved by the removal of a deformed, irreparably damaged, diseased, painful, or ineffectual part of the body.

Types of Amputation (surgical). The surgical amputation is carried out with attention given to the following:

- Types of prosthetic devices available to the patient
- Disability the patient is likely to suffer from amputation at a specific place
- Increased energy the patient is likely to expend in locomotion with the amputation at a specific place
- Appearance
- Amount that must be removed

There are several terms used to designate specific types or conditions of amputation that therapeutic and adapted recreationists should be familiar with. The place at which the amputation occurs is referred to as the level of amputation. Amputation at a joint is called disarticulation. Minor amputation is used to describe surgery to remove small bones, commonly of the hand, the foot, the fingers, or the toes. A major amputation is one that removes large bones like those of the leg and arm. An open amputation is one in which the surface of the wound is not covered with tissue. It is used for the control of gas gangrene or other infections and is followed by surgical closure as the infection is brought under control. In a closed amputation the surface of the wound is closed with a flap of skin so as to create a stump that can be used effectively with a prosthesis.

Amputation of Upper Extremity. The basic concern in amputation of any portion of the arm is to maintain function or to substitute for lost function. In general, most amputations in the upper extremities are designed to maintain the greatest possible length of the extremity. However, in amputation of the forearm, a long forearm stump is usually avoided because it is difficult to fit it with an effective prosthesis. Amputations of bones of the hand are designed to retain the ability to grasp. In amputations near the wrist, the goal is to create a stump suitable for the fitting of a prosthesis. Preservation of the joint, in most cases, increases the possibility for the fitting of an effective prosthesis.

Amputation of Lower Extremity. The most important concern in the amputation of a lower extremity is that the stump be able to bear weight in standing and walking. Depending upon the level of amputation, weight must be borne by the stump, by the sides of the leg, or by the hip. However, most frequently it is the stump that bears the weight; chief exceptions are amputation at the hip in which the weight is borne by the hip bone and amputation at the center of the lower leg when it is borne chiefly by the sides of the leg. The common levels of amputation are at the foot (transmetatarsal), ankle (Syme), below the knee, at the knee, about the knee (supracondylar), and the lower third of the femur (Fig. 7-1).

Bone Injuries. The most common injury to the bone is a fracture, i.e., a break. Fractures may be accompanied by injury to the surrounding tissue.

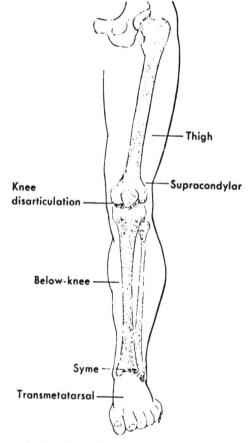

Fig. 7-1 The common levels of amputation of the lower limb.

Fractures are classified as:

- Incomplete fracture—one that does not entirely destroy the continuity of bone
- Complete fracture—one in which the bone is entirely broken across
- Simple or closed fracture—one which does not produce an open wound in the skin
- Compound or open fracture—one in which there is an external wound
- Comminuted fracture—one in which the bone is splintered or crushed
- Impacted fracture—a fracture in which one fragment is firmly driven into another
- Pathologic or spontaneous fracture—a fracture due to weakening of the bone by disease

Successful healing of a fracture is determined by how closely the fractured ends are aligned, the efficacy of the immobilization procedure, and the quality of the blood supply to the fractured bone. The term for bringing the fracture fragments back into alignment is reduction of the fracture.

There are three common means employed to reduce a fracture. One is manipulation or closed reduction. In the closed reduction the fractured ends are brought together by manual traction while the patient is under anesthesia.

Another method is the use of one or the other of two types of traction devices: skin traction and skeletal traction. In skin traction adhesive strips are attached to the skin of the distal (away from point of origin) end of the extremity to a weight that exerts a pull on the extremity. In the skeletal traction a metal pin or wire is inserted directly into the distal end of the bone and attached to a system of ropes and pulleys that exert a pull upon the extremity. When the fragments of the bone have been aligned, they are immobilized to maintain them in contact to ensure a successful repair.

A third method is the open operation in which a surgical incision is made to enable the ends of the fracture to be aligned. Usually, a plate is implanted to hold the bone in place for effective healing.

Healing of Fractures. As a fracture heals, new tissues form at and around the area of the break. This new tissue is called a callus. At first the callus is composed of both cartilage and bone. In successful healing the cartilage becomes bone.

The period of time necessary for healing varies according to the bone that is fractured. The average number of weeks required for the union of various bones is shown in Table 7-1. This information is useful to the recreationist when, in consultation with the physician, a determination is made of how strenuous the recreational program for patients should be. Generally, the patients can be allowed a greater amount of vigorous activity as they approach the end of the healing time. The number of weeks generally increases for older patients due to poorer blood supply to the bone and slower regeneration of tissue.

TABLE 7-1

Bone	Location	Time to Heal
Phalanges	Fingers and toes	3 weeks
Metacarpus and carpus	Hand bones	4 weeks
Clavicle	Collar bone	5 weeks
Fibula	Lower leg (small bone)	6 weeks
Humerus	Upper arm	7 weeks
Tarsus and metatarsus	Foot bones	7 weeks
Radius and ulna	Lower arm	8 weeks
Tibia	Lower leg (shin bone)	10 weeks
Calcaneus	Heel	10 weeks
Carpus	Wrist	12 weeks
Femur	Upper leg	13 weeks

If a fracture does not heal in the usual amount of time, it is said to be a delayed union. A nonunion of a fracture occurs when there is unsuccessful repair of the break. Both delayed union and nonunion may be caused by improper reduction of the fracture, poor immobilization, infection, and poor blood supply to the bone fragments. Poor blood supply is most frequently the cause of nonunion in fractures of the femoral neck in the upper leg; lower third of the humerus of the upper arm; and tibia, the shin bone of the leg.

Nerve Injury. Injury to the spinal and peripheral nerves is a frequent and serious occurrence. Complete severance of the spinal cord results in paralysis of all muscles below the level of the separation. There are three types of paralytic involvement: hemiplegia (one side of the body); paraplegia (lower portion of the body); and quadriplegia (both arms and legs). A lesion in the cervical (neck) area may cause hemiplegia if it involves half of the cervical cord; however, this is uncommon.

Injury to the cord in which it is severed at or above the third cervical vertebra results in death. Partial lesion in the area creates weakness over the entire body. Complete severance of the cord above the second thoracic veterbra (T-2) causes paralysis of muscles of both the upper and lower limbs (quadraplegia). When the separation is complete at the second thoracic vertebra or below the result is paralysis of the lower limbs (paraplegia) (Fig. 7-2).

In addition to paralysis of the voluntary muscles, severance of the cord causes various other serious problems. One of these is exaggeration of the reflexes, a condition called hyperflexion. The symptoms include whitening of the area around the mouth, severe sweating, hypertension, headaches, and feelings of impending doom. Another serious problem is the development of contractures (shortening of muscles) if the joints are allowed to remain in one position for long periods of time. The condition can be avoided by frequent moving of the joint.

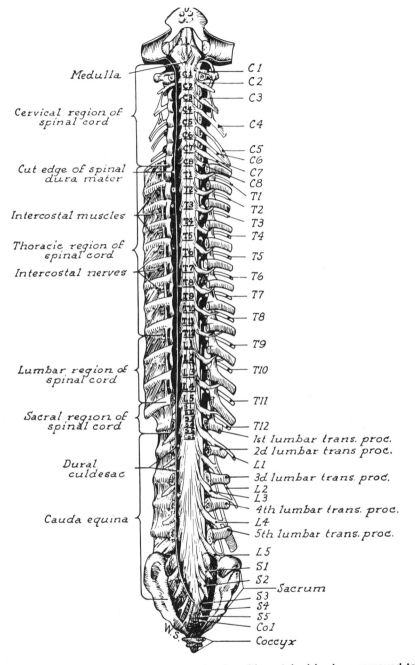

Fig. 7-2 Dorsal view of the spinal cord in situ with vertebral laminae removed to show the relation of the spinal cord segments to the vertebral column. (N. B. Everett, *Functional Neuroanatomy*, 6th ed. Philadelphia: Lea & Febiger, 1971. After Tilney and Riley.)

Urinary infection is common. Individuals with spinal cord severance, since they have lost control of the bladder, must wear a catheter and bag. The catheter is inserted into the urethra (the canal conveying urine from the bladder to the exterior) and empties into the bag strapped to the upper leg. The presence of the catheter and the problem of excreting urine creates conditions in which infection is likely to occur.

Defecation is difficult for those with spinal cord separation. If the problem is severe, surgery is performed to create a small opening in the intestine to permit fecal matter to pass into an attached bag (colostomy bag).

Almost all persons with spinal cord injuries have spasms of the muscles intermittently. When a muscle is in spasm, effective movement is prevented in those parts of the body over which the individual has control.

Injuries of the Brain. Head injuries have become more predominant in recent years. Most head injuries are sustained in either automobile or industrial accidents. Less frequently they are produced by falls. With the rising incidence of criminal violence, more head injuries may be attributed to felonious assault. Penetrating wounds of the brain are comparatively rare. Severe fracture of the skull is related to severe brain injury, but the brain may be damaged without skull fracture and the reverse is also possible. Following injury to the head the victim may suffer from concussion, cerebral contusion, cerebral laceration, or cerebral compression.

Concussion. Concussion is defined as a condition of widespread paralysis of the functions of the brain in consequence of a blow on the head. Often recovery is spontaneous and no gross organic change in the brain substance may be noted.

Cerebral Contusion, Laceration, and Compression. Cerebral contusion is a generalized disturbance of the brain after head injury and characterized by edema (presence of large amounts of blood) and capillary hemorrhages. Cerebral laceration, on the other hand, is used when the contusion is sufficiently damaging to produce tearing in the brain tissue. This may occur either at the site of the blow or by contrecoup on the opposite side of the brain. Cerebral contusion may occur in the absence of concussion. The victim is rendered unconscious by the injury. In severe cases the depth of the coma is increased and the individual dies from medullary paralysis within a few hours of receipt of the injury. In less severe cases, the patient, after recovery from concussion, passes into a state of stupor or mental confusion and other clinical effects. Sometimes disorientation occurs. The condition may last for varying periods of time and in favorable cases gradually passes away. Other involvements may also be produced depending upon the brain structures which have been affected.

Compression occurs when the injury is followed by intracranial hemorrhage.

Results of Head Injury. If, after a head injury, unconsciousness continues more than a few minutes, or if, after recovery from the concussion, mental confusion or other symptoms of cerebral disturbance exist, it must be concluded that structural damage to the brain has occurred. When confusion and drowsiness increase in severity or persist for several weeks, the possibility of hematoma (collection of blood) or a tumor containing effused blood must be considered. Contusion, however, when severe may prove mortal. Acute cerebral compression is almost always fatal.

If there is any reason to suspect brain injury, the patient is kept in bed for at least three weeks, even in the mildest cases. In the early stages, sedatives will be required. When the stage of mental confusion has passed, the patient must remain quiet. In all cases of cerebral contusion, convalescence should be prolonged and return to normal life gradual. Activities for such patients will be limited and strictly controlled by prescription.

Stroke. Stroke refers to sudden vascular lesion (injury of the blood vessel) of the brain. When circulation of the blood to the brain is disrupted, the nerve cells in the involved area die or are damaged. Since the nerve cells of the brain control thought, speech, perception, sensation, and motor movement, permanent or temporary impairment of these functions may occur if circulation is interrupted in the brain areas where the functions are controlled. Inability to use and understand the spoken or written word frequently occurs in the stroke patient. There may be behavioral changes, depending upon the portion of the brain affected; for example, some patients become anxious, fearful, and easily frustrated, while others become overly confident and take chances they would not have prior to the stroke. Control over emotions may be lost and, frequently, responses to the environment may be made in unacceptable ways.

The therapeutic recreationist plays a vital role in the rehabilitation of the stroke victim. Recreational activities are developed to support the work of the other therapists, e.g., the speech therapist, physical therapist, and occupational therapist, who are also involved with the patient. One of the greatest contributions the therapeutic recreationist can make is to foster development of a better self-image by presenting activities the patient will enjoy and participate in with success. In the recreational program opportunities can be offered to enable patients to develop positive interactions and relationships with others giving them a base for reestablishing themselves as social beings, resuming old roles, or exchanging former activities for new ones when necessary.

The nerves in the spinal column do not regenerate so the paralysis is permanent, although much can be done by the rehabilitation team to minimize deformity, improve physical ability, and to strengthen emotional security. During treatment the affected limbs are supported in a position that will prevent deformity. Passive exercise is given by the physical therapist to maintain movement in the joints and active exercise to strengthen remaining unaffected muscles may be provided by recreational activities.

Recent research in bio-feedback training and functional electronic stimulation offers means of providing stimulation of paralyzed muscles caused by injury to the spinal cord. Bio-feedback training is effective in cases where the nerves to the muscles have not been completely severed. The bio-feedback provides the client with information on how an attempt to move the muscles actually affects the muscle. In this way, the client can learn what must be done to stimulate the muscles in the most effective way to produce movement. With sufficient learning and practice, paralyzed clients have been able to walk.

Functional electronic stimulation is a method whereby paralyzed muscles are moved by a muscle stimulator controlled by a computer. The method is used with clients who have suffered complete severance of the spinal cord. At present, the procedure has been developed to the point where a paralyzed client has been able to walk in a controlled situation. It is predicted that in a few years the functional electronic stimulator will be refined to the extent that paralyzed individuals can make all movements that were previously possible.

Peripheral nerve injuries are far more frequent than spinal injuries and may also have serious consequences. Since peripheral nerves do regenerate, the possibility of recovery from injury is greater. The degree of recovery depends on the extent of injury. The treatment for the injury may consist of surgery to repair the injured nerve or the use of supports and braces to maintain the affected muscles in a relaxed position so they will not be stretched by the antagonistic (opposing) muscles.

Congenital Deformities. Congenital deformities are those defects or abnormalities existing at birth. They may occur in any part of the body and vary from such minor abnormality as a slightly deformed toe to such serious defect as the absence of a limb.

Early treatment of congenital deformities is generally desirable, so recreationists offering therapeutic programs in hospitals can expect to have young clients being treated for various kinds of birth defects. Upon their release from the hospital, the youngsters may continue to require adapted recreational activities in the community program or in the school, if the latter offers a recreational program.

Hip Dislocation. One of the most common deformities is congenital hip dislocation. In this condition the head of the thigh bone (femoral head) is partially or completely displaced. In most cases the socket (acetabulum) is much shallower than normal, allowing easy displacement of the head of the femur. Hip dislocation is seen more frequently in the female child than in the male and is more often in both hips than in one. If only one hip is affected, it is more often the left one.

Prolonged malpositioning of the head of the femur produces a chronic weakness of the leg and hip muscles that causes inefficient hip movement.

The treatment is directed toward relocation of the head of the femur through manipulation. When this is not possible, the relocation is effected through surgery. After reduction of the dislocation, the hip is immobilized for six months or more.

Congenital Amputation. Complete or partial absence of a bone or malformation of a bone is a frequently occurring congenital deformity. Partial absence of a long bone is more frequent than is total absence. Congenital defects of the bone of the upper extremity more frequently involve both limbs than those occurring in the lower extremity. A complete absence of the bone of a limb or part of the limb is called congenital amputation. The habilitation, i.e., achievement of function, of the individual with a congenital amputation is similar to the rehabilitation of those who have surgical or accidental amputation.

Spina Bifida. Spina bifida is a congenital deformity that is becoming an important orthopedic problem. The number of children requiring orthopedic care for spina bifida has greatly increased in recent years because advances in medicine have made it possible for more children born with spina bifida to survive. Spina bifida occurs when there is incomplete development in one or more vertebrae leaving a cleft in the vertebral column.

The disability that accompanies spina bifida varies with the severity of the malformation. In some cases there is complete paralysis in the lower portion of the body accompanied by the inability to control the bowels and bladder; in other cases, there is little or no evidence of paralysis. Paralysis and deformity in the lower extremities may require extensive orthopedic treatment with casts and braces.

Osteochondrosis. Osteochondrosis is a disease of one or more of the growth or ossification centers (epiphyses) in children. An epiphysis so affected softens and disintegrates and, consequently, collapses if pressure is applied. Then new bone and cartilage replace the old, often resulting in a deformity.

Although osteochondrosis can occur at any epiphysis that bears weight, it most commonly occurs at the epiphysis in the head of the femur. This condition is called Legg-Calvé-Perthes disease or coxa plana. Treatment consists of preventing the collapse of the bone by corrective bracing that prevents weight from being placed directly upon the head of the femur (Fig. 7-3).

Joint Infection. Joint infection is the invasion of the tissue of the body by disease-producing organisms in such a way that injury results. The organism most commonly infecting bones and joints is a pyogenic (pus-forming) one. An infection of the bone is called osteomyelitis, while an infection that is localized to a joint is termed pyogenic arthritis. The bone may become infected by the introduction of a pyogenic organism through a break in the skin that exposes the bone as in a compound fracture. However, the most common way that infection occurs is by being carried by the blood from a distant area, such as an infected toenail or abscessed

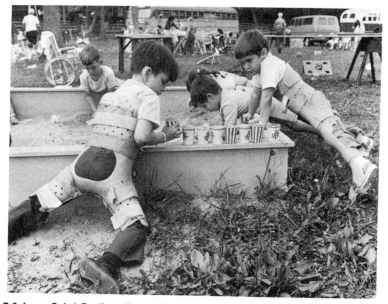

Fig. 7-3 Legg-Calvé-Perthes disease is treated by placing the client in a special brace that prevents the head of the femur from bearing any weight directly. (Newington Children's Hospital).

tooth, to the bone. In a large majority of cases there is a history of injury to the bone at the site at which the infection occurs.

The treatment consists of control of the infection by the use of antibiotics and immobilization. In chronic cases surgery is performed to eliminate the affected area, and often skin grafts are necessary to cover the area at the site of the surgery.

Joint infection requires immediate attention because the infection rapidly destroys the cartilage to a point beyond repair. Treatment consists of aspiration (removal) of the formed pus on the joint and the use of antibiotics. In most cases, this treatment is insufficient and must be followed by surgery, where the joint is opened and thoroughly cleansed. The joint is then immobilized and supported in traction or plaster splint for a period of time.

Degeneration. Degeneration is a term applied to the deterioration of tissue and decline in function. One of the most common of the degenerative diseases is chronic arthritis. Arthritis is defined as inflammation of a joint and is essentially a process resulting from degenerative changes in the surface of the joints (articular cartilage). The etiology of arthritis is rather vague and so there is disagreement on the classification of the disease. Generally, chronic arthritis is divided into two kinds, rheumatoid arthritis and osteoarthritis, although there is not always a clear-cut difference between the two.

Arthritis is usually found in adults, but one form known as juvenile rheumatoid arthritis affects children. It can occur as early as six weeks after birth. Usually the disorder is not as severe as the forms of adult arthritis and the prognosis for recovery is good.

Rheumatoid Arthritis. Rheumatoid Arthritis is characterized by an inflammatory disorder of connective tissue. The disease may affect the skeletal muscles and some of the organs, but it chiefly affects the synovial membranes (connective tissue which lines the joint cavity). The joints most frequently affected in order of their frequency, are: fingers, knees, elbows, feet, shoulders, and hips.

The onset of the disease is often insidious, usually starting in the hands or feet and spreading slowly to the other joints. In some instances the onset may be rapid, often accompanied by a high temperature. In either case, there is at first only a little stiffness in the joints, but this disappears when the joints are used. As the disease becomes established, swelling of the joints occurs and the muscles begin to atrophy (waste away). Pain and tenderness of the joints are severe and muscle spasm makes movement difficult. The skin looks smooth and shiny over the swollen joints. As the muscles atrophy, joint deformity develops rapidly even to the point that the joint may become dislocated.

Since rheumatoid arthritis is a disease of unknown etiology, a curative drug has not been developed. Treatment is directed generally to the health of the patient and locally to the diseased joints. Rest and relaxation, balanced diet, exercise, recreational activity, and maintenance of general good health are basic to treatment. The duration of the rest periods depends upon the acuteness of the attack. Patients are confined to bed if they have a fever; in less acute cases, set periods of rest during the day may be sufficient.

For local treatment of the joint, a number of procedures are used: rest, splinting, exercise, heat, massage, surgery, and intra-articular injection. Rest to the affected joints is essential during the acute stages of the disease. Splinting of the joint provides the necessary rest, aids in preventing joint deformity. As the condition improves, the splints are removed at times to allow the joint to be exercised.

The program of exercise will be conducted by the physical therapist. The exercise is graduated to avoid fatigue and includes all muscle groups. The activity is often performed in warm water which facilitates movement and reduces muscle spasm. Heat and massage are used in the subacute stage; they help to reduce muscle spasm and are comforting to the patient.

As a general treatment, drugs are frequently used. Aspirin is commonly used for the purpose of relieving pain. Often hydrocortisone is injected into the joints for temporary relief. Other drugs are also sometimes used; however, it is generally felt that there are no drugs yet developed that can be relied upon to arrest progress of the disease nor any that can restore damaged joints.

In some joints function is restored or partially restored by operation. If the joint is severely damaged and is not functional, the fusion of the joint surfaces is sometimes performed.

Osteoarthritis. Osteoarthritis is a degenerative disease affecting the cartilage of the joint. The disease occurs chiefly in the weight bearing joints and is, therefore, most commonly found in the lower limbs and spinal column, but it is also known to affect the upper limbs as well.

As the disease progresses, the cartilage of the affected joints degenerates. These joints become painful and stiff with swelling. The pain is brought on by immobility of the joint and is relieved by movement, only to return again if the movement is prolonged. In the early stages of the disease, there is slight limitations of movement, which increases as the disease progresses. In severe cases, there is deformity, but it is not as marked as in rheumatoid arthritis.

Many of the same treatment procedures used for rheumatoid arthritis are applicable in the treatment of osteoarthritis. Keeping active becomes very important for those with osteoarthritis because the joints can be kept mobile only by movement. Prescribed activity is given after the active phase of the disease; too much movement during the active stage can be dangerous. If carefully planned and executed, activities can prevent deformity for a long period in the client's life. Weight reduction is also important for heavy clients with spinal column and lower limb involvement to relieve the joints of undue weight. A recreational program of activities involving suitable movements can assist both the prevention of deformity and the reduction of weight.

Neurologic Disorders

Neurologic disorders is a term used for diseases or dysfunctions of the nervous system. Neurologic disorders differ from psychiatric disorders in that neurologic disorders have as their basis an organic dysfunction, while psychiatric disorders are fundamentally functional, lacking a demonstrable physical basis. The following neurologic disorders, which are those most commonly found in the population, will be discussed in this chapter: cerebral palsy, epilepsy, multiple sclerosis, muscular dystrophy, and Parkinson's disease.

Cerebral Palsy. The types of neuromuscular disability found in those with cerebral palsy are usually classified as spasticity, athetosis, ataxia, rigidity, and tremor. There are many subdivisions of these classifications; and, also, the types may be mixed. Hence, only the two single most common types will be described: spasticity and athetosis.

Spasticity. Most cases of cerebral palsy suffer from spasticity, a condition in which muscular movement in the area involved is restricted due to contracture of the muscles. In the attempt to move a specific joint, other joints in the same limb may move involuntarily due to the uncertain pull of the spastic muscles. Sometimes the movement is slow; at other times, it is explosive. The slightest stimulation—a noise, sudden movement, or slight touch—will evoke a muscular response.

Normally, when muscles are contracted to move a joint, the antagonistic muscles relax. However, when a muscle is stretched quickly, it has a tendency to contract reflexly. This reflex contraction is known as the stretch reflex and is kept under control by various motor centers of the brain. In spastic paralysis many of the connections between the motor centers and muscles are lost, and the stretch reflex is disturbed both in timing and in strength. During times of relaxation, the stretch reflex is not active and the abnormality is not as great.

Spasticity is most common in the antigravity muscles (those holding the body upright), and hence the maintenance of good posture is extremely difficult. Walking gait is disturbed if leg muscles are affected, since overcontraction of certain muscles cause the legs to adduct and the hips to rotate inward. The heels may also draw up, so that walking occurs on the outer part of the ball of the foot and on the toes. This produces the characteristic "scissor gait" of the spastic individual.

If the arms are involved, they are usually drawn up to the body with the elbows bent and wrists and fingers flexed. Balance is usually not disturbed, but contractures in the lower limbs provide poor support and hence poor body balance. Mental impairment is more frequently associated with spasticity than any other type of cerebral palsy.

Athetosis. The person with athetosis, unlike one with spasticity, has no difficulty moving; rather, the difficulty is in moving too much. There is an inability to produce the desired movement; often the movement starts too soon and there is little control over its speed. Sometimes the movement accomplished against tension is slow and at other times it is fast. A voluntary movement of one part of the body produces extraneous movement elsewhere, an action called overflow.

Some overflow is normal and common to nearly everyone, as evidenced in the extraneous contortions of athletes as they put forth maximum effort. Normally, control over such movements is maintained by a certain area of the brain which in an athetoid individual is affected so that control is no longer possible. There is less overflow, however, when the person is relaxed and calm; nervousness and tension increase the overflow. This is an important consideration in programming recreational activities for clients with athetosis.

Because of the absence of control, the body position is constantly changing. There is frequently an overextension and spreading of the fingers, and the toes turn up and foot rotates inward. The arms are often drawn back with the palms held downward. The head is thrown back with the mouth open. A peculiar expression or grimace is usually evident. There is less possibility of mental deficiency than in spasticity.

Treatment. Treatment for spasticity and athetosis generally takes two forms: surgery to reduce the contractures of the muscles and to remove the restrictions on movement caused by the deformities; and education to achieve use and control of the muscles for more effective movements of the limbs. Simple games and movement activities involving locomotion and manipulative skills are presented to encourage development of these skills.

Epilepsy. Medical experts call epilepsy a psychomotor explosion within the cortex of the brain rather than an impairment or loss of cortical function. The explosion can produce a convulsive seizure and the loss of consciousness. The classification of epilepsy is based on its chief causes; however, the specific manner in which a cause operates is frequently obscure and in some instances a single pathological condition may occur in more than one classification:

Specific Causes

- Increased intracranial pressure
- Inflammatory conditions due to infections
- Trauma
- Congenital deficiencies
- Degenerative diseases
- Circulatory disturbances

General Causes

- Exogenous poisons (those from outside the body)
- Anoxemia (deficiency of oxygen in the arterial blood)
- Metabolic disorders
- Endocrine disorders
- Allergic states

Unknown Causes

Seizures. Epileptic seizure take various forms. The two most common are grand mal and petit mal. All varieties have characteristic features such as short lapses of consciousness, spreading convulsions, limited convulsions, spasms of one limb or half the body, tingling sensation, hallucinations of smell or taste, and external stimuli exciting convulsions.

Grand Mal. Epileptic patients frequently exhibit symptoms which precede an attack and which enable them to recognize that a grand mal seizure is likely to occur. These symptoms include emotional changes and aura, which is a peculiar sensation or phenomenon that gives warning of an approaching attack of epilepsy. The aura may take the form of a complex mental state or it may be referred to one of the senses. The aura may, for example, be gustatory, olfactory, visual, or auditory hallucinations.

The convulsion may or may not begin with a harsh scream. Consciousness is either lost immediately or shortly after the onset of the attack.

The first motor manifestation of the convulsion is typically a phase of tonic spasm of the muscles. The upper limbs are commonly adducted at the shoulders and flexed at the elbows and wrists. The lower limbs are extended and the feet turned inward. The initial phase accounts for only a few seconds, rarely sustained more than thirty seconds. This phase (tonic) is followed by a second phase (clonic) in which the sustained contraction of muscles gives way to spasmodic jerking. In the clonic phase, the tongue may be bitten; foaming at the mouth may occur; incontinence of urine, although not feces, is common.

Toward the end of the clonic phase the intervals between the muscular contractions become prolonged until they finally cease. The individual remains unconscious for a variable time. It is not unusual for the individual to sleep for several hours after a seizure. Rarely does the individual exhibit manifestations of mental abnormality after seizure.

Petit Mal. The lightest form of petit mal occurs with the individual experiencing no lapse of consciousness, but rather a sensation of dizziness or of falling into a trancelike manifestation which may last for a few seconds. Next in involvement comes lapse of consciousness, with or without an aura; the motor and postural functions of the brains are apparently so slightly involved that the individual with this seizure maintains his or her balance and does not fall. Although the attack may produce a dazed facial expression that is also associated with staring eyes, recovery occurs after a few seconds. In the more severe forms of petit mal consciousness is lost, resulting in a fall. There may be slight muscular rigidity.

Multiple Sclerosis. The various forms of sclerosis are diseases in which destruction of the myelin occurs. The myelin is the white fatlike substance forming a sheath around the nerve fibers. In multiple sclerosis, the most familiar of this type of disease, wide spread patches of demyelination occur in the nervous system followed by the presence of tumors.

In most cases, the early appearance of the disease is followed by striking improvement, so that remissions and relapses are a characteristic feature of this disorder. The duration of the disease is prolonged. The early symptoms are usually those of localized lesions of the nervous system, while the late manifestations are of progressive involvement which tends to produce limitations of movement. The individual requires assistive devices to be at all mobile.

Treatment. The extremely variable course of the disease may lead to fatal termination in three months, or the individual may be able to work for twenty-five years. There is no specific treatment. The general management of the patient requires tact and judgment. Fatigue is to be avoided but, short of this, every effort must be made to maintain the patient at his or her usual occupation for as long as possible. This will have tremendous significance for the role that therapeutic recreational service will have to play in the latter stages of the disease. Personal encouragement, stimulation, and suggestion may long postpone the bedridden state.

Muscular Dystrophy. Muscular dystrophy is the name applied to a group of progressive, degenerative diseases of the skeletal muscles. The diseases are characterized by deteriorating changes in the muscle fiber, causing muscular atrophy (wasting away) and weakness. There is no agreement among medical authorities on the classification of muscular dystrophy. However, there are two general types that are often recognized by writers: Duchenne or progressive muscular dystrophy and fascioscapulohumeral.

Duchenne is the more prevalent, accounting for over 65% of the cases in children. The disease begins early in childhood and progresses rapidly usually leading to death in the late teens or early twenties. It occurs predominately in males with symptoms in evidence by the age of three or four. Prominent among the symptoms are difficulty in running, climbing stairs, and rising from a sitting position. Calves of the legs and other muscles may become enlarged while they become weaker. Muscular weakness spreads gradually throughout the entire body eventually producing complete dependence and death.

Fascioscapulohumeral muscular dystrophy afflicts, as the term implies, the muscles of the face, scapular region (shoulders and back), and the humerus (upper arm). Onset of the disease is later in life than Duchenne, usually the years of adolescence and early adulthood. Progress of the disease is slow and often interrupted by long remissions; it may be completely arrested at any time.

In the course of the disease, muscles in the area of the face, upper arm, shoulder, and back become weakened. Pelvic muscles may also be affected as the disease progresses. The degree of weakening varies among individuals. In advanced cases, the cheeks sag, the eyes close completely, and the scapulae become winged (one side protruding from the back). Often the upper arm is thinner than the forearm.

Treatment. There is no specific treatment for any of the progressive muscular dystrophies. The factors that are important in the clinical care of those with the disease and of which recreationists should be cognizant are:

- The client should maintain an active life as long as possible, avoiding prolonged bed rest.

- The client should be involved in activities that require a wide range of movement to prevent contractures (shortening of muscles).

- Overweight is to be avoided by the client.

- The client should be introduced to adapted equipment to help maintain independence in work and play.

- Emotional support should be provided

Parkinson's Disease. Parkinson's disease, named after James Parkinson who discovered the disease, is a disturbance of motor function characterized by slowing and weakness of emotional and voluntary movement, muscular rigidity, and tremor. Parkinsonism may be produced by a number of different pathologic states.

In Parkinson's disease the facial muscles exhibit an unnatural immobility. Voluntary movements exhibit some impairment of power, but the slowness is more apparent. Generally those movements that are carried out by small muscles suffer most. Movements of the small muscles of the hands are markedly affected with consequential clumsiness and inability to perform fine movements, such as those of needlework, dealing cards, and playing the piano or other instruments. Tremor is the characteristic involuntary movement of parkinsonism.

Parkinsonism is not necessarily accompanied by any mental change, and the sufferer's intellectual capacity and emotional reactions may continue unimpaired behind the mask in which the disorder fixes the features. When the syndrome is a manifestation of a diffuse pathologic process involving other parts of the brain, there may be mental deterioration leading to aspects of mental illness including a loss of emotional responsiveness, profound depression, and suicidal tendencies.

Programming Recreational Activities

Clients with orthopedic and neurologic disorders require an individualized recreational program determined by the extent of their disability and their interests and needs. Programs in treatment centers will be directed primarily toward complementing the medical treatment and rehabilitation of the client. In community settings, the goal is to provide opportunity, through adaptation of the activities, for clients with these disorders to receive the same benefits from the program as do those who are not disabled.

In treatment centers where there is a rehabilitation team, the medical personnel will provide members of the team the necessary information about each client so that the recreationist will be aware of which muscles need stimulation, the parts of the body that need to be protected, and the movements that are contraindicated. If the prescription is developed only for the physical therapist, the therapeutic recreationist must work closely with the physical therapist to ensure that the recreational program complements that of the physical therapist as well as providing for the development of the positive outcomes of recreational participation.

If the rehabilitation team includes a psychiatrist or psychologist, the prescription may include recommendations for activities for promoting the acceptance of the disability and providing reassurance of ability to cope. The recreationist must then program the activities with a view to strengthening the mental health as well as the physical health of the client.

The recreationist in a community setting, where prescriptions are not developed, has a greater responsibility in interpreting the needs of clients. However, individuals able to participate in community programs will be past the active treatment stage and well on their way to successful rehabilitation; hence, their needs will not be beyond the scope of the recreationist to provide an adapted program. It is necessary, of course, for the recreationist to obtain as much information as possible about the client's disabilities in order to select appropriate activities.

Recreationists in both treatment centers and community settings need to make activity analyses of proposed program offerings as insurance against dangers to the client and failure in successful performance.

There will usually be some activities that the disabled client is able to participate in without modification; but to ensure that the client is not limited to these few experiences, other activities must be adapted. In some cases, the entire activity must be adapted or equipment completely modified as would be necessary for a bilateral amputee to paint a picture or a wheelchair patient to play basketball. In other cases, only portions of the activity need to be modified; a client who cannot stand to engage in a culinary arts activity, for example, can sit in a chair with casters.

Many means of adapting recreational activities for those with orthopedic and neurologic problems are possible. Basically, the adaptations consist of:

- Substitution of a different body position than is normally used, for example, lying or semi-reclining rather than sitting to play checkers.
- Substitution of slower movements for faster movements such as walking for running.
- Modification of the equipment such as a longer handle on sport racquets and gardening tools to extend the reach of a client in a wheelchair.
- Developing new techniques for accomplishing the activity such as changing two-handed skills to one hand or even to the feet or teeth.
- Assisting with part of the skill as in the awl for the client who holds it in place for tooling leather.
- Simplifying the activity, for example, making use of premixed ingredients in cooking activities for clients who lack strength or have restricted movements in the hands.
- Decreasing distances, for example, reducing the size of the court on which a game is played.
- Providing more frequent rest periods than are normally required.

Adaptations for Amputation of the Limbs. One of the major contributions recreational activities can make to those who have lost a limb to amputation is instilling confidence in the ability to execute most of the skills previously performed. Providing recreational activities that offer immediate success is important in developing this assurance. As self-confidence grows, more difficult skills can be introduced.

Amputation can create special problems besides limiting movement. Those with missing limbs perspire more freely during activity because the body's cooling surface is reduced in area. If this becomes a problem in recreational participation, the client can be encouraged to wear lighter weight apparel; also, the coolest possible environment for engaging in the activity can be provided.

Maintaining balance is difficult for amputees during the early stages of rehabilitation because the center of gravity of the body has been altered by the missing limb. Physical recreational activities present the greatest problem, so adaptation will be necessary. For example, if in a dance activity an arm action counter to the leg action is required, changes may need to be made in the movement of the limbs to avoid loss of balance. The nature of the adaptation can be determined by skill analysis.

Amputations of Upper Limbs. The selection of activities depends on the level of amputation and the type of prosthesis. Nearly all activities are possible for clients with arm and hand amputations, even if a prosthesis is not worn. In activities that require the use of both hands, the functional portion of the limb can be utilized or equipment can be devised to substitute for one hand. In playing cards, for example, the cards can be held against the chest with the stump of the amputated arm or a device for holding the cards may be utilized. In all cases of this kind, the recreationist should make careful analysis of the activity and the amputee's potential in order to develop substitute movements or equipment adaptations to enable successful participation by the client.

When an arm prosthesis is worn, the same process of analysis must occur. However, the emphasis is placed on the potential for reproducing natural movement that the prosthesis makes possible.

For many sports and physical recreational activities special prosthetic attachments are available to enhance participation. Examples of these are a special mitt device that enables balls to be caught and another device that holds wood securely for carving. Often the ingenious recreationist can improvise similar helpful devices from readily available materials or adaptation of existing equipment.

Amputations of Lower Limbs. Amputations of the lower limbs pose problems of ambulation. If a prosthesis is not used, the client must move about in a wheelchair or on crutches. Activities require greater modification in these circumstances than when the client has a prosthesis and is more fully mobile. The physical ability and interest of the client dictates the type of physical recreational activities that are offered. Many activities once thought impossible for those with amputated lower limbs are now engaged in by many such individuals: skiing with one limb is now commonplace and wheelchair sports participation is no longer considered an extraordinary achievement for paraplegics; clients have learned to paint holding the brush between the teeth, and crafts have been performed with their feet by clients with no arms. Obviously the possibilities for clients without limbs are restricted only by their own determination and the opportunities available, both of which the recreationist can do much to enhance.

Adaptations for Bone and Nerve Injuries. Fractures of the bone are a common injury and usually cause only temporary disability. In the early stages the area of injury must usually remain immobile so that the recreational activities must be selected or adapted with a view to avoiding movement in the injured area. Table 7-1 offers a guide to the recreationist in planning the program for the client with a broken bone, but these suggestions should not be given precedence over the physician's recommendations concerning the involvement of the area of injury in activity.

Peripheral Nerve Injuries, Spinal Cord Injuries, and Spina Bifida. In programming for clients with nerve injuries, it must first be known which nerves are involved. In treatment centers this information is provided the rehabilitation team along with the designation of movements that are contraindicated. Given this basic information, the therapeutic recreationist can select appropriate activities. Some experimentation will likely be necessary to learn the precise type and extent of movement the client can engage in, that is, a client may have the capacity to play shuffleboard from the wheelchair but not be able to perform the movement required to work in a garden with long-handled hoe, although the two activities appear to be much the same.

Adaptations for Joint Infection and Degenerative Diseases. In developing recreational programs for those with severe arthritis, the recreationist must be in frequent consultation with the client's physical therapist and physician to review the functional status of the client and to develop guidelines for the program activities. Generally, activities that produce undue stress on the affected joints should not be included. Sports are usually contraindicated. Childhood games that require running, twisting, and dodging should not be offered for children with juvenile rheumatoid arthritis.

Frequently, the hands are affected by arthritis. Arts and crafts activities, such as finger-painting and clay modeling, that do not place undue stress on the finger joints, may be included for arthritic clients with hand involvement.

Adaptations for Osteochondrosis. One of the great problems of the recreationist who has a client with Legg-Calvé-Perthes disease is the need to provide active recreational activities while the client is in braces. Those children who have the disease suffer no pain and tend to resent the restraint imposed by the braces. They want to be active, and it is to their benefit to be physically active.

Most clients in braces will be able to walk with the aid of crutches so activities that are appropriate for other users of crutches will be suitable in this instance. The use of low scooters which the child can lie on and propel with the hands pushing against the floor provides mobility in vigorous games. Soccer played in the gymnasium by pushing the ball forward with the front of the scooter is one of many game possibilities.

Adaptations for Neurologic Disabilities. Selecting and conducting recreational activities for clients with neurologic disabilities necessitates some of the same considerations as programming for clients with physical disabilities since both have impaired movement. However, the impairment is frequently manifested in different ways and so requires a slightly different approach in conducting the activities.

Cerebral palsy is one of the most difficult disorders for which to program because of the absence of movement in parts of the body and the lack of control over the movement that is possible. The program for these clients must be individualized and the activities selected by the type and severity of the disability. Regardless of whether the clients are in the treatment center or community setting, the recreationist must work closely with the physical therapist, for this individual will have been involved with the client from the time of the initiation of the therapy and will continue to be involved.

The physical therapy program is directed toward reducing the effects of the pathologic reflexes by manipulation, including passive stretching of the spastic muscles and strength-building exercises for the antagonistic (opposing) muscles. All physical recreational activities should complement this treatment, i.e., the spastic muscles must not be strengthened by participation in the activities offered in the program.

Although clients with cerebral palsy will be more successful in passive activities, the program must not be limited to these. Physical recreational activities are important not only to fill the need for gross body movement, but to provide reassurance that many kinds of activities are possible in spite of the disability.

In providing gross motor activities, those that require a slower response are better than those needing a quick response. For example, catching a balloon, which moves slowly through air, is easier than catching a tossed ball. Large objects are generally more easily controlled and large items of equipment and tools utilized in arts and crafts are more easily managed than small items. Moving objects are more difficult to handle than stationary ones; consequently, activities built around putting stationary objects into motions are more successful than those requiring control of a moving object. Activities that require free gross body movements are more successful than ones that demand finely coordinated movements. Simple repetitive movements are much less difficult to perform than complex movements involving many parts of the body.

An emphasis on the doing of an activity rather than on perfection of performance encourages freer and easier movements because extreme anxiety about doing well often causes a greater spasticity in the muscles. Frequent rest periods are important since the client with cerebral palsy performs better when fresh and relaxed. Rest periods should be taken even though the clients are doing well rather than working until the quality of the performance decreases.

The different types of cerebral palsy cause different responses to activity. Frequently clients with athetosis demonstrate better movement than those who are spastic in the large muscle groups; however, the spastic individual usually can perform fine movements better. Movements that are continuous are frequently easier for those with spastic cerebral palsy while those who are atheoid have more success with movements in which there is a pause or slight relaxation between movements.

No special programming is required for those who are epileptic since they are entirely capable of participation in the regular program of recreational activities. Drugs, primarily phenobarbital and Dilantin, are extremely effective in preventing seizures. The incidence of seizures among the general population of clients with epilepsy is low, but in institutions where individuals with mental retardation and emotional illness are cared for and treated, the incidence is much higher.

In providing recreational services in situations where seizures are relatively high among the clients, care should be taken in selecting and conducting the activities. Swimming is one of the more difficult activities to present safely. Clients must be constantly watched while they are in the water. Other activities that may pose a danger are performing on elevated apparatus and using power tools.

First aid measures to be taken in the event of seizure during recreational activity are:

- Place the individual on the floor away from all possible hazards such as furniture with sharp edges.
- Place something soft under the head and under the arms if the arms are being flailed.
- Loosen any restraining clothing such as shirt collar or belt.
- If breathing is difficult, tilt the head backward to keep the air passage open.
- When the convulsions have stopped, cover with a blanket.
- If the individual is hazy or sleepy, move to a quiet place to rest or sleep.

Muscular Disorders. The loss of motor ability that is caused by the muscular disorders discussed in this section presents a difficult problem for the recreationist in developing an effective program. An equally difficult problem, if not more so, is the motivation of clients to participate in the activities, because for them there is so little hope of regaining the lost strength or movement in the muscles. As indicated in the earlier discussion of the disorders, those with Duchenne multiple sclerosis do not usually live beyond the age of 21. While individuals with fascioscapulohumeral and muscular dystrophy may live to middle age, there is small hope of improvement. Parkinson's disease occurs more frequently in people of advanced years but, again, no improvement can be expected.

Because of the negative prognosis, morale is low. Clients frequently adopt an attitude that since they cannot get better, they will simply sit and await the end. To interest these people in recreational participation will tax the ingenuity of the recreationist, but the effort is worthwhile. Recreational activities are a rich source of enjoyment and draw attention away from morbid aspects of the situation. Moreover, there is evidence that remaining active markedly slows the rate of muscular deterioration. This fact may serve both as motivation to participate and encouragement to continue.

The main focus of the recreational program is to provide immediate enjoyment. Praise and encouragement are vital. Goals must be short term—day to day, and the use of extrinsic rewards may be valuable in promoting achievement of the goals.

The recreationist must be aware that even with the same muscular disorder, clients do not exhibit the same degrees of limitation in movement. Hence, programming requires careful analysis of movement potential so that the activities selected will be ones the individual client will enjoy and be successful in. In general, the activities should be those that provide a wide range of movement for the client but do not overtax weakened muscles. Activities, even mild ones, should be terminated when the client evidences fatigue.

CARDIAC AND PULMONARY DISORDERS

Disorders of the cardiac system, which has the heart as its primary organ, and the pulmonary system, of which the lungs are the chief organ, are different types of disorders with separate symptoms and treatment procedures. They do have a related function, however: both systems are responsible for the delivery of oxygen to the cells and for dispelling carbon dioxide. In referring to the two systems in their joint performance of this function, the term cardiorespiratory is applied.

Cardiopathic Disorders

Cardiopathic or heart disorders are of two general types: organic and functional. A disorder is classified as organic when a definite structural deviation or lesion (injury) is present in the heart. In a functional disorder, no actual deviation or lesion exists, but there is a disturbance in the function of the system.

Symptoms. The symptoms of a heart problem are produced by the failure of the heart to perform properly. The symptoms vary in accordance to the kind of heart disturbance that is present. The following symptoms are often indicative of some type of heart problem:

- Difficulty in breathing
- Edema (swelling) in the feet, ankles, or abdomen
- Dizziness
- General weakness and fatigue
- Indigestion and constipation

- Double vision
- Bluish discoloration of the skin
- Pain in the chest, particularly angina pectoris

Angina pectoris is a sudden and severe pain in the chest accompanied by a sensation of suffocation and a feeling of impending death that is due most often to a lack of supply of oxygen to the heart muscle. The pain may radiate to the left shoulder, down the inside of the arm, and to one or more fingers.

It should be noted that the aforementioned symptoms, with the exception of angina pectoris, are frequently the result of causes other than heart disorders. Contrary to popular belief, chest pains other than angina pectoris usually do not indicate a heart problem; sharp pain accompanying a deep breath inhalation is seldom due to this cause. It should never be assumed that the presence of one or more of the symptoms indicates a cardiopathic problem until a thorough medical examination has been made.

Heart Failure and Other Heart Disorders. The term heart failure refers to a condition of the heart resulting from the heart's inability to maintain an adequate flow of blood to all tissues of the body. Heart failure is divided into two clinical types: coronary occlusion and congestive heart failure. A coronary occlusion is a condition in which there is an obstruction in the flow of the blood in the artery of the heart due to a spasm of the muscle or the presence of a clot. Congestive heart failure occurs when the muscles of the heart fail to function properly.

Treatment. Specific treatment of heart disorders varies with the type of problem. In general, however, these pertinent principles are observed in treating cardiac patients:

- Mental and physical rest. The amount of activity allowed is dependent upon the severity of the disturbance. Effort is made to free the patient from all anxiety, fear, and worry.
- Medication. Drugs are frequently used, including morphine, barbiturates, vasodilators, digitalis, quinidine, and anticoagulants.
- Proper diet. In the early stages, liquid is given, but little food. Later bland food is served for two or three days to help the patient return gradually to a regular diet. Sodium is avoided.
- Exercise and participation in physical recreational activities. Specific exercise and activity may be prescribed, determined by the severity of the patient's condition and the degree of recovery. Exercise is used specifically to strengthen the heart muscles and generally to develop the entire body.
- Avoidance of tobacco and caffeine beverages. Stimulants are contraindicated because they place an additional burden on the heart.
- Utilization of oxygen. Administration of oxygen is routine if there are any signs of difficulty in breathing.

Surgery is being increasingly used in treatment of heart disorders. Surgery is beneficial for those patients who require assistance in innervating the heart properly; in these cases an electrical device known as a pacemaker is inserted into the chest cavity.

New surgical techniques now permit single and simultaneous multiple operations where the closed coronary artery or arteries are by-passed and replaced by other blood vessels. The body's own saphenous vein is used for the grafts. Angiocardiography, an x-ray film of the heart, pinpoints and determines the severity of obstructions. The techniques require the use of a heart-lung machine which takes over the heart's function during surgery. Enabled to work on a motionless organ, the surgeon sews one end of the vein graft to the aorta and the other end to the blocked vessel on the other side of the obstruction. Once surgery, a six-to eight-hour procedure, is completed, the heart is electrically stimulated to resume beating. In any given year, 170,000 surgical bypasses are performed; only 1 to 4% of patients die or suffer complications because of the procedure.

Thrombolysis. Thrombolysis (clot dissolving) therapy is performed by heart catheterization with injection of streptokinase, a substance that helps dissolve clots, into the area of blockage in a coronary artery. If injected soon enough after the onset of a myocardial infarction (heart attack), this material re-opens the clogged artery and renewed blood flow may then revive imperiled cells.

A newer and even more promising procedure is the use of a chemical that is given intravenously to dissolve clots. The chemical circulates in the blood until it comes in contact with a clot. It then acts only on the clot and dissolves it, sometimes within minutes of injection. Although this is still experimental, the initial outcome indicates the procedure holds the best promise for the least complication, trauma, and minimum risk to the patient.

Classification of Patients with Cardiac Problems. The basic consideration in planning the recreational program for those with cardiopathic problems is the functional capacity of the heart. Two commonly used classification systems are shown in Tables 7-2 and 7-3.

Although the information that the classifications provide is somewhat overlapping, the use of both in diagnostic referrals to the therapeutic recreationist provides the most complete picture of the tolerance level of the patient for activity.

Causes of Heart Disease. There are numerous different causes of organic heart disease. Some of the more common of these are infection, rheumatic fever, anemia, hypertension, and coronary accidents.

Infections. Any infection in the body may injure the heart depending upon the vulnerability of the heart and the severity of the infection. Infections that are particularly likely to produce damage to the heart are those of the pyogenic or pus-producing type, e.g., streptococcal and staphylococcal.

Among the common infectious diseases causing injury to the heart are

TABLE 7-2. FUNCTIONAL CAPACITY

Class I:	Patients with cardiac disease but without resulting limitation of physical activity. Ordinary physical activity does not cause undue fatigue, palpitation (rapid beating) of the heart, dyspnea (difficult labored breathing), or anginal (suffocating) pain.
Class II:	Patients with cardiac disease resulting in slight limitation of physical activity. They are comfortable at rest. Ordinary physical activity results in fatigue, palpitation, dyspnea, or anginal pain.
Class III:	Patients with cardiac disease resulting in marked limitations of physical activity. They are comfortable at rest. Less than ordinary activity causes fatigue, palpitation, dyspnea, or anginal pain.
Class IV:	Patients with cardiac disease resulting in inability to carry on any physical activity without discomfort. Symptoms of cardiac insufficiency or of the anginal syndrome are present even at rest. If any physical activity is undertaken, discomfort is increased.

TABLE 7-3. COMPLEMENTARY CLASSIFICATION

Class A:	Patients with a cardiac disorder whose ordinary physical activity requires no restriction.
Class B:	Patients with a cardiac disorder whose ordinary physical activity needs no restriction but who should be advised against severe or competitive efforts.
Class C:	Patients with a cardiac disorder whose ordinary physical activity should be moderately restricted and whose more strenuous habitual efforts should be discontinued.
Class D:	Patients with a cardiac disorder whose ordinary physical activity should be extremely restricted.
Class E:	Patients with a cardiac disorder who should be at complete rest, that is, confined to bed.

pneumonia, meningitis, scarlet fever, and diphtheria. The injury to the heart is caused either by the toxins released by the infecting microorganism or by the microorganism becoming lodged in the heart and affecting it directly. The infection is called endocarditis if the inner lining of the heart is infected, pericarditis if the outer covering is infected, and myocarditis if the inner layer of the heart muscle is infected.

Preventing the infection from attacking the heart is possible through proper treatment of the underlying infection by antibiotics, drugs, rest, and diet. If the heart has been damaged by the infection, bed rest is required until the infection has subsided and signs of the injury, as measured by the electrocardiograph, have disappeared. The prescribed long bed rest is usually accompanied by a mild exercise program in which the amount of activity is gradually increased. Passive recreational activities are an important part of the rehabilitation program during bed rest.

Rheumatic Fever. Rheumatic heart disease occurs most often in children between the ages of six and twelve as a result of rheumatic fever. The etiology of rheumatic fever is not known, but it has been established that a streptococcal infection is related to its development; however, not all individuals who have strep infection develop rheumatic fever. The rheumatic reaction usually occurs two or three weeks after the initial attack of the infection, but no symptoms of rheumatic fever may be present until some time later. It is not communicable.

Rheumatic fever usually but not always causes heart disease, and the heart is generally the only organ seriously affected by the fever. During the course of the disease, the valves of the heart may become inflamed, causing subsequent scarring of the valves and surrounding tissue. The scars can interfere with the ability of the valves to function properly. If the valves are prevented from closing correctly, a back flow of blood— called regurgitation—is permitted. If the valves do not open correctly, the blood cannot flow out easily; the name for this condition is stenosis.

Since streptococcal infection can be controlled by drugs, the main objective in the control of rheumatic heart disease is to prevent the onset of rheumatic fever by early treatment of the infection with drugs, chiefly penicillin. If rheumatic fever has developed, the chief objective becomes prevention of possible heart damage through treatment consisting of bed rest, blanced diet, and plenty of liquids. Drugs, although not highly effective, are used also to control rheumatic fever. During the time of bed rest, passive recreational activities are important in helping young clients to adjust to the need to be inactive.

Anemia. Anemia is a common cause of heart disease throughout the world. It can be caused by several different agents including bacterial infections, chronic hemorrhage, malnutrition, protozoan diseases, and a chronic degenerative state. It is recognized that the anemia interferes with the oxygen supplied to the heart. In addition, it increases the demand on the heart to supply oxygen to the body causing the heart to work harder.

There are three basic procedures used in the treatment of anemia: (1) removing the cause; (2) administering blood transfusions; and (3) providing sufficient rest and good diet. In most cases, the heart disease can be eliminated if adequate treatment is given at an early date.

Hypertension. Hypertension or high blood pressure is another common cause of heart disease. Hypertension is the result of constriction or spasm or accumulation of fatty deposits in the arterioles throughout the body, a condition that necessitates more forceful contraction of the heart to push the blood through the arterioles, causing increased pressure. The heart is affected detrimentally because of the extra workload on the heart due to the increased blood pressure.

Arteriosclerosis (hardening and thickening of the artery walls) often accompanies hypertension in the older patient. The cause of arteriosclerosis is not well-established. It does appear that it is linked to a hereditary factor. Some authorities feel that it is associated with a mode of living in which excessive anxiety, worry, and insufficient amount of rest as well as overeating, consumption of alcohol, and smoking are common, while others feel that cholesterol metabolism and arteriosclerosis are related. Recent research provides increasing evidence to indicate that diet and exercise are factors in the regulation of the cholesterol metabolism, thereby reducing the possibility of arteriosclerosis.

Therapy for hypertension consists of following good health habits. Mental and physical rest and regulated exercises are extremely important. The diet should be well-balanced; usually the physician recommends a decrease in proteins, and sodiums are restricted. Weight reduction is recommended to those who are overweight. Anxiety, fear, and worry must be reduced as much as possible, and sedatives are given if needed to relieve the emotional stress. Medications are now commonly used to help control hypertension.

Coronary Accident. The most serious coronary accident that may occur is occlusion of a coronary artery or rupture of one of the blood vessels which hemorrhages into the muscle tissue of the heart and decreases the blood flow to the heart. When the blood flow is decreased because of a clot in the coronary artery, the condition is called coronary thrombosis. When there is death of tissue caused by coagulation, the condition is known as myocardial infarction.

Treatment for coronary heart disease is related to the severity of the incident. It is now unusual for a stabilized coronary victim to be kept in bed for more than a few days. With continued recovery the physician may prescribe staged movement and exercise, together with a simple stress test. Increased exercise, particularly walking, is typical during the recuperation period. A salt-free liquid or soft diet is usually prescribed and all stimulants of the heart, including coffee, tea, cola drinks, tobacco, and alcohol, are restricted. Patients, if they have difficulty breathing, will be provided with oxygen. Also, specific drugs such as morphine, barbiturates, digitalis, and vasodilators may be prescribed.

Pulmonary Diseases

The more common diseases of the lungs, which will be discussed in this section, are asthma (and hay fever), chronic bronchitis, emphysema, and pulmonary tuberculosis. The incidence of these disorders, with the exception of tuberculosis, is on the increase with emphysema being the disorder increasing at the fastest rate. Tuberculosis has been on the decline for several years, and the tremendous advances made in the treatment and control of the disease indicate that its elimination is within reach.

Etiology and Pathology. A characteristic common to asthma, chronic bronchitis, and emphysema is an increase in the excretion of mucus in the lung area. The greater accumulation of mucus causes frequent coughing. The victims of emphysema experience greater difficulty in expelling the mucus than the sufferers of the other diseases because of loss of elasticity of the lung's air sacs that occurs in emphysema. All four diseases are also characterized by dyspnea (difficulty in breathing) at some stage in the development of the inflammation.

In emphysema the characteristic symptoms may be developing in the early years but not become evident until the middle years of life. Similarly, pulmonary tuberculosis symptoms may be present long before detection of the disease, by which time it has usually progressed to an advanced stage.

Asthma. Asthma is characterized by sudden recurring attacks of dyspnea due to a spasmodic contraction of the bronchi (tubes) of the lungs. The attack is caused by a reflex action of the muscles of the bronchial tubes which produces spasmodic contractions usually precipitated by a substance to which the body is allergic.

Some evidence indicates that emotions play a part in the genesis of attacks of asthma. Although the relationship between the emotional aspects and sensitivity to allergens has not been clearly established, some psychiatrists regard asthma as a psychosomatic disorder and minimize the physiologic influences.

During an attack the patient usually perspires freely, the pulse is weak, and nausea and diarrhea may be present. In an acute attack the patient breathes with great difficulty and frequently experiences the feeling of impending death. Although in prolonged attacks, death due to asphyxiation can occur, this is relatively rare.

Hay fever or seasonal fever is a term applied to asthma that recurs at about the same time each year and is caused by some specific, seasonal allergen (e.g., roses, ragweed, etc.).

General Treatment. If the patient can avoid the substance to which he or she is sensitive, serious attacks may be eliminated. When attacks do occur, drugs are used to reduce their severity. If breathing is especially difficult, oxygen may be administered by a mask or tent.

In most cases patients have less breathing difficulty if they are in a sitting position. A bed table on which to rest the head while sitting up may provide a more comfortable position for the patient. In some cases a vaporizer is used to help loosen the secretion in bronchial tubes so it may be expelled more easily. Since there is an unusual amount of sweating, the patient's bed clothes require frequent changing to prevent chilling. Fluid must be administered in large quantities. If the oral fluid intake is inadequate, fluids may be given intravenously. Elimination of faulty breathing habits through breathing exercises may relieve some of the breathing difficulties. The patient is kept as calm as possible, and frequent reassurance is offered; in this effort, the therapeutic recreationist can play a significant role by offering relaxing activities.

Chronic Bronchitis. Bronchitis is an inflammation of the bronchial tubes caused by allergens, pollutants, and sometimes viruses and bacteria. Sometimes the inflammation is of short duration, leaving no serious effects, as in the common cold. In contrast, chronic bronchitis is an inflammation of long duration, resulting from constant exposure to the causative factors, with possible serious consequences.

Chronic bronchitis is characterized by a marked swelling of the lining of the bronchial tubes, accompanied by increased production of mucus which causes the individual to cough up sputum. The swelling of the tubes and the increased amount of mucus hinder the passage of air through the tubes. In addition, when the bronchial tubes are irritated, the muscles of the tubes tend to contract, further narrowing their diameter. These conditions make breathing, particularly exhalation, difficult.

Attacks of severe breathing difficulty may occur at any time of the year; however, they are more prevalent in winter and are more likely to occur in the night. Air pollution increases the likelihood of an attack. A greater effort is required to exhale because the swelling traps air in the air sacs and the tiny bronchi of the lungs. The force created by the additional effort can cause the walls of the air sacs to become weakened, leading to the development of emphysema.

Treatment. The treatment of chronic bronchitis is directed toward removal of the pollutants or allergens that cause the inflammation. In addition, effort is made to drain the excess excretion in the lungs. The use of a humidifier helps to thin the excretion and so facilitate drainage. Sometimes it is also helpful to place the patient in a position in which the head and shoulders are lower than the rest of the body to assist the draining of the fluids. In cases where the patient has extreme difficulty breathing, oxygen is administered.

Emphysema. Emphysema is a condition in which there is an abnormal inflation of the alveoli (air sacs of the lungs) due to the presence of air. In emphysema the alveoli lose their elasticity and become permanently enlarged, creating air pockets in the alveoli from which the individual is unable to expel all the air. Consequently, oxygen and carbon dioxide cannot be exchanged in the alveoli as is the case in normal respiration. A person with severe emphysema may be unable to cough up mucus, further complicating the exchange. A bluish skin discoloration may result due to lack of oxygen in the blood. As the alveoli become permanently enlarged, the bronchioles (small tubes in the lungs) also lose their elasticity and the muscles of the diaphragm weaken. This causes an increased rate of breathing.

Emphysema may develop early in the patient's life but usually does not become evident until the individual is around 50 years of age. In mild cases, the patient is comfortable at rest but exertion causes shortness of breath. In severe cases the dyspnea is chronic.

Treatment. Emphysema is irreversible; once damage to the alveoli occurs it cannot be repaired. Treatment is directed toward making breathing as easy as possible. Bronchodilating drugs provide relaxation of the bronchial muscles and this makes breathing easier. Drugs that encourage expectoration may be used to encourage the elimination of mucus. Extreme fluctuations in weather are to be avoided. Intake of large quantities of liquids is extremely important; otherwise, the mucus tends to dry up and expelling it from the lungs becomes difficult. In addition to ingestion of liquids, the air the patient breathes must contain adequate amounts of moisture. Humidifiers are used to increase the moisture content of the air.

The patient is not permitted to participate in physical activity that places an undue burden upon the lungs. However, to the extent that it can be comfortably performed, active participation in normal routines—including recreational activities—is encouraged. Slow performance of all motor movements helps to avoid overtaxing the respiratory system.

Often the patient is placed in a position where the head and shoulders are lower than the rest of the body to provide better drainage of the secretion. However, the patient usually breathes more easily in a sitting position. In situations where the patient has great difficulty breathing, he or she may be given oxygen.

Chest physiotherapy may be administered to the patient to help in the removal of secretions from the lungs. For this, the patient is placed in a supine position so that the bronchial tubes may drain to the throat, and an attempt is made to jar the accumulated secretions loose by clapping on the chest with cupped hands.

Programming Recreational Activities

There is a common factor to be considered in programming for clients with heart and pulmonary disorders—control of the use of energy. The energy output for cardiac clients can be monitored by pulse count (see Chapter 14). With clients who have pulmonary disorders, the breathing rate may be estimated by observing the client breathe. Generally, the lungs are not placed in a condition of stress as long as the individual can breathe easily with the mouth closed. However, when the breathing becomes forced and air is taken in through the mouth, activity should be terminated for clients with serious pulmonary problems.

In selecting activities for those with cardiorespiratory problems, consideration should be given to the functional capacity of the individual client and activities selected in accordance to the class the individual's physician has diagnosed the person to be in.

When selecting activities the stress placed on the cardiorespiratory system is not completely determined by the type of activity but by the vigor with which the client participates. Some clients may take part in activity with more vigor than others. For example, one person may fish with tremendous exuberance and so make a moderately vigorous activity of an ordinarily mild one, while another's efforts as fishing are truly mild because of the low level of exertion.

The degree to which a person becomes emotionalized is another factor in determining the workload on the heart. A game of checkers is a mild activity and places little stress on the cardiorespiratory system, but those who play the game so that emotions run high may increase their pulse rate beyond the target rate and so place undue stress on the system. Any competitive play, with its emphasis on winning, may cause an increase in heart beat beyond the desired point. For purposes of comparison of their energy requirements in situations of normal emotional reaction, some typical recreational activities are listed below in order from the least to the most demanding.

1. Table games played while seated
2. Art and craft activities
3. Table games played while standing
4. Woodworking
5. Playing a musical instrument
6. Fishing
7. Walking slowly
8. Billiards
9. Croquet
10. Horseshoe pitching
11. Shuffleboard
12. Cooking
13. Sailing
14. Walking moderately
15. Golf
16. Conditioning exercises

Recreational activities for clients who are confined to bed with cardiac disorders are greatly restricted and close monitoring of stress experienced in participation is required.

Individuals with respiratory disorders can usually participate in most passive recreational activities, and programming this type of activity for these clients presents no problems. However, more physically vigorous activity may require adaptation. Activities like archery and croquet present no difficulty, but a game like tennis would need to be modified to reduce the strenuousness of the movements. This can be achieved by reducing the size of the court.

Those with lung disorders generally must expectorate frequently during activity. Receptacles to receive the sputum should be made readily available for those with this problem.

AUDITORY AND VISUAL IMPAIRMENTS

In the past it was common to consider auditory and visual disorders as similar because both have their origin in a complete or partial loss of one of the senses. However, the etiology and pathology of the two have little resemblance; and certainly the recreational programming varies considerably.

Auditory Disabilities

An auditory disability is one in which the individual is partially or wholly lacking the sense of hearing. Most hearing disabilities are structural in origin. Structural disorders are of two basic types: conductive hearing loss and sensorineural hearing loss. A conductive hearing loss is one that is caused by a physical obstruction, for example, impacted wax or a middle ear infection, that impedes the conduction of sound waves to the inner ear. If the obstruction is removed or successfully treated by a physician, the loss of hearing is usually not permanent; however, if the middle ear is damaged, hearing is impaired to some degree. A hearing aid is beneficial in improving hearing in those cases where there is a conductive hearing loss.

Sensorineural hearing loss is a serious condition, resulting from damage to the cells or nerve fibers that receive and transmit the sound stimuli. It does not generally respond to medical treatment. The loss may be present at birth, in which case the condition is classified as congenital deafness. Sensorineural hearing loss having a noncongenital origin is classified as acquired deafness. The amount of sensorineural hearing loss may range from mild to total inability to hear. If the loss is not complete, a hearing aid may be helpful because the improvement in quality of these devices in recent years now makes it possible for the patients with sensorineural hearing loss, as well as those with conductive hearing loss, to benefit.

Etiology and Pathology of Conductive Hearing Loss. The most common cause of conductive impairment is an inflammation of the middle ear (otitis media). The condition is readily controlled by antibiotics; left untreated, it can result in permanent hearing loss.

Another cause of conductive hearing loss is the disease otosclerosis. This disease affects the bony capsule of the inner ear, turning the hard bone into a spongelike substance. It causes hearing loss through the fixation of the stapes (one of the three bones of the inner ear) as the spongy bone invades the window of the stapes. At the onset, the disease affects the middle ear but in the later stages it can invade the inner ear causing sensorineural hearing loss.

Treatment of Conductive Hearing Loss. Conductive hearing loss responds well to medical and surgical treatment. As indicated earlier, otitis media is alleviated by antibiotics. In addition, the physician may perform a myringotomy, which is an incision in the eardrum, if there is any danger that the drum may rupture spontaneously. The incision is to allow the middle ear to drain. The advantage is that the incision is made in the best place for rapid healing to occur. Spontaneous rupture of the drum may result in perforation of the drum that does not heal, or heals over with scar tissue which can destroy the efficiency of the drum.

When chronic otitis media does not respond to antibiotics, the infection may reach the covering of the brain. When this is the case, surgery is performed to remove the eardrum and some of the bones in the inner ear. The operation is called mastoidectomy, and is performed not to improve hearing, but to stop the infection which may be a threat to life. A simple mastoidectomy is sometimes performed, which is an attempt to stop infection without removal of the bones of the inner ear. A successful simple mastoidectomy does not cause hearing loss as does radical mastoidectomy.

A rupture of the eardrum, in addition to causing possible hearing loss, poses a constant potential hazard to the middle ear because infection could enter it through the perforation. The rupture can be closed by one of several possible surgical techniques.

A procedure called stapedectomy is used to improve hearing loss due to otosclerosis (hardening of the bone). The operation consists of removing the stapes and creating a prosthetic link in its place.

Pathology of Sensorineural Hearing Impairment. Sensorineural hearing impairment can be either congenital or acquired. Some cases of congenital hearing loss are inherited; however, many others can be ascribed to damage to the embryo. Certain diseases contracted by the mother in early stages of pregnancy will frequently injure the embryo so as to produce abnormalities in the child, one such abnormality being deafness.

Acquired sensorineural hearing impairment may occur at any time during the life. The causative agent can be one or a combination of factors such as disease, injury, or the process of aging. The last named is the most common single cause. As an individual grows older, the sensory process of hearing tends to deteriorate. This loss is called presbycusis. It may be manifested in various degrees from a light hearing loss, especially in the higher frequencies, to total deafness.

Causes. Diseases that may cause sensorineural hearing impairment include measles, scarlet fever, mumps, diphtheria, and certain types of virus infection. These diseases often produce a toxic condition that affects the sensitive nerve endings in the cochlea (a tube in the inner ear), causing hearing loss. Sensorineural hearing loss may also occur when fracture to the bone(s) of the temple occurs and the inner ear is damaged.

Exposure to loud noises is another frequent cause of sensorineural hearing loss. Intense sounds can cause permanent damage to the nerve fibers in the cochlea. Exposure for short duration generally produces auditory fatigue, and recovery usually takes place within a day. However, continual exposure usually produces a permanent hearing loss and in some cases results in total deafness.

Visual Disabilities

Visual handicaps vary from total to partial blindness. The degree to which an individual is handicapped is determined largely by how greatly his or her vision deviates from normal. The deviation is measured by visual acuity tests.

Pathology and Treatment. The most common causes of severe sight problems are accidents, diseases, and heredity. When accidents and infectious diseases occur, the eye is treated to promote healing. Vision impairment that results is generally permanent and usually cannot be alleviated.

Accidental Injuries. Accidental injuries to the eye in work situations produce numerous incidents where vision is destroyed. Sharp instruments and hazardous toys cause many of the serious injuries to the eye that children experience. Other common injuries that occur are chemical burns, contusion, and penetrating injuries.

Infectious Diseases. Loss of vision may be caused by the primary infection of parts of the eye: the cornea, eye socket, optic nerve, or conjunctiva. The secondary infection of contagious diseases, such as scarlet fever and typhoid fever, may also affect the eye and cause vision loss.

Other Disorders of the Eyes. There are several eye disorders that have a higher incidence among descendants in certain families; it is thought that a tendency to incur the disorder is the hereditary factor rather than the condition itself. The disorders, which may produce blindness, are retinitis pigmentosa and some forms of glaucoma, cataract, retinal detachment, and retinopathy. The nature and treatment of these disorders are briefly described to enable recreationists to appreciate the problems they present for clients.

Retinitis Pigmentosa. This disorder is not as common as the others, but it is a serious one and, in some cases, can cause total blindness. The cause is degeneration and clumping of the retinal pigment. The earliest symptom is night blindness. As the degeneration of the retinal pigment progresses, peripheral field vision is lost and finally, in severe cases, complete blindness results.

Glaucoma. Glaucoma is characterized by increased pressure within the eyeball and progressive loss of vision. The pressure is caused by the failure of the fluid of the eye to drain. Glaucoma as a cause of blindness can readily be prevented by early detection and treatment. However, after the loss of sight, treatment does not restore the vision. Treatment generally consists of controlling the pressure within the eye by using miotic drops. These drops within the eye cause the pupil to become smaller, thereby improving the outflow of fluid.

Cataract. The cataract is a defect in the transparency of the lens of the eye. The most common cause is an inherited factor that is influenced by the slow degenerative changes of age. However, injury, poisons, and virus infection may also cause a loss of transparency of the lens. Common symptoms of cataract are blurring vision and unpleasant glare in a bright light. The loss of sight is gradual and progresses at different rates in different individuals.

Cataracts can cause total blindness, but most types respond well to surgery. After surgery, the eye is protected for about a month. Protection at night usually consists of a metal shield taped over the eye to avoid accidental rubbing of the eye during sleep. Wearing glasses is recommended as a protective procedure during the day.

Retinal Detachment. This is a condition where the retina, or a portion of it, becomes separated from the choroid. The retina receives nourishment from the choroid so that the part of the retina that is separated is not nourished and therefore causes loss of vision. Most detachments begin from holes in the retina. The fluid contents of the eye seep through the holes and exert a pressure between the retina and choroid which causes the separation.

The most common cause of holes developing in the retina is shrinking of parts of the eye as a result of aging. Some types of myopia (nearsightedness) are predisposed to retinal detachment. In these cases, the young are affected as well as the aging. Frequently retinal detachment is caused by infection of the interior of the eye and injuries to the eye. Unless the retinal holes are repaired, there will be progressive detachment of the retina resulting in total blindness.

Surgery is necessary to repair the retinal holes. The hole is sealed by causing a scar to develop around the hole, thereby closing it. Before and for a day after surgery the patient's head is maintained in a position in which the retinal hole is in the lower part of the eye since gravity has a tendency to pull the torn part of the retina down. Usually by the second day the patient is allowed to be up and assume a normal position.

Retinopathy. Retinopathy is a noninflammatory disease of the retina. A frequent cause is diabetes mellitus, which is an inherited disease. Over half of all diabetic patients have retinopathy and over two percent of these become totally blind. In diabetic retinopathy the capillaries in the retina are destroyed, causing loss of sight. Control of diabetes appears to decrease the possibility of retinopathy.

Programming Recreational Activities

Disorders of vision and hearing involve losses that affect receiving information through sight in the first instance and through oral transmission in the second case. Consequently, one of the major considerations in programming recreational activities for clients with these disorders is how to achieve effective communication.

Communication with Blind Clients. For blind clients, communication will obviously involve oral descriptions to a far greater extent than is usual for most other clients. The tendency for inexperienced recreationists is to give much more information than can be readily absorbed by the listener. In the effort to be helpful, the recreationist often keeps up a steady barrage of comments that confuses rather than helps the client. To avoid this problem, the recreationist should first think through the activity, perhaps several times, isolating the information actually needed at each step of the activity and then formulate minimal descriptive instructions to explain to the blind client how to accomplish each phase.

Another means of communication with those who have vision disorders is the use of kinesthesis. This term refers to the involvement of muscular activity in the performance of movements, and its use employs manual leading of the client's body parts through the movements of the activity. If an activity requires a specific placement of the hands or feet, for example, the recreationist takes hold of each hand or foot and places it in the desired position. When the manipulation is accompanied by verbal explanation, the process becomes an effective method of communicating with vision impaired clients.

There are available several kinds of communication aids that are especially valuable to the client whose vision is too poor to read ordinary printed matter. The best known of the aids is the braille system, which consists of coding words on paper in raised dots arranged in various positions so that they can be read by feeling with the fingers. Braille may be written on a special typewriter or with the use of a stylus. Another aid is the optacon, which is an instrument that converts printed material into impulses that can be read tactually. Also available is the Kurzweil Reading Machine that translates written words into oral ones.

Communication with Deaf Clients. For communication with clients with auditory handicaps, the three most common methods are the use of the written word, signing, and speechreading, frequently referred to as lip reading. At one time authorities felt that those with hearing problems should be taught only speechreading to force them to learn to "read" speech more rapidly and perhaps to learn to talk. However, currently both signing and speechreading are taught to provide the widest possible communication skills, an approach called the total communication system.

The sign language that is usually taught is the American Sign Language (AMESLAN). Because the signs of AMESLAN are closely related to the action being described, recreationists may find they can without formal training communicate with those who use the signs. The use of AMESLAN is accompanied by fingerspelling of words for which there is no sign. The words are spelled out with distinct positions of the hands and fingers for each letter of the alphabet. By learning these positions and some signs, the recreationist can achieve effective communication with clients who have serious hearing loss.

In treatment centers, clients with visual and auditory disorders will be limited to those with acute involvement. Loss of sight or hearing will have occurred recently. Hence, the chief responsibility of the therapeutic recreationist will be to assist through leisure education to enhance the client's adaptability to the new circumstances and to provide reassurance in facing life without full use of the senses.

Those who are blind will be receiving assistance from a mobility and orientation instructor with specific training and competence in this kind of work. Help is given the visually impaired individuals to use their remaining senses to relate their body positions to other subjects and to move from one place to another. The therapeutic recreationist will need to coordinate the programming of recreational activities with the instructor to ensure the selection and presentation of activities of a complementary nature.

Clients in the Community. Upon the return of clients with seeing and hearing impairments to their communities, efforts should be made to engage them in the recreational program as a means of reassuring them that their sensory loss does not affect their re-integration in community life. To enable them to participate in the activities to their advantage, some adaptation will need to occur. For those with hearing loss, if communication has been developed, modifications are relatively simple to achieve. Clients with sight impairments need a greater degree of modification. Emphasis should be placed on utilizing other senses like touch and hearing to receive information needed to perform the activities. Development of kinesthetic sense, awareness of how proper movement should feel during performance, is particularly important in doing motor skills.

More adaptations are needed, also, in equipment and facilities for vision impaired than for hearing impaired clients. Spaces for recreational activities should be large and barrier-free. Non-essential equipment and unnecessary obstructions should be removed. Recreational equipment should be stored in special places where clients can locate the items easily each time they wish to use them.

Playground equipment for children with vision impairments may be the same as that found on any playground, including free form climbing apparatus, swings, and teetertotters. However, greater care needs to be taken to locate the equipment to prevent possible injury to non-sighted participants. For example, swings should be placed in rows of two to avoid a center swing that may be difficult to reach without danger from the other swings. Guard rails and markers are necessary to prevent children from bumping into equipment or being hit by moving apparatus like swings.

Small items of recreational equipment, like scissors, may need to be painted white or yellow to increase their visibility for clients with some vision. Balls and bean bags with bells or buzzers in the interior are very helpful in indicating location to the clients.

Seeing and hearing impaired children of school age are frequently enrolled in special schools offering training in compensatory skills as well as educational instruction. Recreationists employed in these schools provide leisure education as well as adapted recreational programs for the children who are enrolled. With the implementation of PL 94-142, sensory impaired children are more and more being educated in the public school. Recreationists working with these students have similar responsibilities to those in the special schools.

SELECTED REFERENCES

Birkerstoff, E. R., *Neurology,* 3rd. ed. (New York: Arco Publishing, Inc., 1982).

Hamilton, H., ed., *Cardiovascular Disorders* (Springfield, Pennsylvania: Inter-Med Communications, 1983).

Keele, D. K., *The Developmentally Disabled Child: A Manual for Primary Physicians* (Oradell, New Jersey: Medical Economics Books, 1983).

Monk, C. J., *Orthopedics for Undergraduates,* 2nd. ed. (New York: Churchill Livingston, Inc., 1981).

Chapter 8

Mental Retardation and Learning Disabilities

Mental retardation and learning disabilities were once regarded as the same disorder. Today, however, research has clearly demonstrated that they are two distinct and separate disorders. Mental retardation ". . . refers to significantly subaverage general intellectual functioning existing concurrently with defects in adapted behavior and manifested during the developmental period." [1] A learning disability, according to the definition given in Public Law 94-142, ". . . means a disorder in one or more of the basic psychologic processes involved in understanding or in using language, spoken or written, which may manifest itself in an imperfect ability to listen, think, speak, read, write, spell or do mathematical calculations." [2] The term encompasses such conditions as perceptual handicaps, brain injury, minimal brain dysfunction, dyslexia, and developmental aphasia. Not included are learning problems that are primarily due to visual or hearing disorders; mental retardation; or environmental, cultural, or economic disadvantage.

Although the definition by the federal government does not specifically address perceptual motor learning problems, it is recognized by authorities that such problems are related to inability to listen, speak, read, and write, etc. and that, furthermore, they have a profound effect upon perceptual motor performance, which is vital to participation in the many recreational activities that require movement by various segments of the body.

MENTAL RETARDATION

A difficulty in determining the presence of mental retardation is the lack of precise guidelines for establishing "subaverage general intellectual functioning." One of the causes of the imprecision is the incomplete knowledge about the nature of intelligence. Currently a number of theories purport to explain its nature, but there is little agreement among authorities as to what intelligence actually is.[3]

Nature of Intelligence

There are two basic concepts of the nature of intelligence: one regards the nature of intelligence as a unitary phenomenon, the other as a specific phenomenon. An early proponent of the unitary concept was Spearman,[4] who as a result of his studies, concluded that intelligence is one single general factor that is inherited but is, also, influenced by life experiences. He felt that this single factor is involved to some extent in all human behavior and some kinds of behavior are completely dependent upon it. Although he recognized that there are specific kinds of intelligence that influence certain kinds of behavior, he believed that the differences in intelligence between one child and another are chiefly influenced by the factor of general intelligence.

Thorndike[5] has offered another theory of intelligence which is in direct contrast to the unitary concept. From his research, Thorndike concluded that intelligence is composed of highly specific absolutes and that general intelligence is the total of all the specifics. He believed there were many different kinds of specific intelligence, but he grouped them into three categories: abstract, mechanical, and social. Thorndike's concept of intelligence as a specific phenomenon is the most widely accepted theory today.

Measuring Mental Capacity

The confusion that exists about the use of the terms describing mental retardation extends to the means of measuring mental capacity to determine if retardation is present and, if so, to what degree. Procedures for measuring mental capacity generally consist of the evaluation of (1) measured intelligence, i.e., intelligence that can be measured by a test, or (2) impairment in adaptive behavior, the ability to function independently and to meet the culturally imposed demands of the environment. Since measured intelligence is usually related to learning ability, especially academic subjects, this factor often assumes greater importance during childhood, whereas adaptive behavior is generally the more significant determinant of the degree of retardation in an adult. Both are important factors since there is a relationship between the ability in measured intelligence and the ability to adapt and meet the demands of the environment. However, in adulthood the ability to function independently in making a living and handling oneself and one's affairs with some degree of success takes on more importance than the ability to learn.

Measured Intelligence. Measured intelligence is evaluated by intelligence tests which consist of test items that have been selected to represent information which the majority of children in a specific age group will have acquired. Two types of items are used: verbal and performance. Verbal tests require the use of language. It is assumed when this kind of item is used that the child has had an average exposure to the language for his or her specific age and has no hearing problem. Performance test items do not require the use of language to any great extent. A typical example of a performance test is the form board test where the child is asked to fit forms of different sizes and shapes into their proper places on the board. Scores on the two kinds of tests do not correlate highly, which is a likely indication that they are measuring different kinds of intelligence.[6]

A commonly used test for evaluating measured intelligence is the Stanford-Binet Test. The score of this test is expressed in terms of mental age or intelligence quotient (I.Q.). The mental age is calculated by determining which of the test items, arranged according to difficulty, the child has answered correctly. Consequently, a child who correctly answers all of the items up to and including those which the majority of 6 year olds are able to answer correctly—but none beyond this—has a mental age of 6. If a child is able to pass all the items up to and including the age of 6 and also several items beyond that, he or she is given credit in terms of months so that the mental age, for example, may be 6 years and 2 months or 6 years and 5 months or even 7 years and higher.

The maximum mental age is 18 years since it is believed that mental ability as measured by intelligence tests does not increase beyond this age. The I.Q. score expresses the relationship between the mental age and the chronological age. The score is determined by multiplying the mental age by 100 and dividing it by the chronological age (I.Q. = M.A. $\times$ 100 / C.A.).

Interpretation of Scores. Any I.Q. score on a measured intelligence test has to be interpreted in the light of knowledge about the child and the situation in which the test was given. For meaningful results, the child who is taking the test must have the background and experience suitable to the test that is used. In addition the child has to be adequately motivated to take the test, be cooperative, and be physically capable of making the desired responses.

While present tests of measured intelligence are useful, the results are frequently misinterpreted. Test scores are not necessarily stable for children; they frequently fluctuate widely, especially during the first ten years of life. It has been noted that the greater the maladjustment of the child, the more likely it is that test scores will significantly vary.

All aspects of intelligence are not measured by the intelligence tests. Undoubtedly there are a large number of important factors of cognitive function that are as yet unknown and so not evaluated by the available tests. Consequently, a score on an intelligence test for a specific child must be used with discretion in estimating mental ability and must not be considered as an absolute or totally valid measurement of intelligence.

Adaptive Behavior. The procedures for evaluation of adaptive behavior have not been studied as long and as closely as have those for measured intelligence. The most extensive study of the measurement of adaptive behavior has been made by Doll. The test he developed, the Vineland Social Maturity Scale,[7] is a standardized method for quantitative estimation of personal social maturity of the mentally retarded. The scale evaluates the ability to perform everyday activities and the ability to be a cooperating and contributing member of a social group. The principle underlying construction of the scale is similar to that used in the Stanford-Binet test in that the items selected represent experiences common to specific chronologic age level. The items are divided into eight areas of experience: self-help general, self-help dressing, self-direction, occupation, communication, locomotion, and socialization. For example, characteristic test items in self-help general include: sits unsupported, grasps with thumb and fingers, asks to go to toilet, and cares for self at toilet.

A means of measuring motor skills as a component of adaptive behavior of mentally retarded persons has been developed at the University of Connecticut and Mansfield Training School. The test is suitable for use with those who are severely and profoundly retarded. Items in the test measure motor abilities that are basic to many of the movements of daily living. Other tests that are used for evaluating motor ability or phases of it are: Fait's Physical Fitness Test for the Mentally Retarded (Mild and Moderate), AAHPER Special Fitness Test of the Mentally Retarded, and the Lincoln-Oseretsky Motor Development Scale. (See Chapter 6.)

Classification. Mental retardation is classified in a number of ways. The American Association on Mental Deficiency classifies measured intelligence into the following: mild, moderate, severe, and profound. In each classification, scores on the Stanford-Binet Test of Intelligence and the Wechsler Intelligence Scale for Children are placed as shown in Table 8-1.

TABLE 8-1

Stanford-Binet	Weschler	Classification
52-67	55-69	Mild
36-51	40-54	Moderate
20-35	25-39	Severe
00-19	00-24	Profound

In educational circles the terms educable, trainable, and totally dependent are frequently used to classify mental deficiency. States have different classification arrangements for educational purposes; however, most of the states use the Stanford-Binet Test and employ the classification shown in Table 8-2. Familiarity with educational classification is

TABLE 8-2

Stanford-Binet	Classification
50-75	Educable
25-49	Trainable
00-24	Totally dependent

desirable for recreationists working with school personnel in developing the Individualized Education Program (IEP) and conducting recreational programs for mentally retarded students.

The American Association of Mental Deficiency divides adaptive behavior into four levels of impairment: mild, moderate, severe, and profound. Those whose impairment is regarded as mild are able to develop acceptable social and communication skills but experience slight retardation in sensorimotor skill development. They frequently need supervision and guidance under social stress. Moderately retarded individuals are able to learn with special help to communicate with a fair degree of success. They develop motor skills at a slower rate than mildly impaired youngsters. Supervision is usually required under mild social stresses. Severely impaired individuals have poor motor development; however, they can learn simple tasks and are able to profit from training programs. Their speech is not fully developed, and they are able to achieve only minimal communication skills. Those classified as profound have a minimal capacity for development of motor skills and are totally incapable of self-maintenance. For measurement of motor skills as a component of adapted behavior related to gross body movements common to many profoundly mentally retarded individuals, the Texas Revision of the Fait's Basic Motor Skills is an effective tool (see Chapter 6).

From the medical standpoint, mental retardation is divided into two large groups: primary or endogenous and secondary or exogenous. The former consists of mental defects due largely to chromosome abnormalities, e.g., multiple genes as in the case of Down's syndrome (mongolism). In the other group are those cases of retardation caused by environmental factors such as infection, trauma, and intoxication, for example.

Causes of Mental Retardation

Well over a hundred causes of mental deficiency have been identified, but these account for only about one-quarter of all cases diagnosed as mental retardation. The various causes are categorized by the American Association on Mental Deficiency into these eight groups: (1) infection, (2) intoxication due to poisons, etc., (3) trauma, (4) disorder of metabolism, growth dysfunction, and poor nutrition, (5) new cerebral growths, (6) unknown prenatal influences, (7) unknown with structural changes, and (8) presumed psychologic with no known structural changes. Each of the types of causes is briefly examined in the paragraphs which follow.

Infections. Infection plays a major role as a cause of mental retardation. A prominent example is certain infectious diseases, that when contracted by the mother during pregnancy, can cause mental retardation of the child. It is not known if mental deficiency is caused even if there is no direct infection of the fetus; but if the fetus does become infected, the chance of some degree of mental retardation in the child is high.

Also, it is possible for the fetus to be infected even though there are no recognized symptoms of an infectious disease in the mother. Some of the maternal diseases known to produce mental deficiency in offspring are: syphilis; German measles (rubella) if contracted by the mother during the first three months of pregnancy; toxoplasmosis (caused by a genus of parasite, usually mild in the mother but can produce serious types of mental retardation such as hydrocephalus and microcephalia).

Postnatal infections of the brain are responsible for a large number (10 or more percent) of all cases of mental retardation. Evidence indicates that a substantial number of these are youngsters who have residual brain damage secondary to the common infections of childhood but the damage is not recognized at the time. Childhood diseases that are capable of producing encephalitis (inflammation of the brain) which may cause retardation are: measles, mumps, and chicken pox.

Intoxication. Intoxication produced by certain toxic agents is another cause of mental retardation. Although it is not a common type of intox-ication, one source is prolonged toxemia of pregnancy, a condition pro-duced by metabolic disturbances of the mother. Other sources of maternal intoxication are carbon monoxide, lead, and quinine. Kernicterus, a con-dition associated with a high level of bile pigment in the blood that may follow severe jaundice in the newborn child, is another example of in-toxication that can cause mental deficiency. The condition is frequently due to blood incompatibility, especially Rh incompatibility, between mother and fetus. Kernicterus can also be the result of prematurity or any con-dition producing a high level of bile pigment.

Trauma. Trauma to the brain during the birth process accounts for numerous cases of retardation. Lesions that are commonly produced by birth injuries include tears of the meninges (membranes that envelop the brain), blood vessels, and brain tissue. The degree of retardation is dependent upon the extent of injury.

Although not clearly established, there is some evidence to indicate that even when the brain produces no deficit in intellectual ability, trauma may result in psychologic disturbances that produce mental retardation. These disturbances may be evidenced in subtle disorganization and de-fects in performance in motor, sensory, perceptual, or emotional behavior. Children suffering from such disturbances may function at a lower intel-lectual level although they may possess average or better ability in specific areas of intelligence.

Although not common, mental retardation can develop if the mother is exposed during pregnancy to large amounts of irradiation, which causes organic disturbances of the brain. Prenatal anoxia (lack of oxygen) also causes injury to the brain that usually results in mental retardation.

Brain-injured children may be either hyperkinetic or hypokinetic, i.e., either extraordinarily active or lethargic. The greater number, however, are restless and engage excessively in motor activities. Difficulty with balance is usual and tends to manifest itself in general uncoordination of movements. Special difficulty is experienced in all balancing activities, such as walking a beam and standing on one foot. The perceptual process may also be impaired so that the child has difficulty in visualizing the difference between figures in the foreground and in the background. The brain-injured child often has problems in perceiving spoken and written words. Behavior often deviates considerably from normal due to the frustration and confusion engendered by the disability.

Disorders of Metabolism, Growth, or Nutrition. There are various metabolic disorders that cause mental retardation. Particularly prominent is dysfunction in metabolism of proteins, carbohydrates, and fats. Phenylketonuria (PKU) is a well known example of dysfunction of protein metabolism while hypoglycemoses and Tay-Sachs disease are common types of dysfunction of carbohydrate and fat metabolism, respectively.

Other disorders included in this group are Marfan's syndrome, a condition where there is a defect in connective tissue metabolism; Hurler's disease, which is characterized by deformed bones throughout the body; and hypothyroidism, which is caused by a deficiency of thyroid activity.

New Growths (Neoplasm). Within this group of causes of retardation are various tumors, nodules, and other growths in the cerebrum. Usually the conditions are hereditary. It is common with these conditions for other abnormal growths to be present in various parts of the body; discoloration of the skin in certain parts of the body is also common. Examples of neoplasm are Van Recklinghausen's disease, Sturge-Weber-Dimitri disease, and tuberous sclerosis.

Unknown Prenatal Influences. Included under the heading are all causes that are of unknown origin and evidence structural deviation at or prior to birth. It is assumed that these disorders are hereditary or familial in nature. Examples are absence or partial absence of the cerebrum, malformation of the cerebrum, craniostenosis (characterized by a steeple-shaped skull), and hydrocephalus (enlarged skull) that is not classified in other categories of causes.

Presumed Psychologic Causes. This group includes those cases of mental retardation for which there is no clinical or historic indication of organic disease or pathologic condition that could result in mental deficiency. The specific cause in these cases is generally assumed to be a factor within the inheritance of the individual, the influence of environment upon mental development, or both.

There is presently considerable controversy concerning the influence of inheritance and environment on the development of intelligence. It has been well-documented that either can, in some instances, be totally responsible for arrested mental development. The extent of their respective influences in other instances is debatable due to contradictory evidence supplied by researchers. There does appear to be support, however, for the conclusion that a deprived environment can hinder the development of intelligence as measured by standardized tests and that the level of intelligence can be raised by exposure to superior learning opportunities.[8] Future research will undoubtedly establish more clearly the degree of influence of inheritance and environment and the specific circumstances under which environment exerts a decisive influence.

Selecting or Setting the Environment

Public Law 94-142, the Education of Handicapped Children's Act of 1975, emphasizes that mentally retarded students must be educated in "the least restrictive environment". (Leisure education is included in the areas in which education is to be provided.) The least restrictive environment is interpreted to mean that setting which is most conducive to learning. The question often arises as to whether mainstreaming (integrating) in the regular recreational program or the separate recreational program is the least restrictive environment for the mentally retarded student. The key for the recreationist in answering the question is which provides the better leisure educational experience.

Many mentally retarded individuals can if given proper assistance benefit greatly from being mainstreamed in the recreational program. Attention must be paid to the child's response and the responses of others in the program to ensure that the child feels good about the program and enjoys the activities and that they are of recreational value to the individual. One of the greatest contributions mainstreaming can make is providing an opportunity for mentally retarded clients to learn to fit into the peer group. In addition, the nonretarded peers have the opportunity to gain a better understanding of those handicapped by mental limitations.

Programming Recreational Activities

The degree of retardation and the adaptive ability of the retarded individual exert an influence upon the kinds of recreational activities that are appropriate. Classifications of mental retardation based upon measured intelligence can be used as a guide only in planning the program generally. As with other disabled clients, such person's capability must be considered individually in selecting the activities.

Severely and Profoundly Retarded. Severely and profoundly retarded individuals are difficult to interest in any activity and, if they do become interested, it is only for brief periods. The ability to perform motor movement will vary from random, meaningless movements to simple skills such as walking and tossing and catching an object.

The possibilities of recreational activities for these individuals are limited. However, this does not mean that they cannot participate in some type of activity. Their recreational experiences must be closely supervised; and, for effective results, there should be one supervisor for each retardate. This ratio can usually be obtained only if there are numerous volunteers available.

The selection of activities should be made from those that are motor in nature since it is generally only in these activities that the severely and profoundly retarded are successful. Furthermore, since many of these clients are inactive, any opportunities for them to participate in muscular activity will be to their advantage. In encouraging them to perform motor activities the recreationist will need to utilize manual kinesthesis, a technique in which the individual is led through the desired movements. For example, in throwing, the recreationist helps the person to grasp the object to be thrown and then moves the arm through the desired movement. Use of verbal description to accompany action is desirable even though the client is nonverbal, for it is possible that he or she may learn to associate the words with the actions from hearing them repeatedly.

The following motor activities are appropriate for those who are severely and profoundly retarded: crawling on the hands and knees, on the belly, and on the knees only; rolling; walking up and down stairs; running; grasping objects with the hand; throwing; catching; balancing; jumping off objects; stepping over and into objects; bouncing; climbing; and kicking.

Moderately and Mildly Retarded. The moderately and mildly retarded clients have potential for learning to participate in a wide variety of recreational activities. One of the important responsibilities of the recrea-

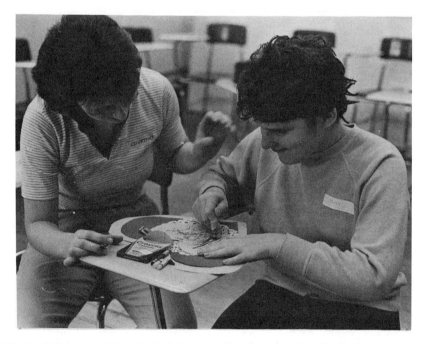

Fig. 8-1 Helping mentally retarded clients to develop recreational skills that they can pursue on their own is an important objective of the special recreational program.

tionist is to develop skills to enable them to seek or provide their own recreational activities when they are placed in the community.

In choosing the activities for the program, the recreationist must give consideration not only to the mental and physical disabilities, but to chronologic age level as well. Older children and adults, particularly the adolescents, resent being treated like children and are likely to reject simple activities that younger children engage in. However, generally these clients will not be able to participate in complex activities. The following guide is offered for selecting appropriate activities and presenting them to ensure acceptance of the activities and successful participation in them by the client:

- Reduce the activity to basic elements.
- Have several patients performing the same activity.
- Reduce choices that must be made to as few as possible.
- Select problem solving activities that have simple solutions or in which the solution to different problems is the same.
- Choose activities that have repetitive movements.
- Repeat activities frequently.
- Assure the participant that the quality of the performance brings no penalty.
- Maintain the same personnel in the activity.
- Limit complex motor skill requirements.
- Reduce the amount of information that needs to be memorized in order to participate.

Multiple Disabilities. Many handicapped persons are afflicted with two or more disabilities. It is not uncommon for a mentally retarded person to have epilepsy as well, or for the cerebral palsied individual to be blind also. The reason for the occurrence of multiple disabilities is that the factor that produces a disability in one part of the body often affects another part or parts of the body in a way that produces a handicapping condition.

In programming for those with several disabilities, the recreationist must consider how the combination of disabilities affects the total person. However, knowledge about each specific disability and the limitations it imposes can be utilized to formulate a number of recreational possibilities that the client can participate in successfully.

LEARNING DISABILITIES

Although a learning disability is defined by the federal government as a disorder of the psychologic process involving the use of the spoken or written word, there are other common characteristics that those with learning disabilities frequently exhibit. Tavar and Holahan have identified a number of such characteristics based upon the frequency of mention in the literature on learning disabilities;[9] of these, the following appear to have the most significance in recreational program planning: "(1) hypertension, (2) perceptual motor impairments, (3) emotional liability (moodiness, anxiety), (4) general coordination deficits, (5) disorders of attention (distractibility and perseveration), (6) impulsiveness, (7) disorders of memory and thinking."

Expectations are that due to the regulations of PL 94-142 recreationists will be working to an increasing extent with school personnel in providing recreational services for learning disabled students. As indicated in earlier discussions, if the assessment procedures identify deficiencies in a student's recreational skills and overcoming the deficiencies becomes an objective in the IEP, the recreationist should be involved. Therefore, it becomes important for the recreationist to have background knowledge about the nature of learning disabilities, especially the perceptual motor problems which influence performance of many recreational activities.

Perceptual-Motor Learning

Perceptual-motor is a term applied to the relationship between sensory perception and motor responses in the performance of movement. Perception is, of course, involved in all volitional movement. In preparation for moving, specific stimuli are generated by the sense modalities of the body. The modalities are identified as the eyes, ears, touch receptors, vestibular system (balance organs in the inner ear), and proprioceptors (sensory receptors located in muscles and joints). The stimuli from these sense modalities are relayed to specific parts of the brain, where interpretations are made about the nature of the movement. In consequence, muscular contraction is initiated or altered to achieve the required movement.

Most children experience no problem in the interpretation of the sensory input and in achieving the appropriate motor response. They are able through trial-and-error experimentation to achieve the appropriate motor match required by the perception. However, a large number of children do have difficulty making appropriate motor matches. Some of these are youngsters with learning disabilities; others experience no academic learning problems. Both types need specific assistance in interpreting sensory input and responding to it with the most suitable motor movement. Additionally, there are a substantial number of children who, while they do not experience severe perceptual problems, are sufficiently affected to be hampered in making successful motor responses. Such children may be benefited by work in perceptual-motor activities designed to improve interpretation of sensory input. The recreational program can offer a variety of interesting motor activities to promote the development of perceptual-motor learning for children with problems.

Perceptual-Motor Learning Problems and Activities

Inadequacies in perceptual-motor learning ability manifest themselves in the specific difficulties they create. These have been categorized as: (1) non-specific awkwardness or clumsiness, (2) problems of laterality and/or directionality, (3) lack of body awareness, (4) poorly developed kinesthesis and (5) inadequate visual and auditory perception.

Non-Specific Awkwardness. Motor awkwardness appears to be general in nature; however, upon closer examination the awkwardness is frequently limited to only specific movements. The awkwardness may, for example, appear in the skills of running or dodging but not in throwing or catching. Furthermore, there may be varying degrees of awkwardness in different movement patterns.

The first step that must be taken to assist clumsy children to improve their motor performance is to determine the movement skills that are awkward. To make such a determination, the child must be carefully observed performing various movement patterns. Having identified a specific skill, the teacher must isolate the components of that skill which contribute to the awkwardness.

After identification of the movement fault(s), components are selected for remedial work based on their importance to proper execution of the movement and the ease with which they can be improved. The child is taught how to perform each component properly and how to incorporate it into a well-coordinated performance.

Children who are slow in developing a well-coordinated movement will require many repetitions. To assist the child in more readily developing the "feel" of the correct movement, the recreationist encourages the child to concentrate on the way the movement feels when the body is being manually guided through correct performance of the skill. The manual guidance should first be applied slowly through several repetitions while the child gives full attention to the sensations of the movement. Then the speed of manipulation is gradually increased over several performances, with the child continuing concentration on the feeling, until the proper speed of the movement is reached.

In some cases it may be of value to the child to be shown the errors being made that result in awkward movement and the ways in which they should be changed to achieve successful movement. However, the emphasis should be on the way the correct movement is accomplished and how the correct movement feels when it is being made.

One of the more difficult problems for the awkward child in achieving effective skill performance is synchronizing the various components in coordinated total movement after the correction of errors in the components has been accomplished. This difficulty can be alleviated to some extent by having the client attempt to perform the total movement at intervals during practice on the components. Then when the components have been mastered, the total movement is performed repeatedly in gradually acclerated cadence.

Laterality and Directionality. Problems in laterality and directionality are common manifestations of perceptual-motor inadequacies. Laterality is defined as internal awareness of the two sides of the body, i.e., an understanding of which is the right and the left side of the body. Laterality is important to the ability to move the body in specified directions, so that a child with deficiencies in awareness of the right and left sides of his or her body experiences great difficulty in responding to directions that involve moving to his or her right or left.

Directionality is, like laterality, a function of body awareness; and the two terms are often used in conjunction. Directionality can be said to be the cognizance that objects and other people have their own left and right sides; it is, therefore, a determinate in the association of direction of movement that is made with such terms as up, down, over, and under. Lack of good directionality hinders a child in moving in the appropriate direction when instructed to make a movement involving the relationship of an object or person to the child.

The more opportunities a child has to develop awareness of which side of his or her own body and that of other people and of things is the left and the right, the greater is the possibility of overcoming problems of laterality and directionality.

Folk dancing is an example of a recreational activity involving laterality that can be presented so as to offer opportunities to work on identifying right and left. In response to the direction of movement called by the recreationist, children slide a foot along the floor. For practice in utilization of directionality, any activity is suitable that requires children to select an object and then respond by moving their body to the left or right, above or under the object.

Body Awareness. Body awareness, the ability to cognize the body in the space it occupies while at rest or in movement, is frequently poorly developed in children with perceptual-motor deficits. Inadequacy of body awareness is manifested by difficulties in the location and identification of body parts. Lack of body awareness is also indicated by an inability to move specific parts of the body in synchronization with the rest of the body as well as an inability to balance the body effectively.

It does not necessarily follow, however, that a child who cannot verbalize identification of his or her body parts and how they move is unable to conceptualize the different parts and their movements. This observation relates particularly to children who are mentally retarded or have a language disability. But with children who are able to communicate verbally with effectiveness, an inability to identify body parts and describe body movements does suggest the presence of body awareness problems.

Activities that give children experience in identification of body parts and in becoming aware of the body's movements are readily provided in recreational education. Popular, familiar games like Simon Says can be adapted to offer the desired experience as, in this case, having all the actions that Simon says to do consist of touching parts of the body. Or while observing their reflections in a mirror, children move various parts of the body. They identify for the recreationist the movement and the parts of the body executing the movement, for example, "My hand is moving over the top of my head."

Balancing. Inadequately developed body awareness, as pointed out above, affects the ability to balance the body. Because poor balance is so detrimental to success in the daily routines and play of childhood and because physical recreational activities can make such an important contribution to alleviating balance problems, the subject will be discussed in some detail.

To be able to balance in any of a variety of possible positions, the child must be able to utilize stimuli originating from the sense modalities and translate the input into motor action that will maintain the balance of the body in the desired position. The sense modalities contributing to achieve-

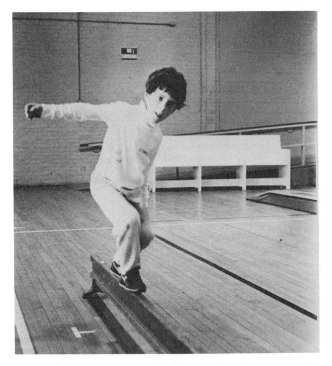

Fig. 8-2 Balancing activities need to be included in the school recreational program for the learning disabled child who is deficient in body awareness.

ment and maintenance of balance are the eyes, vestibular system, proprioceptors, and the nerve endings that provide the sense of touch and pressure. The eyes provide input about the adjustments of body parts required to maintain equilibrium. Information about the movement of muscles and joints is provided by the proprioceptors. The inner ear, which includes the vestibular system, supplies information concerning the movements of the head and gives indication of how the head is held in relationship to the force of gravity. Information concerning how the body contacts the surface it is balancing on is provided by the touch receptors.

In addition to the contributions of the balance modalities, muscle coordination is important in maintaining balance in any position. Therefore, the ability to balance the body depends upon the proper interpretation of the input from the balance modalities and coordination of the muscles to maintain the body in a position of equilibrium.

Learning to Balance. Moving the muscles appropriately to maintain a balance in any given position, is in part a "specific" skill, i.e., the learning acquired to coordinate the muscles to achieve successful performance in one position of balance does not necessarily aid to any great extent the learning of a different balance activity. On the other hand, there is some evidence to indicate that improvement in perception of balance does aid in maintaining balance in various positions. A case in point: If perception of input from the vestibular system is improved, all balance skills that involve the system are more easily learned. If a deficiency exists in the perception of stimuli from the balance modalities, all balancing skills are difficult to learn. If the perceptions are improved, balancing is more readily learned. However, because of the important role muscle coordination plays in balancing, the learning of one balance skill does not necessarily improve all balancing ability.

Principles of Balance. In teaching children to balance in various positions, development of an understanding of the principles of balance is of the utmost importance. Knowledge of and the use of the principles given below help children solve many of their balance problems:

- Lowering the center of gravity improves stability;

- Increasing the size or width of the base of support enables greater stability to be achieved;

- Placing the center of gravity over the base creates greater stability.

The principles can be established through demonstration by the recreationist and experimentation by the students in applying them in various balancing positions. For very young children, simplification of the principles and their application will be necessary.

Utilization of all Balance Modalities. Children who have difficulty learning to balance need to be encouraged to utilize all of the balance modalities. For example, balance will be more easily maintained if the eyes are focused on a spot at about eye level in the distance rather than on the feet. Also, removal of the shoes allows the sense of touch in the feet to provide more useful information on the contact of the feet with the base.

When it is known that a child has a deficiency is one of the balance modalities, such as poor vision or vestibular system damage due to meningitis, the recreationist should encourage the child to rely more heavily upon the other modalities. To do this with a child with either of the two kinds of deficiencies just cited, the following activity is suggested: The child is aided to take a balancing position, such as standing on a narrow balance beam, and held in place. Instructions are given the child to concentrate on the way the body feels as balance is lost and then on the movements that must be made to regain balance. Slowly the support is withdrawn while the child concentrates on the sensation of losing balance and experiments to determine which muscles must be contracted to return the body to a position of balance. The recreationist remains close at hand to supply support if needed.

Repetitions of this activity will strengthen reliance on the unimpaired modalities to achieve effective balance. Success in doing so will encourage the child to make use of these modalities in other situations requiring balance of the body.

The possibilities for activities that promote learning to balance are nearly limitless. The simple balancing activities described below serve as examples of the opportunities that can be offered.

- Children stand on one leg, then move the raised leg to various positions, eventually accompanies by movements of one or both arms.
- Placing one foot directly in front of the other, children walk along a stripe of several inches width painted on the floor.
- Children balance a book or like object on the head while walking across the floor. Later they perform the activity on a balance beam.

Kinesthesis. Kinesthesis is another form of perceiving the relationship of the body's parts and the orientation of the body in space. Kinesthesis is chiefly dependent upon the proprioceptors, which supply information to the central nervous system from the muscles and joints. As a result, the individual is made aware of the position of the parts of the body, their relationship to one another, and the force and extent of muscular contraction, among other important information essential to effective movement. When kinesthesis is not fully developed, problems arise in such activities as moving through a small space and positioning the tennis racquet to make contact with the ball because no "feel" for the proper performance of the skill is present.

A child who has difficulty performing motor activities, but shows no evidence of deficits or damage in the other sense modalities, may reasonably be considered to have poorly functioning proprioceptors. Such a child may be helped to improve the "service" of the proprioceptors by offering recreational activities that increase reliance on the modality. One possibility is an activity in which children make drawings on paper while holding their eyes closed.

Visual Perception. Visual perception is the interpretation of the nerve impulses provided to the brain by the eyes. It involves at least four components: visual discrimination, figure-ground discrimination, depth perception, and object consistency. All play a role in the learning of motor skills.

Visual Discrimination. Visual discrimination is involved with determining the size, shape, color and texture of an object. The first four named characteristics are used fairly early by children in identifying objects. Texture becomes an aid in visual discrimination somewhat later. In many cases the quality of discrimination varies in each area, i.e., the child may have a high level of ability in discriminating size but not in shape. On the other hand, the ability to discriminate in all areas may be nearly equal with the child possessing a high, average, or low level of discrimination in each area.

Children who have deficiencies in visual discrimination are not usually successful in recreational activities. There are few activities that do not require some degree of ability to discriminate in size, form, color, and texture. Since these children are unable to make the distinctions, they make faulty choices and inappropriate decisions that produce failure. Recreational opportunities can be created for children to work with objects of different sizes, colors, forms, and textures. When the activity also requires differences to be identified, additional opportunities are created to enhance discrimination.

Figure-Ground Perception. Figure-ground perception is the ability to differentiate a specific object from its background. The ability develops slowly throughout childhood, reaching maturation in adolescence. The ability to identify and focus attention upon a single object or figure in a cluttered or complex background, such as identifying and locating the "it" in a game of tag relies upon figure-ground perception. Following the path of a ball in the air is another illustration of the utilization of figure-ground perception.

Activities can be designed for presentation in the recreational program to help children strengthen their figure-ground perception. Three examples are given below:

- Children closely watch a brightly colored ball suspended in front of a distracting background in order to catch it.

- Children roll balls along the floor in an attempt to place them between objects located a short distance away.

- Children play tag in a small space that facilitates focusing attention on the one being chased.

Depth Perception. Depth perception is the ability to judge accurately distances between objects or points and to perceive the three dimensions in proper perspective. Underdevelopment of depth perception, while having limited effect upon the development of academic skills, has a profound effect upon the development and performance of motor skills. For example, in catching a ball it is imperative that the distance between the ball and the hands be judged accurately so that the hands do not over or under reach. Dodging objects or another player while running is another example of the use of depth perception in motor activities.

In developing depth perception the child should be provided various experiences that offer an opportunity to utilize modalities other than sight alone to determine the dimensions of an object or the distance of one object in front of the other. For example, a child may be asked to verify his or her interpretation of a cube by feeling it to determine which surface of the cube is closer to him or her, which surface slants away from him or her, etc. Use of a ruler or tape measure to help establish which object is closer or farther away offers another kind of experience.

Object Consistency. This term refers to the ability to identify an object from any direction that it is viewed. Such ability permits objects in the environment to be recognized even though viewed from a different side from that in which they were originally identified. For example, the child recognizes a set of swings when viewed from the side as well as the front, the direction from which identity of the swing was first learned.

A deficit in object consistency obviously causes many problems in school and out. Even a small degree of deficit puts the child at a disadvantage in such recreational activities as using free form play equipment and playing with such items as bean bags that consistently change their shape.

In developing the perception of object consistency the child needs to have experiences in viewing an object from different viewpoints and then determining the features of the object that give clues to its nature when viewing it from different angles. Most children will learn readily how to identify a simply formed object, even though they have not been conscious of how it looks from all angles. For instance, it is easy for most children to identify a softball bat or a climbing ladder.

Auditory Perception. Auditory perception, the interpretation of sound, includes various factors: discrimination of different pitches, intensities, and tonal qualities; figure-ground discrimination, directionality of sounds; and temporal or rhythmic reception. It is difficult to differentiate between difficulties in auditory perception and disturbance in the hearing apparatus. Only after a complete hearing examination and medical and educational analyses are made can a determination of cause be made.

As with visual perception, auditory perception is usually self-learned at an early age. However, for some children special instruction is required to provide experiences in the specific factors of auditory perception where deficits exist.

The recreationist has a unique opportunity to assist in the development of auditory perception through rhythmic activities. Different pitches, intensities, and tonal qualities of sound can be used with movement by the skilled recreationist. Even without extensive training in dance, the recreationist can help students to develop rhythm and appropriate tempo in movement.

All movement patterns require rhythm in the execution as well as the monitoring of tempo. Participation in movement patterns encourages this development. In addition activities focusing on rhythm and tempo may be developed; for example, marching to cadence, skipping to music, clapping in time to a swinging ball suspended from the ceiling.

Overall Motor Performance. A number of activities have been suggested for development of perception in specific modalities to enhance motor performance. It is important to recognize that, in general, there is limited transfer of learning from one kind of perceptual motor skill to another kind. For example, learning to adjust the hand properly in catching balls of different sizes has limited influence on the ability to learn to dance or walk in rhythm to a cadence. Therefore, to help children develop "perceptual-motor skills" the recreational program must offer a wide variety of activities that provides a myriad of experiences in utilizing the various sense modalities. In this way the child builds up a large repertoire of movement patterns to draw upon when meeting new challenges in motor performance, ensuring greater success and enjoyment of recreational activities.

REFERENCES

1. Herbert J. Grossman, ed., *Manual on Terminology and Classification in Mental Retardation,* 1977 revision (Washington, D.C., American Association on Mental Deficiency, 1977) p. 5.
2. Federal Register, *op. cit.,* p. 42478.
3. Herbert Grossman, ed., *op. cit.,* p. 5.
4. C. Spearman, *The Abilities of Man* (New York: The Macmillian Co., 1927) *passim.*
5. Edward L. Thorndike et al., *The Measurement of Intelligence* (New York: Bureau of Publications, Teachers College, Columbia University, 1926) *passim.*
6. Max L. Hutt and Robert G. Gibby, *The Mentally Retarded Child—Development Education and Treatment,* 4th ed. (Boston: Allyn and Bacon, Inc., 1979) p. 20.
7. Edger A. Doll, *Measurement of Social Competence* (Circle Pines, Minnesota: American Guidance Service, Inc., 1953) p. 16.
8. Glen Van Etton, et al., *The Severely and Profoundly Handicapped Programs, Methods, and Materials* (St. Louis: C. V. Mosby Co., 1980) p. 62.
9. S. Traver and D. P. Hallahan, "Children With Learning Disabilities: An Overview" in J. M. Kauffman and D. P. Hallahan, eds., *Teaching Children With Learning Disabilities: Personal Perspectives* (Columbus, Ohio: Charles E. Merrill Publishing Co., 1976) p. 18.

SELECTED REFERENCES

AAHPER, *Physical and Recreational Programming for Severely and Profoundly Mentally Retarded Individuals* (Washington, D.C.: American Alliance for Health, Physical Education and Recreation, 1974).

Arnheim, Daniel D. and Sinclair, William A., *The Clumsy Child,* 2nd ed. (St. Louis: C. V. Mosby Co., 1979).

Cratty, Bryant J., *Perceptual and Motor Development in Infants and Children,* 2nd ed. (Englewood Cliffs, New Jersey: Prentice-Hall, Inc., 1979).

Grossman, Herbert J., *Manual on Terminology and Classification in Mental Retardation* (Washington, D.C.: American Association on Mental Deficiency, 1977).

Lerch, Harold, et al., *Perceptual-Motor Learning—Theory and Practice* (Palo Alto, California: Peek Publications, 1974).

Moran, Joan and Kalakian, Leonard, *Movement Experiences for Mentally Retarded or Emotionally Disturbed Children,* 2nd ed. (Minneapolis: Burgess Publishing Co., 1977).

Wallace, G. and McLoughlin, J. A., *Learning Disabilities: Concepts and Characteristics,* 2nd ed. (Columbus, Ohio: Charles E. Merrill Publishing Co., 1979).

Wehman, Paul, *Helping the Mentally Retarded Acquire Play Skills* (Springfield: Charles C Thomas, 1977).

Chapter 9

Mental Disturbances

Mental disturbance is any emotional response of sufficient severity to cause maladjustment or inability to function in a socially acceptable manner. The condition is often referred to as mental illness. Treatment of mental disturbances occurs largely in hospitals and institutions, so therapeutic recreationists will be involved to a far greater extent than the community adapted recreationists with those who are mentally disturbed.

Knowledge about mental disturbances enables the therapeutic recreationist to obtain and provide valid information about the patient that might otherwise be obscured or ignored. As a result, the patient receives more precise service and, consequently, should recover and/or be rehabilitated more quickly. Only if the therapeutic recreationist is capable of exchanging worthwhile and meaningful information about the patient will medical personnel begin to rely upon the recreationist as a knowledgeable member of the rehabilitation team. Of necessity, then, the recreationist will have to understand basic medical psychologic procedures, as well as the origin and course of a variety of disorders, and their residual effects. In this way, the recreationist will be more competent to deal with patient needs, will understand the dysfunctions which occur as a consequence of mental illness, and will be in a better position to arrange a therapeutic recreational regimen as one aspect of the treatment or rehabilitation program.

With better orientation to client problems and the ability to provide pertinent information which can be of therapeutic use to all members of the rehabilitation team, the recreationist may well become a primary adjunct in the fight to provide optimum care during a client's institutionalization as well as after re-integration in the community.

CLASSIFICATION IN PSYCHIATRY

Classification is the means by which complex phenomena may be more easily understood by organizing them into groups according to some recognized standard. The classification of mental disorders consists of groups of particular mental illnesses categorized on the basis of some common characteristics. The official classification system as outlined in the American Psychiatric Association's "Diagnostic and Statistical Manual of Mental Diseases" (DSM) [1] attempts to make an inclusive identification of the clinical features of the mental disorders. The DSM listing, given in Table 9-1, is used here to show the range and extent of mental disorders. However, the specific psychologic disturbances are limited to the common manifestations of mental illness typically observed within treatment centers where therapeutic recreationists are employed.

Disorders and Subgroupings

The official diagnostic manual of the American Psychiatric Association as developed in Table 9-1, lists key groups of disorders and a variety of subgroupings. For purposes of clarity only a brief description is offered below to assist in understanding these diagnostic categories.

TABLE 9-1. CLASSIFICATION OF MENTAL DISTURBANCES

I. Disorders Usually First Evident in Infancy, Childhood or Adolescence
  (a) Mental retardation
  (b) Attention deficit disorder
  (c) Conduct disorder
  (d) Anxiety disorders of childhood or adolescence
  (e) Other disorders of infancy, childhood or adolescence
      1. Reactive attachment disorder of infancy
      2. Schizoid disorder of childhood or adolescence
      3. Elective mutism
      4. Oppositional disorder
      5. Identity disorder
  (f) Eating disorders
      1. Anorexia nervosa
      2. Bulimia
      3. Pica
      4. Rumination disorder of infancy
      5. Atypical eating disorder
  (g) Stereotyped movement disorders
  (h) Other disorders with physical manifestations
      1. Stuttering
      2. Functional enuresis
      3. Functional encopresis
      4. Sleepwalking disorder
      5. Sleep terror disorder
  (i) Pervasive developmental disorders
II. Organic Mental Disorders
  (a) Senile and presenile dementias
  (b) Substance-induced
      1. Alcohol
      2. Barbiturate or similarly acting sedative or hypnotic
      3. Opium, opium alkaloids and their derivatives
      4. Cocaine
      5. Amphetamine or similarly acting sympathomimetic
      6. Phencyclidine (PCP) or similarly acting arylcyclohexylamine
      7. Hallucinogen
      8. Cannabis
      9. Tobacco
      10. Caffeine
      11. Other or unspecified substance

III. Schizophrenic Disorders
   (a) Disorganized
   (b) Catatonic
   (c) Paranoid
   (d) Undifferentiated
   (e) Residual
IV. Paranoid Disorders
   (a) Paranoia
   (b) Shared paranoid disorder
   (c) Acute paranoid disorder
   (d) Atypical paranoid disorder
V. Psychotic Disorders Not Elsewhere Classified
   (a) Schizophreniform disorder
   (b) Brief reactive psychosis
   (c) Schizoaffective disorders
   (d) Atypical psychosis
VI. Neurotic Disorders
   (a) Affective disorders
       1. Mixed
       2. Manic
       3. Depressed
       4. Single episode
       5. Recurrent
   (b) Other specific affective disorders
       1. Cyclothymic disorder
       2. Dysthymic disorder or depressive neurosis
   (c) Atypical effective disorders
       1. Atypical bipolar disorder
       2. Atypical depression
   (d) Anxiety Disorders
       1. Phobic disorders or phobic neuroses
   (e) Somatoform Disorders
       1. Somatization disorder
       2. Conversion disorder or hysterical neurosis, conversion type
       3. Psychogenic pain disorder
       4. Hypochondriasis or hypochondriacal neurosis
       5. Atypical somatoform disorder
   (f) Dissociative Disorders or Hysterical Neuroses, Dissociative Type
       1. Psychogenic amnesia
       2. Psychogenic fugue
       3. Multiple personality
       4. Depersonalization disorder or depersonalization neurosis
       5. Atypical dissociative disorder
   (g) Psychosexual Disorders
       1. Gender identity disorders
          a) Transsexualism
          b) Gender identity disorder of childhood
          c) Atypical gender identity disorder
       2. Paraphilias
          a) Fetishism
          b) Transvestism
          c) Zoophilia
          d) Pedophilia
          e) Exhibitionism
          f) Voyeurism
          g) Sexual masochism
          h) Sexual sadism
          i) Sexual paraphilia
       3. Psychosexual dysfunctions
          a) Inhibited sexual desire

        b) Inhibited sexual excitement
        c) Inhibited female orgasm
        d) Inhibited male orgasm
        e) Premature ejaculation
        f) Functional dyspareunia
        g) Functional vaginismus
        h) Atypical psychosexual dysfunction
    4. Other psychosexual disorder
        a) Ego-dystonic homosexuality
        b) Psychosexual disorder not elsewhere classified
VII. Factitious Disorders
IX. Disorders of Impulse Control Not Elsewhere Classified
    (a) Pathologic gambling
    (b) Kleptomania
    (c) Pyromania
    (d) Intermittent explosive disorder
    (e) Isolated explosive disorder
    (f) Atypical impulse control disorder
X. Adjustment Disorder
    (a) Depressed mood
    (b) Anxious mood
    (c) Mixed emotional features
    (d) Disturbance of conduct
    (e) Mixed disturbance of emotion and conduct
    (f) Work (or academic) inhibition
    (g) Withdrawal
    (h) Atypical features
XI. Psychologic Factors Affecting Physical Condition
XII. Personality Disorders
    (a) Paranoid

1. Disorders of Infancy, Childhood or Adolescence. These disorders usually manifest themselves in early childhood and might properly be considered by clinicians when diagnosing adults. There are five minor classes of disorders associated with such disturbances: (1) intellectual (mental retardation); (2) behavioral (attention deficit disorder, conduct disorder); (3) emotional (anxiety disorders); (4) physical (eating disorders, stereotyped movement disorders, other disorders with physical manifestations); and (5) developmental (pervasive developmental disorders, specific developmental disorders).

2. Organic Mental Disorders. These disturbances are the result of psychologic or behavior disorganization that is the result of temporary or permanent dysfunction of the brain. Characteristic of the disorders are various intellectual impairments, personality distortions, and abnormal emotional responses.

3. Substance Use Disorders. Disorders which occur because of ingestion of substances affecting the central nervous system fall in this category. Behavioral changes are noted in the individual's inability to function in a social or occupational situation, and with a pathologic pattern of use.

4. Schizophrenic Disorders. Schizophrenia includes a group of psychotic reactions in which there are essential disturbances in reality relationships, and in emotional and intellectual processes. Although there are an infinite number of particular symptoms and patients show various signs, there are certain commonalities which can be observed in all schizophrenics. There is quite observable apathy or complete indifference to the normal course of human events as well as a disassociation of thought from its normal affect.

This disorder is of insidious development. Frequently the earliest signs are not at all clear and represent a considerable difference from their appearance during the later stages of the disease. The early clinical feature is chiefly that of neurotic symptoms. At a more developed stage, the significant symptoms generally include a gradual withdrawal from reality, emotional blunting and warping, disintegration and splitting of thought processes, in combination with grotesque delusions and hallucinations. In addition, various stereotyped behavior patterns, a distinct deterioration of personal habits related to personal appearance and hygiene, and the lack of moral controls are also encountered.

5. Paranoid Disorders. Paranoid reactions are systematized delusions that have no association with personality deterioration. Paranoia may be of the type that focuses on delusions of grandeur or persecution. Another form manifests itself through hallucinations but lacks the usual systematization. Paranoid disorders are infrequently seen within hospital populations because individuals afflicted with this disturbance are sufficiently in control to avoid hospitalization. It is only when their behavior becomes a threat to public tranquility that paranoids are noticed and segregated for treatment.

Paranoid reactions are the gross exaggerations of suspicions that all people have about their bad luck or their unfortunate life situation which places them in inferior positions and permits them to be dominated by others. The paranoid starts with this theme and makes an extreme case out of it. Thus such individuals feel that they alone are being singled out for punishment and ridicule, plotted against, or otherwise maltreated by known and unknown enemies and even by all of society. The nature of the delusion is such that it centers around a particular idea, such as vocation, marital life, religion, or similar theme on which the individual fixes.

Although ideas of persecution predominate in paranoid reactions, many paranoiacs develop delusions of grandeur in which they endow themselves with magnificent qualities, outstanding abilities, or messianic exaltations.

6. Affective Disorders. The disorders of affect consist of a prominent trait which is displayed as a conspicuous alteration of mood, usually either in the direction of depression or euphoria. The profoundly depressed person sees the world pessimistically and is absolutely convinced that everybody, including himself, is, in the Augustinian sense, "depraved" or evil. The disturbed individual who tends toward elation is unnaturally optimistic and views the world as completely free of trouble; is singularly joyful; and anticipates nothing but exuberant experiences. In such disorders, disturbances of thought and action are also present, but they are of secondary concern and are directly related to the prevailing mood or affect.[2]

Attempts to categorize affective disorders have had a long history. It was Kraepelin, in 1899, who coined the term manic-depressive psychosis. The suggestion of such a term is that mania and depression form a single entity, i.e., together they form a pathologic process that is one of fluctuations between extreme degrees of elation and depression.

The manic phase is characterized by incessant and furious excitement. The individual verbalizes constantly, exhibits bizarre behavior, and during the episode is likely to experience vivid hallucinations. The depressive phase is manifested by a mood of dejection, insomnia, and somatic (body) preoccupation.

7. Somatoform Disorders. In this category is grouped all of the disorders involving physical symptoms implying problems for which no organic basis can be sufficiently demonstrated to explain the symptom. In fact, direct evidence, or at least a strong premise, suggests that the symptoms are connected to psychologic factors or conflicts. Among the disturbances in this group is somatization disorder, a chronic disorder with multiple symptoms that starts in early life. Another problem included in this category is psychogenic pain disorder for which there is no attributable physical or mental origin. Hypochondriasis, or preoccupation with the belief that one has a serious disease, is still another somatoform disorder.

8. Dissociative Disorders. The outstanding characteristic of these disorders is an abrupt, temporary change in the normally integrated functions of consciousness, identity, or motor behavior. This category includes psychogenic amnesia (orientation disorder), psychogenic fugue (flight from reality and identity), multiple personality, and depersonalization disorder.

Loss or diminishment of memory may result from emotional disturbance as well as from some precipitating incident such as trauma. Thus psychogenic amnesia might occur after a wretching emotional shock or accident, particularly if cranial injury were sustained by the individual. Frequently, such memory loss is also accompanied by the inability to clearly identify situation, people, and time; it is compounded by a general state of confusion. In some instances, the confused individual not only is disoriented but may also tell completely fabricated experiences, honestly believing them to have occurred. Amnesia, together with physical flight from known surroundings, is termed a fugue state. Here the individual roams from accustomed haunts and may take up an entirely new life. This psychoneurotic reaction may be terminated quite suddenly days, weeks, months, or years later with the individual being unable to recall anything after the event that caused the shock: there is total amnesia from the onset of the fugue.

Depersonalization occurs when the individual feels that personal identity has been lost and may be hard pressed to identify others who are well known.

9. Psychosexual Disorders. The essential feature of these disorders is the individual's feelings of discomfort and inappropriateness about his or her anatomic sex. Hence, the person engages in behavior generally attributed to the other sex and in a variety of other aberrant patterns with regard to sexual objects.

10. Factitious Disorders. In disturbances of this type, physical or psychologic symptoms are produced voluntarily by the individual with the sole objective of becoming a patient. The client's control over his or her symptomatology is determined by eliminating all other causes for the behavior.

11. Impulse Control Disorders. A disorder of impulse control features behavior that causes harm to the person or others. Tension is heightened prior to the act and there are feelings of intense gratification during the performance of the act. Kleptomania and pyromania are two examples of such behavior.

12. Adjustment Disorders. These disorders are maladaptive responses of excessive stress to common experiences. One consequence may be depression of mood.

13. Personality Disorders. This classification includes basic characteristics which are deeply imbedded, inflexible, and maladaptive with respect to perception of and thought about oneself and the environment. These disorders are of such severity as to cause considerable inability to adapt to distress. The sensation of having seen something prior to actual experience is frequently observed in the disturbed personality. Both visual and auditory *déjà vu* is a common experience.

Symptoms and Syndromes

The whole approach to categorization and classification of abnormality has been open to question because of the tendency to place a patient exhibiting some of the symptoms in a diagnostic niche. It is now appreciated that a combination of diagnostic classification and dynamic appreciation of individuality is necessary if the best in client care is to be rendered. Symptoms of several different disorders and syndromes may be present simultaneously. Currently, diagnosis is seen, not as a static label rejecting all other chronic syndromes, but as a statement about the pattern of symptoms at a specific time.

In this connection, it should be pointed out that symptoms are not syndromes. A syndrome is a cluster of symptoms, often observed, and may overlap several categories. All living human beings react holistically, i.e., in totality. One cannot artificially reduce such patterns of symptoms into particular categories except to make them more susceptible to examination. Furthermore, one symptom may appear in several completely different psychologic disturbances. The symptom, in and of itself, may be almost inconsequential, unless it is taken together with other factors comprising a syndrome.

DIAGNOSIS

The single essential reason for diagnosis is the selection of the optimum applicable treatment pattern. With the advent of newer techniques, including chemotherapy and other therapeutic methods, it has become more important than ever to identify, adopt, and employ the appropriate regimen for each syndrome. Precise diagnoses of patient's syndromes may not be forthcoming due to differences of diagnostic technique, individual variables of behavior, and differences of symptom evaluation or interpretation. Despite the imprecision of diagnostic technique, it is still necessary to attempt to identify abnormality so that treatment of the mental disturbance can occur.

The same argument which is presented against categorization of illnesses and disabilities, i.e., that one cannot really categorize because all individuals are unique and have specific needs which are peculiarly their own, also applies to the issue of diagnostic approaches to mental illness. Thus, there is a desire on the part of those who view diagnostic classification as meaningless to seek other means for establishing treatment programs. Those who oppose diagnosis often emphasize the significance of a psychodynamic rather than a preconceived approach to the patient. It is urged, therefore, that patients should not be labeled by syndrome, but should be understood as unique individuals with distinct experiences, patterns, behavioral conflicts, anxieties, and potential goals. Recognition of the patient as an individual is thought to be diametrically opposed to classification.

We do not accept the purported inimicality between the two orientations, rather we accept a median view that accommodates both aspects. No real contradiction exists between the two concepts. A patient has certain behaviors common to a diagnostic category and has, as well, those unique and peculiar features which characterize him or her as an individual. One orientation forms the basis for prescriptive analysis and the other reinforces the patient as an individual.

ATTITUDES TOWARD MENTAL DISTURBANCES

Of all the diseases with which humans have to cope, those which are classified as psychiatric seem to arouse the greatest fear. Of course, people have great anxiety about physical diseases for which there is no cure and which lead to agonizing death. But for most people, the thought of mental illness produces a fearfulness that is not difficult to understand although it is hard to explain. Mental disturbances do not appear to have any physical symptoms, at least none that the layman can readily recognize. Afflicted individuals simply behave in a manner that is totally at odds with the environment and sometimes act so bizarrely as to become a threat to themselves or others. It is this inability to anticipate the responses of victims of psychotic episodes that may account for the palpable fear that occurs when the average person is exposed to mental disturbance.

Of course, the entertainment industry has spawned and reinforces stereotypes of the mentally ill. The classic Hollywood melodrama invariably depicts the "psychopathic" killer as either an ice-cold expressionless and remorseless monster or as a wild-eyed raging "maniac" destroying everything in its path and striking out in all directions. If people see enough of this nonsense, they begin to believe it.

People's attitudes toward mental disturbance is also formed by the lack of physical manifestation; if some organic deficiency or obvious disease effect was evident, the condition could be more easily accepted as an actual disease. For most laymen, mental illness is a fearsome problem that appears to strike from nowhere and is indiscriminate in its victims.

As more is being learned about neuroscience, however, a different attitude and approach are being shaped by professionals who deal with every aspect of mental disturbance. Attitudinal changes have demonstrated remarkable shifts from an earlier time, when the mentally ill, the "lunatics," were thought to be affected by moonlight and needed to be mechanically restrained, beaten, or otherwise traumatized in order to drive out whatever demons possessed them, to the real beginnings of modern-day psychotherapy based on the pioneering work of Sigmund Freud.

Changes in Medical Practices

In the twenty-five years between 1930 and 1955, the use of insulin and electroconvulsive therapy reached a peak in the treatment of some emotional problems as did prefrontal lobotomies, in which surgery was performed on a portion of the brain to alter the individual's personal or behavioral patterns. Although electroconvulsive therapy is still used, there is a greater reliance upon drug treatment, known as chemotherapy. Among clinical psychologists there are those who espouse the concept that mental illness is environmentally stimulated and that stress or pressure may lead to chemical changes which produce deviant behaviors in an attempt to adjust to whatever problems precipitated the stress. Accordingly, some psychiatrists are convinced that the introduction of chemicals (drugs, medication) will correct the imbalance thereby enabling patients to profit from other treatments that can eventuate in their return to community living.

Drug Therapy. Another concept, resulting from recent advances in brain research, holds that mental functions can be defined in terms of activities of the brain at the cellular level. Many disorders formerly regarded as purely psychologic are now being viewed as a consequence of organic brain tissue disorder in terms of synaptic response or sensitivity. As current research clarifies the role of neurotransmitters (chemicals in the brain that transmit impulses) in mental illness, such understanding may lead to the development of drugs that surpass anything now available in specifically treating chemical abnormalities associated with brain disorders; the increased precision will permit greater potency with fewer side effects. Neuroscience is on the threshold of producing drugs that can alleviate many problems once thought to originate from warped psyches, but which are actually caused by imbalances in brain chemistry.[3]

There are, however, a number of psychiatrists who are concerned with the use of drugs in mental illness. Particularly is this true of those psychiatrists who believe that psychotic disorders are caused more by experiences than by faulty brain chemistry. In fact, they are afraid that many drugs used to treat psychotic disorders cause "chemical lobotomy." Many of these drugs are brain-disabling agents and they are widely misused to control people in mental hospitals, prisons, homes for delinquent children, and nursing homes. Another pressing concern is the possibility of severe side effects from such drugs. For example, one of psychiatry's most distressing problems is tardive dyskinesia, a condition characterized by uncontrollable slow writhing that sometimes accompanies long-term use of widely prescribed anti-psychotic drugs.

In answering such charges, psychiatrists who favor drug use admit that psychiatric drugs may be misapplied. Nevertheless, for many disorders there is no other effective treatment. An example may be severe depression. Severe depression afflicts approximately eight million persons in the United States at any given time, and is described by many patients as being the worst of all pain, far more devastating than any they have ever known. In fact, the death rate from the disorder, frequently due to suicide, was once nearly as high as for heart-attack victims. That death rate plummeted when electroshock and drug therapies were developed to treat the disorder.

Schizophrenia, a disease accompanied by delusions, incoherent thoughts, paranoia, and emotional disturbances, is tremendously benefited by drugs specifically designed for its treatment. Similar far-reaching effects on the treatment of other types of mental illness can be expected as the public becomes more accepting of the therapeutic value of psychiatric drugs. With continual advances in neuroscience, there is a greater realization that many psychologic disorders are biochemical problems. The general public will come to recognize that it is proper to take a drug to treat mental illness in the same way that it is appropriate to treat high blood pressure or other physical problems with drugs.

Mainstreaming Psychiatric Patients. Among the changing attitudes within the field of psychiatric care has been the shift of treatment from impersonalized institutionalization to that of the community, in effect, mainstreaming psychiatric patients as quickly as practicable. This attitude has been fostered by the acceptance of the social origins of mental illness and takes its cue from the need to understand the socio-cultural environment of each patient. The approach considers mentall illness in such broad terms as to include sociopathic or deviant behavior, substance abuse, and mental retardation.

When it works, community-based psychiatric service is delivered through decentralized mental health facilities that offer day treatment programs, crisis intervention, after care follow-up, and, where necessary, the use of drugs for maintenance purposes. The primary function of these services is to prevent the institutionalization of clients or to assure the rapid rehabilitation of clients back into the community setting. Great support is given by a number of occupational, family, religious, and recreational organizations operating within the community. Through the use of such groups, it is rationalized, the deterioration in consequence of social isolation and refusal of treatment that may often take place when the individual is hospitalized can be reduced to negligible proportions. At least as important to the kind of treatment received by disturbed individuals is the education of the public to the reality of mental illness and the need to modify long held stereotypes about the mentally ill.

TREATMENT METHODS

The methods of treating mental disturbances at a particular treatment center depend upon the basic philosophic premise of treatment accepted by those in charge of the treatment. Consequently, the emphasis may be on psychologic support, medication, group and individual approaches, or a combination of two or more of these.

In the past treatment of mentally disturbed patients relied heavily on psychologic support utilizing the method known as psychoanalysis. Now, however, this form of treatment if used at all is given as part of a combination of treatments.

Currently the major method of treatment is chemotherapy or the use of drugs. However, it is frequently used with psychoanalysis or behavior therapy. Chemotherapy has proven an effective treatment to control psychotic episodes or to reduce relapse through maintenance medication. Through its use patients can be helped to reach a stabilized level of behavior where they are capable of functioning in an acceptable manner outside of the treatment center.

Antipsychotic drugs are often indicated for the patient's acute psychotic condition. Among the major tranquilizing drugs are chlorpromazine, thioridazine, trifluoperazine, fluphenazine, or haloperidol. Of course there are other drugs which are utilized depending upon the psychologic state of the individual. Some drugs may be anti-depressants (euphorics). Physicians prescribing such drugs will take into account the patient's previous reaction to medication, if any, and physical condition. Of extreme importance is the necessity to watch for any negative side effects that might occur. For this reason, the physician will prescribe a small test dose and if no major harmful side effects develop, the dose can be gradually increased until therapeutic benefits occur.

Behavior therapy differs from psychoanalytic therapy in that behavior therapy gives little regard to the relationship between the conscious and subconscious mind and to understanding this relationship as a means of modifying behavior. Rather, behavior is regarded as being governored by the perceived consequences of the behavior. (A discussion of this concept appears in Chapter 3.)

Other treatment methods used in many institutions for treating the mentally disturbed are group therapy and milieu therapy.

The group therapy approach focuses on interpersonal relationship within a small group situation. The group approach centers on social functioning, rather than psychopathology. Generally, this method promotes self-maintenance and rewards the patient for exhibiting socially readaptive behaviors. Patients are expected to assist in planning their own treatment regimen and to assume responsibility for themselves.

In milieu therapy the emphasis is on the social environment since the mental disturbance is viewed as having been caused by the individual's inability to deal realistically with this environment. Patients assume the major responsibility for improving their condition, but all staff members of the treatment center assist the patients in developing and carrying out an appropriate program of socializing activities. (For a more complete discussion of group and milieu therapies, see Chapter 3.)

DEVELOPING THE THERAPEUTIC PRESCRIPTION

Once a diagnosis has been made, the patient within the treatment center is provided with an appropriate treatment regimen designed to counteract the mental disturbance which has caused institutionalization. The regimen may be a combination of chemotherapy coupled to psychotherapy and other pertinent modalities. When the patient's physical and mental assessment has been made by a physician, a prescription will be written dealing with the patient's needs insofar as positive behavioral adaptations and recuperation are concerned. A treatment or rehabilitation team, including specialists from the fields of social work, occupational therapy, psychology, therapeutic recreational service, and possibly other appropriate personnel is organized to carry out the treatment goals. At this point, the medical prescription serves as the behavioral objectives which the patient is to achieve.

Typically, a patient assessment will have been made by one or more rehabilitation team members to determine the capability of the patient to perform and participate in a diverse program established to assist in ameliorating the mental condition. The assessment is extremely important in terms of understanding the patient's previous recreational experiences, talent, interests, current abilities, appreciations, and expectations. Of considerable significance is the patient's general behavior during any interview or the ability of the patient to fill out activity forms. Thus, posture, energy output, eye contact, hand / eye coordination, interactional style, ability to complete tasks, and other aspects of the individual's potential are noted. It is as a result of any initial interviews and diagnostic procedures that primary treatment goals are devised and recommended activities are implemented. The physician's prescription, based upon examination as well as the patient's maladaptive or bizarre behaviors, will identify major areas of concern.

As an example, let us say that an individual has been diagnosed as showing signs of involutional psychotic reaction. This disorder typically features such problems as extreme tension, anxiety, agitation, and acute insomnia. Strong feelings of guilt are characteristic, as are somatic (body) concerns, either of which can develop to delusional dimensions. There is an absence of prior incidents and, although individuals may be delusional, they do not display the intellectual and association disorders which distinguish the schizophrenic. Occurrence is most common in the involutional period of life.

The involutional period is commonly conceded to take place in the 40- to 55-year-old age group of women and the 50- to 65-year-old age group of men. The incidence of involutional psychotic reaction is found three times as often in women as in men. Its frequency has been increasing in recent years, probably due to an increase in the aging population in general.

In both sexes, the involutional period features various potentially stressful physiological and psychological changes and conditions. In women, the onset of menopause may carry with it a sense of loss, a feeling of uselessness, and a decline in self-esteem. In men, identical feelings may occur because of retirement or diminishing sexual capacity. There are typical experiences of declining health, strength, and intellectual ability, specifically in intellectual efforts requiring speed. Women particularly are vulnerable to feelings of worthlessness after their children have matured and left home. The involutional psychotic reactors have little or no outside recreational interests to occupy them when their chief functions, as perceived by them, are taken away or are no longer available.

Anxiety about death is common during this time; the individual senses that he or she has a finite period remaining and time is running out. Additionally, there is frustration about present accomplishments and the thought that there is no longer any opportunity to achieve the goals that once beckoned. The involutional period requires some major behavioral modifications if the individual is to escape psychologic disruption. However, the personality pattern of the involutional melancholic may be too rigid and compulsive to adjust. The individual is convinced of his or her own failure, is overwhelmed by a fixed belief that such failure is due to personal inadequacies, and lapses into a depression. The more inflexible, restricted, and guilt-ridden the pre-illness personality of an involutional psychotic reactor is, the worse the prognosis for complete recuperation.

With such a diagnosis and prognosis, the chief concern will be avoidance of painful and intolerable feelings of depression, isolation, and unhappiness and changing behavior that tends toward reflexive, impulsive, and self-destructive actions. The treatment goal, based on the prescription will be to modify the client's behavior so that reliance on adjustment mechanisms (hostility, withdrawal, projection, rationalization, fantasizing, etc.) is no longer excessive, thereby avoiding depression and associated affects. All modalities will be brought to bear. Among the definitive behaviors to be changed is the client's anti-social conduct, which can be affected by requiring conformity to institutional rules and limits. Obsessional preoccupations can be modified by guiding the client toward active interpersonal contacts. Oral aggressive behaviors will be reduced while ambiguous moods are returned to a more constant state. This is accomplished through the use of or withholding of privileges for acceptable behavior in appropriate situations.

PROGRAMMING RECREATIONAL ACTIVITIES

A planned program of therapeutic recreational activities for the mentally disturbed patient will probably be undertaken in the following sequence, or some such similar procedure will be effected. The physician's order is written for therapeutic recreational service prior to the initiation of treatment. A comprehensive file on the patient's current behavioral status and capabilities is compiled before the rehabilitation team meets for the first time. The client assessment plus the information compiled on therapeutic recreational service potential is utilized to establish the goal and treatment plan. Selection of suitable recreational activities or experiences intended to reach the objectives set by the treatment plan and to promote particular behavioral standards is the primary function of the therapeutic recreationist.

A variety of activities or experiences may be necessary if the client is to obtain the greatest benefit from the planned sequence of actions developed in response to the prescription. All such recreational activities will be planned for a cumulative effect and are consistent with the concept of the therapeutic milieu. Continuous assessment of the client or patient is essential as well as program evaluation so that basic objectives are met.

Informal program evaluation is conducted on a daily basis. This includes direct observation by therapeutic recreationists working with the patient or client. These data are examined on a daily basis and incorporated into material used for weekly supervision purposes and ultimately for any recommendations for activity modification or continuance. Documentation of activities and experiences of a recreational nature carried out by the therapeutic recreationist assigned to the patient or client as well as progress notes dealing with observed patient behaviors, either positive or negative, are recorded for future reference when updating treatment goals or making other necessary program adjustments. Patient or client problems are identified and examined and recommended solutions are undertaken in accordance with rehabilitation procedures.

Quality Assurance

The rehabilitation team serves as the overall program quality assurance body. With respect to the therapeutic recreational service, the team evaluates the outcome of recreational activity participation to determine whether the client's behavior and insights have been appropriate for the situation and environment; whether there has been sufficient advancement toward better mental health; and whether the client is able to deal with emotional stresses in ways that are indicative of progress in ability to adjust and respond rationally.

Each member of the team operating within a given specialization provides feedback to the team in terms of what the client said, how the client reacted to different activities and conditions, and any significant forward or retrograde movement that the client may have manifested during the course of activity or experiences in attempting to cope with small group interaction, individual skill learning, or any other phase of the program developed from the original prescription. If, for example, the prescription calls for the sublimation of aggressive impulses or the re-socialization of individuals whose typical behavior is so hostile that they are dangerous to themselves or others, certain activities will be undertaken which can assist the individual to learn adjustive skills, decrease hostility to socially acceptable levels, or strengthening the self-image to a point of toleration of situations that usually trigger abnormal or unstable emotional outbursts. Through the use of therapeutic recreational experiences, clients are enabled to adjust to social situations, learn required skills, come to grips with perceived threatening situations so that they can cope in a rational manner.

Although each rehabilitation team member may bring his or her own perspective of the specialization and the client to the team proper, each has something of significance to contribute to the overall output. What may be of considerable value to the team's evaluation of the patient's progress may stem from the recreationist's close observation of the client in a variety of activities which reveals certain penchants for action or habitual ways of solving problems. From this information, suggestions and specific activities can be developed—if warranted.

All such information which flows back to the team in its periodic meetings will be applied to a developing program which has as its objective the restoration of the client to a level of functioning where it is possible for the person to leave the treatment center and re-establish himself or herself within the community.

Individualized Program

Following the prescription and the recommendations of the rehabilitation team, an individual program is established to satisfy the treatment
goals which have been defined. The program is based upon individual
client's needs, extent and degree of mental illness, the objectives of other
therapies being utilized, and the prognosis.

The therapeutic recreationist may be assigned to and be responsible
for one or more patients within the treatment center. Since clients must
remain institutionalized for some period, it is possible to determine what
treatments will be available for the client and which recreational activities
or experiences may prove most beneficial either individually or within
small groups. Among the functions which the therapeutic recreationist
has is to assist the client's recuperation and return to healthy behavior
by encouraging an interest in normal occupations and in activities of a
positive nature. Moreover, the therapeutic recreationist has the responsibility to offer counseling and guidance to the client during recreational
activities for achievement of more emotionally balanced and healthful
outlook and behavior.

Activity Selection

Activities are selected for clients on the basis of analyses that indicate
successful performance is possible to satisfy a particular objective. Each
type of activity is used to provide a specific kind of condition to test the
client's skill, emotional control, response, and personal mannerisms or
habitual procedures in attacking a problem or answering some confrontation. Usually, although not in all situations, stress is laid upon activities
or experiences that have an emotional base or an affiliational association.
In every instance there is great emphasis on self-worth, self-expression,
and self-discovery.

Activities may range from elementary motor skills to complicated physical activities requiring strength, coordination, flexibility, patience, stamina,
and a willingness to persevere for remote satisfaction despite frustration.
The planned program will also contain, judged by client assessment and
current needs, group or individual activities of a social or aesthetic nature
that can be expected to have a positive effect upon the client's mental
health.

Programming might conceivably include a full range of recreational
activities limited only by the number of recreationists and volunteers and
necessary space to make possible a comprehensive series of recreational
experiences. Activities designed to enhance a client's mental health may
have to be repeatedly offered to the client before a response is elicited.
In the repetitions, the activity may take almost any camouflaged form if
the end result is, indeed, client participation; whatever resources that
must be used to gain client compliance should be applied. It is more

important for the client to achieve rehabilitation than be entertained or amused. In the final analysis, unless the client actually participates, the program is unrealized and any rehabilitative effort becomes futile.

Of course, clients may spontaneously choose recreational activities from among those available for independent participation. However, such activities should not preclude experiences that are designed to produce certain positive effects and require patient participation. The question of whether or not such requirement destroys the recreational aspect of the activity should not intrude here. Some authorities find prescribed intervention unsatisfactory while others are of an opposite opinion.

Activities will be programmed in terms of the degree of risk involved for the specific client insofar as emotional control or ability to tolerate frustration is concerned. Among the criteria for selection should be the development of interpersonal relationships within a small group setting, ability to make judgments that are appropriate to the occasion, improved attention span, and enhancement of self-esteem, self-confidence, and personal identity. Additionally, there is the need to maintain the client's physical fitness or to improve it. Activities of a physical nature may be utilized to overcome feelings of inadequacy and to gain a sense of mastery, by offering experiences that demand both competition and confrontation in a controlled situation. Under such circumstances the client is encouraged to recognize the significance of participation in vigorous activities for physical conditioning and psychomotor, affective, and social interaction.

Activities that promote aesthetic appreciation and performance in the various art forms may have unparalleled value in enabling the client to assume responsibility for the completion of a task and to experience a sense of achievement, thereby improving self-image. Such activities also serve a cathartic function, stimulate communication both at the verbal and non-verbal level, and improve intra-group action.

Client Participation. As always, the therapeutic recreationist will attempt to involve clients and patients in developing programs based upon their own personal interests, desires, skills, talents, and experiences. The use of client councils or committees in setting up or devising activities is extremely useful in engaging patient attention; gaining patient identification with a project, issue, or activity; enlisting their efforts and, perhaps, expertise, so that the success of the activity reflects upon them and provides another base for sound personal enhancement. Despite mental illness or emotional disturbance, whether in an institution or as an outpatient, clients may often have a degree of technical skill, knowledge, or experience upon which to draw that can rescue a routine recreational program from boredom and create opportunities for clients to experience peer recognition, individual achievement, and self-satisfaction, as well as enjoyment.

The selection of activities for institutionalized patients or clients residing in the community will be based upon the extent to which the client is benefitted by the activity; the degree to which the activity carries out the prime directive of the rehabilitation team's goals; and the ability of the client to understand the function within a recreational setting. The recreationist should be able to affirm that the selected activities do indeed provide support in ameliorating problems, redirecting behavior, conducing to effective interpersonal relationships, and reducing the incidence of emotional disturbance or disruptive and unproductive behaviors.

Program Evaluation

Since behavioral objectives as well as activity application are the subjects of any evaluation process, certain performance values are anticipated and recommendation is made in consequence of how the client responds to activities. As always, progress notes and observations are centered about self-concept and personal identity, adaptation in situations dealing with group interactions and interpersonal behaviors, decision-making, problem-solving, recognition of maladaptive behaviors, and understanding of one's place within the social milieu. Evaluation also seeks to determine whether the program has actually achieved the stated goals and objectives for which it was established. Equally important is the outcome of evaluation which causes program adjustment in order to improve the possibility of the client's adherence to treatment goals and more rapid rehabilitation.

The concentration on readjustment processes focuses attention on the building or re-learning of skills around which a structured program may be built. Wherever the client is deficient insofar as attitude, performance capacity, or cognition is concerned, remedial activities are instituted. Client assessment indicates both ability and dysfunction insofar as recreational activities are concerned. To the degree that a client can participate in one or more recreational activities or group situations, that existing ability must be protected and maintained. Both the supportive environment provided by the recreationists and programmed activities should be of such caliber and attraction that clients' current capacities, appreciations, skills, and interests will be sustained or enhanced.

Finally, it is the function of the therapeutic recreational service to assist clients to assume responsibility for themselves in social, cultural, and physical activities, thereby realizing one of the primary objectives obtained from any evaluation, i.e., the re-integration of the client into the community. The essential treatment goal of rehabilitation should be a constant part of the recreational program whose intent is to move the client toward a level of personal adjustment that permits a return to autonomy within the community. If complete rehabilitation is not the outcome of such a process, then it may still be possible for the individual to cope with the stress of modern society, get along with others, and make a reasonable effort to live a relatively satisfactory life, despite some emotional disturbances.

Community Based Recreational Services

In the past decade, there was a move toward deinstitutionalization, i.e., removing those patients from hospitals and treatment centers who were not considered acutely ill or dangerous to themselves or others and placing them in half-way houses, group homes, or other community based facilities where they could receive some supervision and medical maintenance as necessary. Ideally, it was thought, mental patients who could be re-integrated into community life, with slight assistance, would be less of a burden on institutions which were invariably understaffed and poorly funded. When hospitals began to discharge up to half their patient populations, it was planned that such individuals were to be given continuous support in terms of community-care centers and group homes or similar residences. Unfortunately, the needed supervision of community placement was sharply curtailed by federal cutbacks of funds and the community's unwillingness and inability to care for discharged former patients. The result was an upsurge of homeless outcasts living, and sometimes dying, on the streets of America's cities. It is estimated that at least one-third of the one million people living in the streets have emotional problems—some suffering from psychotic episodes.

The concept that community mental health centers and after-treatment support programs can be made available is unquestionably valid. Therapeutic recreational service within treatment centers dealing with mental illness has had an excellent record in continuing support to clients after release. The same cannot be said for community mental health centers—where they exist. It is probably also true that therapeutic recreationists employed by community recreational service departments have not been able to program for the average ex-patient to any degree, much less organize and direct adaptive recreational activities for those who must either live in the streets or reside in questionable housing. It is obvious that much can be done and much remains to be done.

REFERENCES

1. American Psychiatric Association, *Diagnostic and Statistical Manual of Mental Diseases,* (DSM III) (Washington, D.C.: APA, 1980).
2. Joseph Zubin and Fritz A. Freyhan, eds., *Disorders of Mood* (Baltimore: The Johns Hopkins Press, 1972).
3. David Stipp, "Open Mind," *The Wall Street Journal* (Monday, December 19, 1983), Vol. CCII, No. 119, pp. 1, 17.

SELECTED REFERENCES

Bean, Philip, *Mental Illness: Changes and Trends* (New York: John Wiley & Sons, Inc., 1983).
Goldberg, David and Hurley, Peter, *Mental Illness in the Community* (London: Tavistock, 1980).

Grusley, Oscar and Pollner, Melvin, *The Society of Mental Illness* (New York: Holt, Rinehart & Winston, 1980).

Insel, Paul M., ed., *Environmental Variables and the Prevention of Mental Illness* (Lexington, Massachusetts: Lexington Books, 1980).

Meyeu, Robert G. and Osborne, Yvonne H., *Case Studies in Abnormal Behavior* (Newton, Massachusetts: Allyn & Bacon, 1982).

Miles, Agnes, *The Mentally Ill in Contemporary Society* (New York: St. Martin's Press, 1981).

Talbott, John, ed., *The Chronic Mentally Ill: Treatment, Program Systems* (Port Washington, New York: Human Science Press, 1981).

Chapter 10

Aging

"Do not go gentle into that good night" is the way poet Dylan Thomas wrote about the final struggle of human beings with their ultimate adversary. The manner of life and the time, place and condition of demise will probably be influenced by many factors. Most people have a life expectancy of a specific number of years. Barring accident and catastrophes, there seems to be no reason why that expectation should not be fulfilled. But as the last of life approaches, many people go into a decline that is as often mental attitude as it is physical deterioration.

The poetic line implies that such decline should be resisted. Such resistance by aging men and women carries important implications for the field of recreational service in general and for the adaptation of activities in particular. Resistance here is conceived as the maintenance of personality integration, mental alertness, physical capacity, and intense interest in the world for as long as possible. This is the ungentle struggle to be waged up to the final hour, and recreational service can be an important ally.

The probable life span of an infant born today is nearly twice that of baby born during the 18th century. The number of aged individuals in the general population has increased dramatically, due in part to better medical care and services, but due also to a sounder physical constitution resulting from nutritionally enriched diet and attention to good health practices. At least 11% of the people in the United States is 65 years of age or older, and the percentage has every prospect of continuing to climb. This, too, has important implications for recreational service.

THE PROCESS OF AGING

Aging begins at birth. However, the process of changes that occur over the subsequent years is considered desirable until well into the middle years of life. It is only when the changes that aging brings cause a decrease in abilities of performance that the process is considered in terms of its effects on the individual. Physiologic and psychologic changes do occur, and they do influence many aspects of the lives of older people, but their effects are not well understood and so are often greatly overestimated by both those who are elderly and by those who provide services for them. The recreationist needs to be familiar with the nature of the changes and their causes and to give them the same consideration in programming of recreational activities as is given to the limitations caused by disabilities and illness.

Physiologic Changes

The process of aging is not completely understood, but certain physiologic changes are known to take place. Among the changes that occur are cellular atrophy, retardation of cell growth and tissue repair, degeneration of the nervous system, gradual reduction in basal metabolic rate, and reduced capacity to produce immune bodies. Hence, older people are more susceptible to chronic disabling diseases, cardiovascular ailments, malignant neoplasms (growths), and cerebral vascular accidents. The decrease in immune bodies in many instances produces greater likelihood of infections. Bones are more prone to fracture and repair following injury occurs more slowly. Diminished acuity of the sense organs is a common occurrence of aging; hearing ability diminishes and vision becomes impaired. There is an increased tendency for the development of farsightedness, which if the individual has been nearsighted in youth, sometimes effects an improvement in vision.

With advanced age certain aspects of the homeostatic process, which are vital for the maintenance of life, begin to deteriorate. After the age of 40, regulation of body temperature, blood sugar level, and acid-base balance of the blood becomes increasingly difficult generally due to tissue changes which produce capillary degeneration, sweat gland deficiency, and arterial rigidity. This may account for the fact that many old people travel south during the winter, shiver more readily, and dress more warmly. The loss of subcutaneous fat also contributes to the fact that older people chill more easily. In hot weather older people have greater difficulty in dissipating heat through the skin, a factor in the incidence of death from heat stroke.

Among other effects of later life, there is a progressive lessening of tolerance to glucose and a higher incidence of kidney impairment. With vigorous exercise the pulse rate increases less with the concurrent limited ability to adjust to such physical stress. There may be modified reactions to various drugs. In summary the human organism shows reduced ability to maintain stability in the internal process of adjustment. Furthermore, the body shows a marked disability toward recuperation whenever homeostatic processes are disturbed.[1]

A decrease in motor efficiency is also experienced as the years advance. Speed, strength, endurance, coordination, and flexibility are gradually reduced. How much of this decline is dependent upon the aging process and how much upon decreased muscular activity is not clearly established. However, it has been demonstrated that those who continue to participate extensively in physical activities lose their motor abilities at a much slower rate than those who are inactive. Some of the physical degeneration that occurs in the aging can be duplicated in the young by enforced inactivity: decrease in muscle size and strength, endurance, coordination, and flexibility; deterioration of bone cells; and poor digestion are common symptoms of lack of exercise in any age group.

The slowing of reactions with age has always been one of the more obvious manifestations. Most slow behavior attributed to age is probably intimately connected with the time required by the central nervous system in interceding with the stimuli and responses necessary in behavior. Usually, not a great deal of the slowness of the aged can really be ascribed to poor motility of joints or muscular contraction or to restrictions of sensory information.

Studies indicate that older people can perform almost all of the things they did at a younger age, but not as speedily. There is good reason to believe that a rather broad-based condition develops with age and sets a specific limitation on the quickness of all behavior controlled by the central nervous system. With advancing age people appear to manifest a specific trait of slowness of response no matter what the task might be. The slowness of behavior with increasing age implies less the presence of neurologic damage, which can be connected to disease, than a major change in the nervous system.

Effects on Mental Capacity. Physiologic changes within the brain can affect mental capacity. Alzheimer's disease and Pick's disease are disorders in which there is brain deterioration that produces a form of senility.

Other organic brain diseases have been identified in the older patient. Such diseases may be related to the brain's dependence upon oxygen nourishment. The brain is extremely shocked by oxygen deprivation and its cells cannot survive for more than a few minutes if circulation is inhibited or stopped. For this reason, arteriosclerosis, which diminishes blood flow to the brain and thereby affects oxygen transmission, is a serious condition in older persons. However, cerebral circulation deficiency does not account for most of the instances of organic brain deterioration in later life. Age itself is not presumptive of a decline in cerebral blood flow and nourishment.

Psychologic Changes

Psychologic changes in aging follow an even less uniform pattern than physiologic changes and, as a rule, do not usually occur as early. Loss of memory of recent events is a psychogenic phenomenon of aging.

Speed in recall and organization of thoughts is diminished in some older people. Conservatism is a characteristic mental attitude commonly ascribed to older people, although this may be true only to the extent that anyone hesitates to change a mode of conduct that has formerly offered satisfaction and security.

It is not true that intellectual capacity and the ability to make discriminating judgments is lost in old age. The older person is just as able to learn new ideas and make valid and accurate decisions based on value judgments as can younger persons. There may be some loss in fluid intelligence but not in crystallized or judgmental intelligence.[2] The former is involved with recall of information like names and telephone numbers, and the loss is more a nuisance than a threat.

Talkativeness accompanied by increased meticulousness and impertinence are exhibited by some elderly individuals. In many instances there is a decided egocentricity and preoccupation with bodily functions. When these various changes become extreme and are associated with periods of obvious confusion and loss of touch with reality, they may be indicative of mental illness.

Senility. A form of mental disability most common to aged individuals is senility. In this condition the individual typically shows inappropriate emotional behavior; for example, talk may be excessive or actions peevish, secretive, and childish. Frequently, the mind becomes foggy, the thinking unclear, and short-term memory diminished.

All senility is not necessarily related to known organic brain diseases or deprivation of oxygen to the brain. Furthermore, research indicates that there is no evidence to implicate hardening of the arteries in the brain, degeneration of brain tissue, or toxins and poisons as causes of all senility. Many forms of senility are functional disorders without diagnosed organic basis.[3]

Why some individuals develop senility and others do not, why some cases are severe while others are mild remain to be discovered. Likewise, further research is needed to explain why senility is common among the aged, yet a large percentage of individuals show no signs of the condition at advanced ages.

Although means of prevention of senility are not known, some authorities feel that individuals who remain active throughout their later years have less possibility of early senility. The procedures of remotivation, resocialization, and reality orientation, described in Chapter 3, have been used with some success in programs for aged individuals to retard the development of senility.

THE SOCIAL DIMENSION OF AGING

In a society which is oriented toward a youth cult, old age is held in low esteem. Many people regard age as a time of loss. Indeed, loss of status and sense of usefulness do accompany the move out of the work-centered life and into the mandatory retirement. Of course, many people long for retirement, but these are individuals whose conceptualization of life and its challenges have long since been distorted by the incessant clangor or dehumanizing conditions of their work life. Farm, factory, and industrial employees are often subjected to such stressful and hazardous working environments that they become used up rather quickly and long for the day of retirement.

Other types of workers, however, view their work as their life. It is this latter group that finds it so hard to concede the passage of time and for whom the loss of the employment contact may cause a distressing decline in status as well as economic level. For such men and women, retirement is a time of great loss. Naturally, one cannot generalize that all older adults fall within either of the two groups.

Attitudes Toward Aging

Studies of attitudes toward various age groups in American culture suggest that the so-called middle years, about 40 to 50, are supposed to be the years of greatest status, security, income, social effectiveness, and power—at least for middle-class society. The inferred loss of status as people pass into older adulthood, a reflection of a culture which is not particularly sympathetic to aging, is unquestionably a significant component in differences in personal adjustment of individuals of various ages. In our society, aging is something to be dreaded; indeed, there is a highly developed mythology about the aged and aging in American society which provides a series of false pictures deeply imbedded in the American psyche.

One of the most dehumanizing situations is that of the older American woman. In an essay on this, Susan Sontag presents a horrendous picture of the female relegated to a lesser status in the stratum of society because of sex and age. A woman rapidly becomes obsolete as a personality in American society where aging, in all of its manifestations, is considered to begin just after adolescence. That such a myth has been perpetuated and reinforced by the mores and manners of society and that it continues even to this day to be accepted by so many as fact is incredible. More importantly, it contributes to the degradation of the female half of the population and this is the greatest injustice of all.

> One of the attitudes that punish women most severely is the visceral horror felt at aging female flesh. It reveals a radical fear of women instilled deep in this culture, a demonology of women that has crystallized in such mythic caricatures as the vixen, the virago, the vamp, and the witch. Several centuries of witch-phobia, during which one of the cruelest extermination programs in Western history was carried out, suggest something of the extremity of this fear. That old women are repulsive is one of the most profound esthetic erotic feelings in our culture. Women share it as much as men do.[4]

All problems which affect the aging have interrelated social dimensions. Economic ability, health, psychologic involvement, housing, social attitudes, resources available are a part of the pattern of life which makes up the life style of the aging in America. The issue is not one of simple black and white commentary. There are those who suffer untold horrors simply because they are old and there are others, fortunate in their declining years, who will never want for anything. They not only have a place, but are revered, served, and will live out their lives in relative contentment. It is between these two extremes that most people will find themselves. A wide range of problems beset the aged just as they do for any age group, but somehow the deterioration of age makes the individual just that much more vulnerable to the deficiencies of society and susceptible to inroads of waning strength and mental acuity.

Among the existing and overlapping problems of aging are those of health care, housing, and financial resources. This is in part directly due to continued inflation and its resultant effect on the cost of living and in part due to an abrupt change in the way people have stopped caring for their aged relatives. Formerly, aged people were protected against insecurity and neglect by their closest relatives. Today, sons and daughters who have obligations to their own children are not inclined to accept responsibility for care and comfort of the aged. This is a grave reflection upon the essential humaneness of a social order which is supposedly based on the concepts of equality and equal protection.

In some ways, even more important than the material and health care needs is the feeling of isolation and loss of personal dignity experienced by many older adults. In the American culture older people tend to be shut out as useless, economically, physically, culturally, and socially. No person should ever be made to feel useless; this tends to destroy self-concept and the very reason for existence. But often meaningful activities in which older people can engage are lacking.

Two emotional experiences of later life often force a change in the social roles of the aged person: the death of the spouse and retirement. Death is a critical event for either spouse but particularly for the widow, who often finds herself at a complete loss without the one person upon whom she has concentrated energy and love. Redirecting this psychic energy may be a long and painful process. In addition to having lost companionship, the widow no longer has a social status, frequently gained through her husband's economic and community role. She must develop a separate identity, founded on her own needs, interests, talents, economic ability, and social skills. At a time of life when physical and mental capabilities are diminished, forging a new identity is distressing and difficult for either the aged widow or widower.

Retirement is also a time of crisis for working men and women. If retirement has been planned and is completely voluntary, much stress is eliminated and the transition period is facilitated. If, however, retirement is forced by some corporate or governmental policy, the wrench is a drastic separation from status, economic level, and vocational identity.

Even where the separation is expected, a feeling of loss is sustained. Inevitably, there is a diminution of status identity developed through affiliation with economic and functional roles in the community; ties with a particular peer group are also severed. Some men, in particular, are incapable of moving into a purely social role, if this has been the exclusive domain of their wives. Focus of social contact by men is more often oriented toward occupational peer groups than is the case with women, and the forfeiture of these groups through retirement creates an emptiness with few essentially social skills to occupy it.

RECREATIONAL SERVICES FOR THE ELDERLY

Whether for the 5% of old people who are annually institutionalized in treatment centers or the 95% who remain within the community, recreational services can be highly beneficial to those who participate. Therapeutic recreational service may be offered to the aged institutionalized client on the same prescription basis as it is offered to any individual who is limited by physical or mental incapacity. To the extent that the individual is capable, participation should be stimulated and developed.

As recreationists increasingly come into contact with older adults in the community setting, they must program activities that will make significant contributions and not be mere time fillers. Recreationists, operating in treatment centers or within the community, must begin by

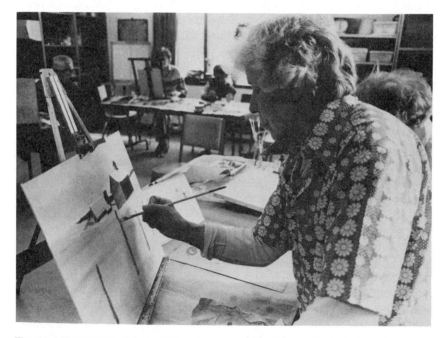

Fig. 10-1 The successful recreational program for elderly clients is based on considerations of their capabilities and their interests.

considering both what their clients are capable of and what they are interested in. Where there is no physical restriction, the older adult may participate in nearly every kind of recreational activity, but because of the benefits of vigorous exercise, participation in active game and sport activities should be particularly encouraged. Of course, moderation and safety measurements are observed.

To the extent that the individual is not suffering from psychologic deterioration, there is nothing of an intellectual nature which cannot be programmed. The enjoyment of learning new things, reading, participation in discussions ranging over every conceivable event from contemporary to ancient history and all of the subjects in between should not be omitted from the intellectual diet of elderly clients. All the various possibilities in the graphic and performing arts should be offered. Thus, any physical, mental, social, or cultural activity in which the older adult client can engage should be enthusiastically encouraged, programmed, and supported. Voluntary activities should not be overlooked as program possibilities. Assisting as a volunteer in the recreational program or performing a community service provides great personal satisfaction and enjoyment and does much to restore pride and status lost upon retirement.

Recreationists who work with aged clientele, especially in nursing homes, report that their most difficult problem is motivating them to participate in anything but the most undemanding activities. This is not surprising in view of the known fact that a slowing of the pace of active involvement commences at the age of 25. The decline in participation in activities that require great expenditures of energy, strength, and stamina continues, unless intervention occurs, until infirmity. Considerable ingenuity and experimentation may be required to discover ways of stimulating the hard-to-motivate to become more active participants.

Community centers especially designed for older adults play an important part in developing social contacts. Such centers have traditionally remained the main arena for cultural and recreational activities in communities. A small percentage of the retired population takes part in activities offered at centers. Recreationists will have to find better methods to gain increased attendance. Perhaps the most successful approach toward the expansion of participation and support is to develop activities that are meaningful to the potential client.

Bingo and similar games and activities, which are sometimes the major activities for older adults, may still have a place; but to attract people and hold their attention and appreciation requires programming that includes the full range of possibilities and has a comprehensiveness which makes many choices available.

The recreationists, either in the treatment center or in the community, have an important role to play in the delivery of certain services to the elderly. While recreational activity is no panacea for an individual's failure to adapt to the circumstances that prevail at any age, it is one social instrument which can enhance the life of the individual. The ability of the older adult to adapt and grow optimally is predicated on physical health, personality, earlier life experiences, and on the societal supports the individual receives. Among the supports society provides are adequate recreational services which can do much to preserve the individual's strengths, offer lifetime skill development for leisure use, and reinforce associations that lead to greater self-realization and self-actualization.

REFERENCES

1. A. I. Lansing, ed., *Cowdry's Problem of Aging* 3rd. ed. (Baltimore: Williams & Wilkins, 1952) p. 660.
2. Daniel Goleman, "The Aging Mind Proves Capable of Lifelong Growth," *The New York Times,* Thursday February 21, 1984, page C1, C3.
3. D. D. Stonecpher, Jr., *Getting Older and Staying Young* (New York: W. W. Norton & Company, Inc., 1974) p. 45.
4. Susan Sontag, "The Double Standard of Aging," *Saturday Review* (September 23, 1972) p. 37.

SELECTED REFERENCES

Barosh, D. P., *Aging: An Exploration* (Seattle: University of Washington Press, 1983).

Barrow, G. and Smith, P., *Aging, Ageism, and Society* (St. Paul, Minnesota: West Publishing Co., 1979).

Hamil, C. and Oliver, R. C., *Therapeutic Activities for the Handicapped Elderly* (Rockville, Maryland: Aspen Systems Corporation, 1981).

Robbin, A., *Aging: A New Look* (Circle Pines, Minnesota: American Guidance Service, Inc., 1982).

Shivers, Jay S. and Fait, Hollis F., *Recreational Service for the Aging* (Philadelphia: Lea & Febiger, 1980).

Simson, S., ed., et al., *Aging and Prevention: New Approaches for Preventing Health and Dental Problems in Older Adults* (New York: Haworth Press, Inc., 1983).

Zarit, S. H., *Aging and Mental Disorders* (New York: Free Press, 1983).

Chapter 11

Socially Deviant Behavior

Socially deviant behavior is defined by sociologists as any behavior that departs markedly from standards or norms of a given society. A fairly wide range of illegal and antisocial actions could thus be included, but in this chapter use of the term will be limited to criminal activity in violation of the law that results in incarceration. More specifically, the chapter will discuss special recreational services in adult penal or correctional institutions (prisons and jails), juvenile correctional settings (training schools and juvenile delinquent homes), and halfway houses.

THE CRIMINAL JUSTICE SYSTEM

The criminal justice system consists of three parts: police, courts, and corrections.[1] The police have the responsibility of arresting the violators of the laws. In the courts, the violators are tried and, if found guilty, are fined or sentenced or both. The sentence may be suspended and the offender placed on probation, which is a conditioned release. When the sentence is imposed, it is served in a minimum, medium, or maximum security correctional institution, depending upon the severity of the crime and other factors such as the potential danger of the prisoner to others and to himself.

Juvenile offenders are often released or placed on probation; sentencing to a term in a correctional facility is generally regarded by the courts as a measure of last resort for youthful violators of the law. Sentences, when they are given, are served in juvenile delinquent or training schools, formerly called reform schools. Some states allow juveniles to be incarcerated in adult correctional institutions, but many prohibit their being placed in prisons and jails where they will be in contact with adult criminals.

Even though corrections is the word used by criminologists to describe the third phase of the criminal justice system, it is in many instances not as accurate as the older term, penal, referring to punishment. The term corrections refers to the legal system's attempt to bring about change in the behavior of offenders so they will not break the law again. However, the focus of correctional institutions over the years has primarily been enforcement of society's punishment for violations of the laws or incarceration of habitual criminals to prevent their further commission of criminal acts rather than correction and rehabilitation of the criminal offenders.

Historically, the basis of treatment of criminals has been retribution: the offender made to suffer punishment to "pay his debt to society." Punishment in this view produces regret for having committed the crime and resolve to reform. Repentence is reinforced by fear of even more severe future punishment so that the individual never again engages in criminal behavior.

This concept of the effect of punishment in deterring criminal behavior was not seriously questioned until the 1900s. Then research in the field of criminology began to offer evidence that incarceration did little to rehabilitate criminals. The severity and length of punishment was found to have no positive relationship to a decrease in criminal activity of prisoners after their release. In fact, most studies indicated that released prisoners participated in criminal activities at a higher rate than before their incarceration.[2]

The evidence of the studies, supported by strong humanitarian concerns, encouraged forward looking criminologists to recommend rehabilitation rather than punishment to bring about changes in the behavior of those in correctional institutions. Although this idea has received much verbal support, in actuality few effective programs of rehabilitation have been established. The chief reasons for the scarcity of such programs are: (1) lingering attitudes that prisons should be places of punishment; (2) perception of rehabilitation programs as ineffective; and (3) insufficient funding.

THERAPEUTIC PROGRAM

Where there are serious attempts to rehabilitate, the approach is therapeutic in nature. The programs are usually staffed by some, if not all, of these professionals: medical doctor, psychologists, psychiatrists, educators, occupational therapists, and recreationists. The procedures for implementing the therapeutic program are similar to those of therapeutic programs in treatment centers (discussed in Chapter 3). Usually there is a rehabilitation team that includes a recreationist, and recreational activities are prescribed to fit the overall objectives in rehabilitating the client. Some broad categories of need that might be identified in the prescription are:

1. Assertiveness
   a) aggressive activities
   b) passive activities

2. Self-motivation
   a) work
   b) leisure
3. Homeostatis (release of tension)
   a) recreational participation
   b) leisure
4. Goal Setting
   a) work
   b) recreational activities
   c) leisure
   d) after release

To plan an effective program, information about the client is needed. Much may be obtained from the rehabilitation team, e.g., physical disabilities, emotional stability, social interaction with other prisoners. In addition the recreationist can secure specific program information in interviews with the client concerning recreational interest, present ability in recreational activities, reaction to participating in recreational activities. From this information a therapeutic recreational program is developed that provides those kinds of recreational activities that promote the objectives identified by the prescription.

DIVERSIONAL OR REGULAR PROGRAMS

As remarked previously, there are few recreational programs in prison with a therapeutic orientation. Most recreational programs are diversional in nature. This does not mean that they have no value for such activities do offer enjoyable occupation of prisoners' idle time. However, the recreational program can and should do more than this: it should contribute to the clients' welfare during incarceration and to preparation for reintegration in society upon their release.

Because prisoners live in an artificial environment where the former life patterns undergo considerable alteration, there is a desperate need for them to have some activities that bridge the gap between life in the prison and life on the outside. The recreational program can provide this bridge and so aid in reducing feelings of alienation, anxiety, and insecurity. Equally important, recreational activities are often the only acceptable means of release of tension in the maintenance of homeostatic equilibrium.

For the activities of the recreational program to be of greatest benefit to clients, the recreationist must know as much as possible about the institution and about the people incarcerated there. Without the sources of information about the prisoners available to the therapeutic recreationist on the rehabilitation team, the recreationist in this case has to glean information from such records as the correctional institution maintains; there will usually be records of physical examinations and perhaps also the results of other tests and diagnostic procedures that prisoners undergo upon entering the system.

With respect to information about the particular correctional institution, the recreationist needs to know the general operating philosophy and the rules and regulations applying both to prisoners and staff. It is important to be informed about the facilities, personnel, and equipment available to the recreational program and the schedule of free time and/or time designated for recreational activities.

PROGRAMMING RECREATIONAL ACTIVITIES

The selection and presentation of recreational activities for clients in prison is similar to programming recreational activities in any institutional setting, but there are certain concerns unique to the prison environment that must be addressed if the program is to be effective.

In developing a recreational program in a correctional institution, the purpose that the program is to serve must first be considered. Whether the emphasis is to be on recreational service for therapeutic benefits or for the values of occupying leisure in worthwhile activities determines programming choices. The space and equipment that are available, and these may be minimal, are other important program considerations.

Developing objectives and establishing how they are to be achieved are as important, if not more so, for recreational programs in prison as for any other program. Since recreational programs are frequently not wholeheartedly accepted by all those in authoritative positions, evidence of a carefully conceived list of desirable goals and objectives and indication of the ways they are to be achieved can do much to win support for the recreational programs.

The selection of activities to be included in the program must be based on attitudes and interests of the clients. These may be determined by seeking direct responses from the clients. Written questionnaires can be used but they are usually not as effective in the suspicious atmosphere of a prison as interviews or face-to-face exchanges between clients and recreationist. Many times consultation with particularly responsive individual prisoners is the most effective means of gaining ideas about which activities are best to present.

Programming Considerations Unique to Prisons

In conducting a program in prison recreationists are often surprised that the clients are much like those on the outside. A basic difference, however, is that they are confined and under supervision 24 hours a day, and this colors their outlook and their responses. Imprisoned clients differ also because they are individuals who have committed a crime (or as with many, a string of serious crimes) and had been found guilty. Consequently it cannot be expected that the level of morals or ethical responses to any given situation will be the same as that found in society generally. The recreationist must be prepared to witness a wide divergence of behavior from exemplary conduct to extremely antisocial behavior. Moreover, behavior is often unpredictable from one situation to the next.

Another fact of prison life that must be addressed, particularly where long-term prisoners are concerned, is the hierarchy of authority that frequently develops among prisoners, which often has as great an effect upon prison conduct as that of the prison guards. While an undesirable feature, if such a hierarchy does exist, the recreationist can perhaps utilize it for the development of the program by persuading the hierarchial leaders to support or at least not oppose participation in the activities. Other prisoners, no longer afraid to show an interest in the program, will be more likely to follow any inclinations they have to take part in the activities.

Security. Security is an ever present program where individuals are incarcerated. The recreational department must plan activities with attention to strict compliance with the security procedures of the prison. Certain types of recreational equipment may pose problems in security, e.g., baseball bats, carving knives, pool cues, or any material or equipment that can serve as or be modified for use as a weapon. When such equipment is used, extreme care must be taken that it is not stolen and that it is readily removed from the prisoner's possession in case of an emergency. Eliminating from use equipment that may be utilized as weapons prevents the offering of many valuable recreational experiences; however, prudence may dictate such limitations in the interest of avoiding use of potentially dangerous equipment. When this is the case, greater emphasis must be given to other activities. For example, the game of baseball may be contraindicated because of the danger implicit in the bat and the hard ball, but a catch-throw game using a softball may be substituted. Or rather than woodcarving with a knife, gluing and sanding of pre-cut objects may be substituted. Making substitutions of this kind can be difficult because they are activities that are not generally looked upon with favor by the clients as worthy substitutes. Efforts directed toward changing the attitude about the activities are then imperative.

Use of Volunteers

Because the recreational service staff in correctional institutions is usually inadequate in size for the number of clients to be served, the use of volunteers could be extremely helpful. The need for security, however, creates problems in utilizing volunteers from outside the institution on a regular basis. Initially there must be careful screening of the volunteers to eliminate friends, relatives, and others who might be tempted to provide illegal assistance or substances to the prisoners. Thereafter, adequate measures must be taken to prevent volunteers from bringing contraband into the institution or otherwise violating the rules and regulations. Because of these difficulties, it is often easier to develop volunteer leadership within the institution. Guards with special skills in specific recreational activities may be interested in helping with the planning and conduct of these activities. Also, individuals among the ranks of prisoners who demonstrate unusual interest or quickly develop skill in an activity are good prospects for training as volunteer assistants in that activity.

Programs in Youth Correctional Settings

In institutions to which delinquent youths are sentenced, a greater emphasis on rehabilitation is generally found than in correctional institutions for adults. An attitude that these young people may still be saved from a life of anti-social behavior shapes the policies and practices in most youth correctional settings. Hence, programs in these institutions are directed toward training in job skills for employment after release, developing basic educational skills, improving social attitudes and behavior, and preparation for re-integration in society. Medical and psychiatric treatment are provided as needed. The recreational program is regarded as important to the entire rehabilitative process, and its value in sustaining morale is recognized. Consequently, recreational services in youth correctional settings are more comprehensive in scope and better funded than is usual in adult correctional facilities.

In the programming of the recreational activities for youthful offenders, many of the suggestions and precautions discussed in the foregoing section on programs in adult correctional institutions are applicable. The situation is comparable to an adult minimum security institution. Therefore, it is both possible and desirable to plan participation in recreational activities in the outside community. Attendance at movies, dances, sport events, and similar entertainment events becomes an integral feature of recreational programming. Proper preparation and adequate supervision are, of course, vital to the success of the trip outside the correctional setting.

Leisure education receives special attention in the recreational program. Misuse of leisure is frequently a contributing cause of delinquent behavior. With greater knowledge about recreational opportunities and development of the skills needed to take advantage of these opportunities, delinquents may re-enter their communities better equipped to avoid the problems inherent in filling the free hours of the day.

Programs in Halfway Houses

Halfway houses are centers used to house prisoners who are going to be released in the immediate future. The halfway house program is designed to ease the adjustment of the criminal to the new status of freedom. The program emphasis is on employment, return to family and friends, and introduction to changes that have occurred during incarceration. Recreational services can make an important contribution to helping criminal clients make the adjustment to their prospective new life. The recreational program by recognizing the new freedom that the halfway house provides the client can offer experiences that enable the client to adapt behavior to the new circumstances. For instance, the client may be allowed to go certain places for recreational pursuits with the time for return set at a specific hour. An itinerary of recreational activities may be developed that allows gradually more freedom of choice and discrimination in time for the client to attend movies, go to the library, and participate in YMCA or YWCA activities, etc.

Leisure education becomes an important part of the total recreational program of the halfway house. Clients are made aware of the recreational services available in the area to which they will be returning and given skills to select recreational activities within their budget, to use these activities as a means of meeting new friends, and in general to use leisure for personal satisfaction and benefit.

SUGGESTED ACTIVITIES

To increase the possibilities of meeting the objectives of the recreational program, a wide variety of activities should be offered. Various circumstances in the correctional institution, as we have seen, limit the types of activities that can be presented. Activities that do lend themselves readily to inclusion in the program are suggested below.

Sports

Sports of all kinds should be included in the recreational program to the extent allowable by the space, available equipment, and funds for supplies. There are usually no great problems of motivation to participate because of the enthusiasm for sports that both male and female clients bring with them from the outside world, and there are such benefits and pleasures to be had from playing.

Of the team games, softball, volleyball, basketball, and soccer present the least difficulties in organization and control. It is essential that in these activities, and in any sports that are included in the program, the competitive element be minimized. The highly charged atmosphere of competitive play can easily become volatile and, therefore, potentially dangerous. The necessity is again stressed to keep watch over the equipment during play and to collect all of it immediately after the game to prevent any of it from being secreted for future use as a weapon.

Since not everyone can play at one time, spectators usually outnumber the players. The recreationist needs to work out a rotation system that allows everyone to play as often as to watch. There may be a few clients who because of fear of body contact or other reasons do not wish to participate in team play; great effort should be made to ensure that these individuals find some other recreational outlet that they do enjoy.

Sports other than team games should be included in the program for their greater carry-over into recreational activities in life after release. Bowling, golf, badminton, tennis, and table tennis are games that have a high probability of being played by prison clients after their release. Most of the games of this kind, however, require specialized equipment and/or courts or other facilities which may not be available and which because of fund limitations cannot be required. However, modified versions and improvisation of space and equipment enable the skills of the game to be learned and fun to be had from playing the game. Modifications of the kind suggested in Chapter 14 to allow physically disabled clients to participate in these games can be utilized to overcome space and equipment limitations.

Because they are relatively easy to present in the recreational program for male clients, boxing and wrestling are often included. One of the values of contact sports like these is the release of pent-up emotions, but this presents a danger of loss of control that may result in injury. Close supervision is, therefore, recommended for recreational boxing and wrestling.

Activities of great benefit that have no potential dangers and require nothing except appropriate shoes (and even these are not essential) are jogging and physical fitness exercises. The two can be combined for an interesting and self-motivating recreational experience by developing a fitness course like those found in many parks and beaches. Figure 11-1 suggests a possible layout for such a course.

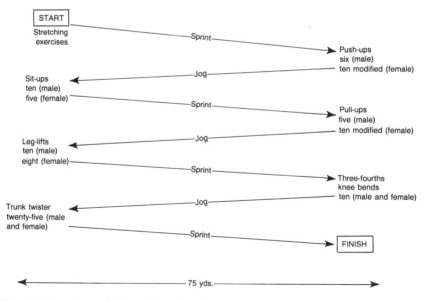

Fig. 11-1 Jogging and Fitness Exercise Course

Another good physical fitness activity is weight lifting. When machines like the Universal and Nautilus are available, their use avoids the problems of time-consuming setting up of equipment and the potential weapon danger of the bars and weights. However, in the absence of machines, bars and weights can be effectively utilized with careful supervision. A course or circuit similar to that suggested for jogging and physical fitness exercises can be developed for weight lifting with bars and weights. A plan for such a circuit is given in Figure 11-2.

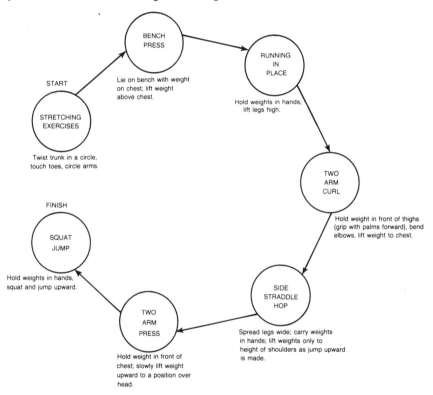

Fig. 11-2 Weight Lifting Circuit

Performing and Graphic Arts

Activities in the arts should have a prominent place in the recreational program because of their acknowledged therapeutic value. Especially noteworthy is the opportunity for personal satisfaction and prestige. Moreover, from the standpoint of the recreational staff, the amount of supervision and security precaution is less than for most other activities.

In the area of music, it is desirable to provide for both active and passive participation. So if space and funds permit, a suitable area should be set aside for listening to recorded music and another area for use as a practice room for individual and group instrumentalists and vocalists.

The development of a band and a chorus is particularly recommended because of the large number of clients who can be involved in a common endeavor that is satisfying and enjoyable. Where the talent warrants it, the possibility of public concerts outside the institutions can be investigated. Certainly performances by the band and chorus can be arranged for special events inside the correctional facility.

Similarly exhibits of art and craft products of inmates in these areas of the recreational program can be arranged. The exhibit may take the form of an arts and crafts fair or bazaar where the items are displayed and possibly sold with the money either paid to the individuals who made the items or going into a fund for expansion of the recreational program. Some correctional institutions have a permanent store for the sale of inmates' products to other inmates and also to visitors to the institution.

Dramatic Productions

Productions of plays and other forms of the performing arts are still another possibility for the expression of talents and interests in the wide variety of onstage and behind-the-scene activities. When a play is being selected for production or even for dramatic reading, consideration should be given to the subject matter of the play. Plays on subjects of an emotionally charged nature may carry actors and audience beyond the point of healthy release of emotions and frustrations. Hence, a careful review of plays being considered for production with this possibility in mind is essential. The review may well be carried out by a committee of recreational staff members and inmates. Committees of this kind are frequently formed in correctional institutions to review movies to be shown to the prison population.

Few plays have casts entirely of one sex so the reactions of males or females, as the case may be, to playing roles of the opposite sex must be considered. There are usually no problems if the recreationist approaches the matter with the attitude of seeking help from the group in resolving a slight difficulty.

Writing Activities

The most usual form of recreational writing activity is the prison newspaper. A newspaper offers such possibilities as developing news and feature articles, editorials and commentary, cartoons, and photography, as well as the mechanical production of the paper. Although creative writing by inmates can also be placed in the paper, a separate publication of poems, short stories, essays, and reproductions of art work should be provided if at all possible, to give recognition to the creative talents of a larger number of prisoners.

Other Activities

Equipment for some passive recreational activities will likely be available: television, radio, movies, cards, and table games like checkers and Monopoly. The recreationist should be aware that in some institutions, activities of this kind are permitted in the cells; elsewhere they can be participated in only at a central location during a limited time, often necessitating return to the cells before the end of the movie or television program.

Reading matter is also sometimes permitted in cells. However, libraries in correctional institutions are often inadequate and the materials outdated. The possibility of a local bookmobile making regular visits or of other loan arrangements with the local library should be considered to offset the limitations of the institution's library. Loans of equipment and other types of assistance from the community recreational program should also be investigated to enrich the program offerings at the institution.

REFERENCES

1. Marion and Carrol Hormachea, "Recreation and the Youthful and Adult Offenders," in *Recreation and Special Populations,* 2nd ed. by Thomas Stein and H. Douglas Sessoms (Boston: Holbrook Press, Inc. 1977) p. 107.
2. Ibid, p. 112.

SELECTED REFERENCES

Douglas, J., *The Sociology of Deviance* (Boston: Allyn and Bacon, 1984).

Goode, E., *Deviant Behavior,* 3rd ed. (Englewood Cliffs, New Jersey: Prentice-Hall, Inc., 1984).

Higgins, P. C. and Butler, R. R., *Understanding Deviance* (New York: McGraw-Hill Book Co., 1982).

Hills, S. L., *Demystifying Social Deviance* (New York: McGraw-Hill Book Co., 1980).

Little, C. B., *Understanding Deviance* (Itosca, Illinois: F. E. Peacock Publishing, Inc., 1983).

Section 3

Activities—Selection and Adaptation

Chapter 12

Special Program Considerations

The programming for special recreational services involves selecting appropriate activities for the program and planning the presentation of these activities to the clients. The selection of activities is dependent to some extent upon the resources available, i.e., the amount and kind of space and equipment, the financial allocation, the number of trained personnel and volunteers, and the scheduling possibilities. The other major factor to be considered in the selection of activities is the clients themselves and the nature of their illnesses and disabilities.

Planning the presentation of the selected activities is based on such consideration as the interests, motivation, and needs of the clients as well as of their abilities and limitations in performing various kinds of recreational skills. Foregoing chapters have presented the general information for providing for these considerations in programming therapeutic or adapted recreational activities. This chapter will deal with other important factors that must be considered in selecting and presenting the special recreational programs. Much of the discussion is applicable to programming in both treatment and community settings; where it is not, the information is presented in relation to the program in the kind of setting in which it is chiefly utilized.

PRESCRIPTIVE VERSUS DIVERSIONAL ACTIVITIES

Prescription for recreational activity is uniquely a part of treatment center programming, except in those rare community programs that are prepared to receive recreational prescriptions from medical personnel and to interpret these into program needs. The development of prescription depends on whether the recreational activities are to be an integral part of the treatment and rehabilitation of the ill or disabled client or are to be only diversional.

It is important that hospitalized patients, whether or not they are receiving therapeutic recreational services, be provided diversional recreational activities during confinement. These activities help to fill endless hours during their recovery with worthwhile and pleasant occupation and in this way may prevent patients from dwelling on morbid thoughts and self-pity. As they engage in recreational activities, patients often begin to reason that if they can do these things, they must not be so ill. Since there is some evidence that the mental attitude of patients has a great deal to do with the course of the disease,[1] it may be postulated that pleasant diversional experiences which produce feelings of well-being do promote recovery from illness.

MOBILITY AS A FACTOR IN PROGRAMMING

A particularly important consideration in selecting and conducting recreational activities for clients with physical problems is the degree to which they are able to move about. Severe limitations on mobility reduce the range of program activity possibilities. Likewise, the cause and current status of the limitations affect the kind of activity that can be offered and the manner of participation by the client. For purposes of further examination of mobility as a factor in programming, clients' conditions are categorized as:

Bedridden   —confined.to bed
Ambulatory   —able to walk with or without assistive devices
Preambulating—Unable to walk and requires a wheelchair or similar device for getting from place to place
Outpatient   —receiving periodic treatment at the hospital
Homebound   —confined to the home

Bedridden

Rest is necessary for recovery of the body from fatigue, illness, or injury. Bed rest has always been considered an important phase of the medical treatment of a patient. However, the use of bed rest for extended periods of time has ceased due to recognition of its serious consequences. Extended bed rest causes deterioration of the body functions which is most conspicuous in the muscles where strength, endurance, and power are lost through enforced inactivity. The heart and blood vessels become less efficient in maintaining good circulation with the result that cardiorespiratory endurance decreases. Lack of muscular activity results in mineral changes in bones that can create problems of bones breaking from even such slight pressure as musuclar contraction. The appetite becomes poor, and defecation and urination are often more difficult and painful without the stimulus of activity. To improve and maintain the physical health of the bedridden patient as well as to keep spirits high, active recreational experiences are essential.

Capabilities of Bedridden Patients. The recreationist should understand something about the capabilities of bedridden patients to move about within the confines of the bed. Patients in bed demonstrate various degrees of mobility depending upon their age, attitude, and illness or disability. The young are generally more mobile in bed than older patients. They usually can and will assume a variety of positions even when restricted by hospital equipment necessitated by their illness or injury. They are more active and twist and turn their bodies or portions of the body much more frequently and with greater range of motion than older patients. Elderly patients seem to avoid certain positions and to favor others. This may be attributed in part to general stiffness of the body produced by pain, but it is also frequently due to a lack of desire to move from a position to which they have grown accustomed or which they find comfortable. Older patients have a tendency to lie on the back with a flexed position of the neck, trunk, and legs and to be reluctant to move from this position. In most cases, patients who do not move much should be encouraged to be more mobile in bed in order to overcome the deterioration of body functions that occurs from enforced bed rest. Precautions must always be exercised, of course, to avoid movements that would aggravate an injured area of the body.

Nearly all patients can and should participate in some form of recreational activity while bedridden. However, there are certain times when all but the absolutely essential activities of hospital routine are contrain-

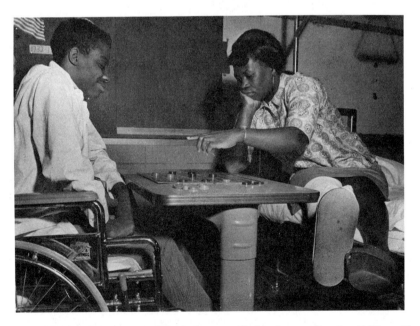

Fig. 12-1 Bed patients can participate in many kinds of recreational activities with simple modification. (Newington Children's Hospital).

dicated. These situations include those when the patient is in shock, under sedation, or has a high temperature. Also included are treatment procedures of immobilization, including traction.

Oxygen Administration. Bed patients have mobility limitations specific to their disability. Some congestive heart failure patients, for example, are not permitted to turn in bed because they must avoid even such minimal consumption of energy. Other patients with congestive heart failure or respiratory disease are given oxygen. During the time that a patient is being administered oxygen, most activities that increase the need for oxygen are contraindicated; therefore, if any recreational activity were to be offered to the patient receiving oxygen, it would need to be extremely passive and not raise the level of oxygen requirement.

Other Cardiovascular Emergencies. Cardiac emergencies, such as myocardial infarction, often require complete bed rest; however, the length of time of the bed rest varies with the opinion of the attending physician. Some doctors prescribe complete bed rest for a week or more, while others allow their patients to participate in mild activities while confined to bed. Patients who have a thromboembolic disease, that is, one in which there is clotting in the blood vessel, are, in some instances, as severely limited in movement as are patients with congestive heart failure.

For patients with cerebrovascular accidents (strokes), the length of time they must remain inactive depends on the type of accident and on the judgment of the physician. Some physicians prescribe a period of bed rest for their patients, whereas others prefer their patients to participate in mild activity soon after their accident.

Other patients, even though confined to bed, may be allowed a considerable amount of activity including prescribed bed exercises. The amount of recreational activity that is made available to the patient must be coordinated with the other necessary activities required of the patient so that the total amount of activity will not exceed that prescribed by the attending physician. The position in the bed that is most comfortable varies for each heart patient. However, most patients with congestive heart failure are more comfortable when the head of the bed is raised 18 to 20 inches and a pillow is placed lengthwise behind the shoulders between the shoulder blades, allowing full expansion of the rib cage.

Surgery. Bed rest may be prescribed for patients who have undergone surgery. The extent and degree of rest required depends upon the type of surgery and the doctor's judgment of the condition of the patient. For example, for a patient who has had a laminectomy (removal of a part of a vertebra) some doctors prescribe bed rest of up to 10 days' duration while other doctors have their patients get up on the operative day. In open heart surgery, most doctors start early exercises while the patient is in bed. Recommended are arm and leg exercises, executed passively initially, and then, as the patient becomes stronger, self-initiated. For those who have had abdominal operations, complete bed rest may be just a matter of several hours, as in the case of appendectomy, or several days, as in the case of sigmoid colostomy (surgery of the colon).

Spinal Injury. Spinal injury patients must be confined to bed for many weeks. They are generally placed in a Stryker frame or Foster bed, which are beds with parts so designed that the frame to which the patient is strapped can be reversed to move the patient from back to front without altering the alignment of the spinal column. Another type of bed for patients with spinal injuries is the Circolectric bed. It is designed so that the frame moves around in a circle, allowing the patient to be prone or supine or even held in an upright position.

The kinds of recreational activity offered to paralyzed patients are determined by the amount of paralysis. Quadriplegics will be severely limited since they do not have the use of either hands, arms, feet or legs. In cases of complete paralysis, the recreational offerings must be limited to such passive activities as reading, singing, and viewing of television, films, and slides. Other possibilities are games of mental skill, such as quizzes and riddles, and table games like checkers and Monopoly if assistance is given the player in manipulating the pieces. If patients have some limited use of an arm, as is often the case with quadriplegics, they may be able to perform the movements of the game by themselves. In acute cases of spinal injury, all recreational activity must be of the kind that does not encourage altering the alignment of the spinal column during the treatment period.

Excessive Pain. Most patients suffer pain from surgery. The pain begins soon after recovery from the anesthesia and generally lasts from 24 to 36 hours but frequently continues longer, depending upon the kind of surgery performed and the pain threshold of the patient. In this period, excessive pain is usually controlled by prescribed administration of a narcotic. Patients who are heavily sedated will not be involved in the recreational program.

Sutured Wounds. In most cases, surgical wounds are sutured, but in some cases the surgeon leaves an operative wound open to expose it to the air for the promotion of healing. In the former, the sutures are removed some time during a period of 3 to 21 days after surgery, depending upon the nature of the wound and its location. The sutures for surface wounds are removed on or about the 4th day, while sutures of heavy wire used in deep muscle tissue are not removed until the 21st day or later. The union of the suture line becomes well established after 3 or 4 days. Although the union of the line is not strong until the 3rd or 4th day, the patient can move and get out of bed without danger of the wound opening soon after the operation.

Most surgical patients will be permitted to participate in some form of recreational activity on the 2nd day after surgery. Some patients will be eager to do something even before then, and recreational activity of a sedentary nature may be offered to these patients. As strength is regained and the surgical wound heals, the patient will be able to take part in more vigorous activities.

Drainage Tubes. Drainage tubes (usually some type of tubing) may be placed in an incision at the time of surgery to allow fluids to drain from around the wound. The drain may come directly from the wound or through a separate incision made near the wound. In some cases where the discharge is profuse, the drain may be attached to a container; in other cases, the fluid is absorbed by bandages. Some bed patients require the use of a catheter, a tube placed in the body for the purpose of withdrawing urine. It may be placed in the urethra or directly in the ureter (the passageway conveying urine from the kidney to the bladder).

Drainage tubes limit the movement of the patient to a degree. The amount of restriction is determined by the kind of drainage tube. Short tubes in surgical incision offer no special problems or limitations. However, with longer tubes care must be taken so the tubing does not become obstructed by kinking or from the patient lying on part of it. The recreationist must select activities for the patient that do not encourage maintaining the body in a position that interferes with the functioning of the drainage tube.

Respiratory Disease. Some patients will be bedridden due to respiratory disease. These patients may have great difficulty breathing. Some, when they experience increased breathing difficulty, become apprehensive and even panicky, which makes the problem worse. The most comfortable position for most patients with breathing difficulties is a sitting or semi-reclining position. With the body in this position, the lungs are not cramped and greater ease in breathing is provided. The patient is usually propped in bed by pillows placed lengthwise at his or her back; a bed table is placed over the bed in front of the patient with a pillow on top as a resting place for the head and arms when the patient becomes tired. Special care must be taken in selecting recreational activities for patients with breathing difficulties so that no additional burden is placed on the respiratory system or the level of oxygen consumption increased.

Arthritis. Bedridden patients will include those suffering from arthritis who have an elevation of temperature. As long as the temperature remains elevated, the patients are usually required to remain inactive. When the temperature returns to normal, participation in appropriate activities while in bed is permitted. Usually the physician of arthritic patients wishes them to be as active as possible. The recreationist should be mindful of this need to be active and select activities for such patients that require action within the range of movement possible for them.

Traction. In cases of fracture where traction is necessary, the patient is almost always confined to bed until traction is no longer required. The restriction upon movement in bed is determined by the location of the fracture and the method used in reducing the fracture.

Patients suffering from a fractured leg may also be placed in traction. In this case, the weight is attached to the foot. The injured leg may also be in a cast in which case the weight is usually attached to the cast. Casts and tractions both limit movement; however, the patient in a cast will usually not have as much limitation as the one in traction. Recreational activities selected for these patients must be ones that allow maintenance of the proper position in traction.

Ambulatory

Patients who are receiving treatment or convalescing from an illness or injury and are able to walk with or without assistance provided by another person or a mechanical aid are considered ambulatory. Their medical problems will range from physical illness and disability to mental and emotional illnesses.

Surgery. In general hospitals, the most common ambulatory patients will be those who have undergone surgery. The time from surgery to the time of ambulation varies with the patient. If the patient has responded well to the surgery and is not excessively fatigued, ambulation is permitted within 24 hours. The patient is usually prepared for walking by mild exercising in bed followed by sitting up in bed with the feet hanging over the side. After becoming accustomed to the upright position, the patient tries standing and walking. Help may be provided during the initial attempts. It is generally considered inadvisable for the patient to move only from the bed to a chair because merely sitting in a chair tends to encourage the pooling of blood in the lower extremities at a time when good circulation is important. The recreationist should be aware of this fact and plan activities that will promote good circulation rather than ones that require the surgical patient to sit in a chair during the early days of convalescence.

Cardiac Problems. Patients suffering acute congestive heart failure or recovering from heart surgery must begin ambulation gradually to avoid overburdening the heart muscles. When the patient is allowed to get up and how much activity is permitted vary according to each doctor and his evaluation of the condition and needs of the patient. The amount of activity desirable for each patient will be prescribed by his or her physician, and the recreationist should plan the program cooperatively with the physical therapist, nurse, and/or occupational therapist if they are involved in providing physical activity to the patient so that the total effort required of the patient will not exceed the prescribed amount.

Since heart rate is a convenient guide to stress of the cardiorespiratory system due to activity, physicians frequently prescribe the workload by indicating a pulse rate that should not be exceeded while engaged in an activity. The prescription may identify a "target rate," that is, a pulse rate to be reached but not exceeded.

Casts. Patients with casts may be allowed out of bed. Casts on arms do not, of course, affect mobility as do leg casts. Patients with leg casts who are allowed up from bed may be fitted with a walking cast. Such a cast is constructed with a metal strip on the bottom of the foot so that weight can be borne on the foot of the cast.

The selection of recreational activities for those wearing casts depends upon the portion of the body involved. In addition to the lack of mobility of the limb that is in a cast, certain other restrictions are imposed. Standing for long periods of time, walking at a rapid rate, and running are restricted for the patient in a walking cast. Activities that produce excessive perspiration should be avoided by patients in any kind of cast. Perspiration causes dampness and soiling of the cast. Continuous wetness softens the cast and reduces its effectiveness, while the soiling of the lining causes irritation to the skin and unpleasant odor. A partial solution to the problem is placing patients in casts in a cool room for the more active kinds of recreational experiences.

Assistive Devices

Ambulatory patients may require mechanical assistance in walking. Among the types of assistive devices available are canes, crutches, walkers, ortheses and prostheses. The use of these requires the development of specific skills.

Canes. The simplest assistive device used in walking is the cane. Its primary use is to help maintain balance while standing or walking and to reduce the pressure or weight carried on one of the feet. There are two common types of canes: the straight one-leg wooden cane with the C-curved handle and the cane with 3 or 4 feet. The cane with 3 feet is called a tripod cane, the one with 4 feet a quad cane. Both are made of metal and have handles of various styles that offer a stable grip. The greater stability the canes provide make them much more helpful to individuals with severe balance problems than the one-leg cane with the C-curved handle.

For greater efficiency in use, any cane is held in the hand opposite the involved limb and is brought forward as this limb is moved forward. The cane should be advanced the same distance as the involved limb; otherwise balance is affected. Holding the cane so far from the body as to cause leaning toward the cane also adversely affects balance.

Crutches. There are several varieties of crutches. The most common is the wooden crutch which is placed under the arm with the support being taken by the hands which are placed on the hand pieces. The hand pieces are adjustable for appropriate height. Other types of crutches are the Lofstrand or Canadian crutch, the adult ortho crutch, and the forearm support crutch. All of these are made of metal and designed for either forearm or upper arm use rather than underarm like the wooden crutch.

They are adjustable by depressing a small button in the lower portion of the crutch.

The physical therapist in the treatment center is usually responsible for teaching the skills of the use of crutches, braces, etc. However, it is valuable for the recreationists to understand the techniques so that they can modify activities that require mobility most appropriately to the client's gait.

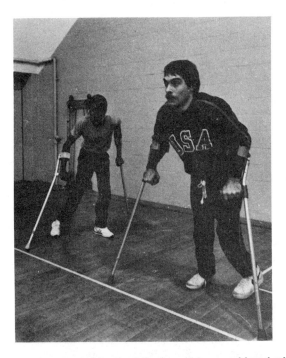

Fig. 12-2 The type of gait used by the client must be considered when adapting recreational activities for clients on crutches.

There are several different crutch gaits, each requiring a specific skill. The gait used by a patient depends upon his or her ability to take steps, the speed he/she wishes to go and his/her own particular condition.

The four-point alternate gait is one of the simplest and also one of the safest because there are always three points of support on the floor. The crutches and feet are moved in this order: (1) right crutch, (2) left foot, (3) left crutch, (4) right foot. The two-point alternate gait is a much faster gait but requires more balance and control because there are only two supports on the floor at any one time. The sequence of this gait is: (1) right crutch and left foot together, (2) left crutch and right foot together.

Either the tripod gait or swing gait is used by the patient who cannot place one foot in front of the other. In the tripod gait both crutches are swung forward together or are placed in front one at a time; then the body and legs are dragged forward to the crutches. The tripod formed by the two spread crutches and the feet must have a large base and the body must be leaned forward to keep the center of gravity in front of the hips or balance will be lost and the patient will fall backward. In the swing gait both crutches are placed forward together and the body and legs are swung forward. The legs may be swung up to the crutches or beyond them. The swinging of the body and legs requires perfect timing for, as the body swings forward, the back is arched; then the pelvis is rolled forward to place the center of gravity in front of the hips. The patient must fall forward onto the feet at just the right moment so that both crutches can be raised to repeat the sequence of movements.

Walkers. Walkers are four-legged stands about waist high that enable a patient who could not otherwise walk to be ambulatory. To walk with the stand, the patient grasps the top portion of the stand and pushes or lifts it forward a short distance and then walks up to it, repeating the sequence over the distance to be traveled. Some walkers have casters and the patient stands inside the frame. This type of walker has adjustable underarm supports and the patient uses the walker in a manner similar to underarm crutches except that the walker is rolled forward as the patient walks.

Ortheses and Prostheses. Two other mechanical devices worn by some types of patients to enable them to walk are the orthesis (brace or any device that assists movement) and the prosthesis (an artificial substitute for a missing part of the body).

Ortheses. An orthesis may be applied to both the upper and lower extremities and / or to the spinal column. Ortheses for the lower extremities may be of several different types, either aiding movement in the ankle, knee, and hip or acting as a weight bearing device. Springs are used in some ortheses to assist in moving part of the legs when there is insufficient power in the muscles. Locks are provided at the joints for rigidity there when necessary.

There are various types of spinal ortheses but chiefly they are all designed to limit motion in the spinal area. Each type is constructed to prevent a specific type of motion in a specific location. For example, one type may be used to prevent motion in the thoracic (upper back) area, while another prevents mediolateral (sideways) motion in the lumbar (small of the back) area. Most upper extremity ortheses are designed to aid in the use of the thumb with a finger or fingers. Some are made just to maintain the hand and wrist in a position of function. Others are designed not only to maintain the hand and wrist in a functional position but to aid in the movement of fingers and thumb.

Prostheses. Patients who have had limbs amputated can usually be fitted with a prosthesis. A lower limb prosthesis consists of an artificial ankle and a foot with a socket for insertion of the stump. If the amputation level is above the knee, the prosthesis is equipped with an artificial knee joint. It is manipulated by movement of the trunk and stump. The tilting table prosthesis is used by individuals with little or no thigh stump; the hip fits into a socket of the prosthesis and is held by means of a harness resembling a girdle. The socket in articulation with the lower portion of the prosthesis forms a table-like hip joint with a lock that stabilizes the hip for standing and walking and unlocks for sitting.

An arm prosthesis may be of two types: a cosmetic prosthesis, which is a dress hand or arm not designed for use and work prosthesis which is designed to enable the wearer to perform various tasks. The work prosthesis can be fitted with a split utility hook that substitutes for the hand effectively in various situations. Some prostheses are rigged with steel cables and a shoulder harness so that the wearer, by moving the shoulder, can manipulate the utility hook for use in grasping objects. This arrangement is also used with a prosthesis for amputation above the elbow to enable the movement of the shoulder to flex and extend the

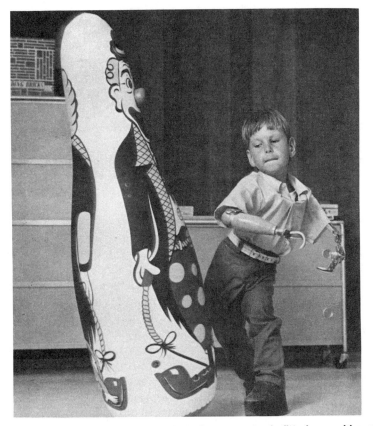

Fig. 12-3 The work prostheses with which the youngster is fitted serve him well in the serious business of play. (March of Dimes).

artificial elbow joint. An electrical device, powered by a small battery is being used with some success. It is manipulated by the shoulder muscle or, in some cases, by controls inserted in the shoe where it is manipulated by the heel and toes.

The prostheses described above may be replaced in the future by the myoelectric prosthesis, a device that utilizes electrical signals given off by the muscles. The signals are picked up by electroids and transmitted to a small battery-operated motor that activates the prosthesis. For example, the thumb and fingers of a below-the-elbow arm prosthesis respond to the signals originating in the arm muscles. In both movement and appearance the prosthesis closely simulates an actual hand and lower arm.

In developing programs for those who are wearing orthoses or prostheses, concern should be given to the limitations of the individual. However, the recreationist should always think of the patient's potential when selecting suitable activities. The patient should be continually encouraged to experiment with various possibilities in order to develop compensatory skills that will broaden recreational opportunities.

Other Problems. Ambulatory patients with sensory handicaps, neurologic problems, psychologic disturbances, and mental deficiencies do not need safeguards to avoid over-exertion unless they also have an illness, injury, or additional physical disability that requires them to avoid heavy expenditure of energy. Obviously, they will require special planning that gives consideration to their physical, mental and emotional limitations.

Perambulating Patients

Some patients will not be confined to bed but will be unable to walk. Wheelchairs, scooters, or similar propelled equipment are required to move these individuals about. In moving from the bed to a wheelchair, some patients require help while others are able to transfer themselves by shifting their bodies from the bed to the chair. A trapeze or overhead sling, which patients may grasp for support while sliding from the bed to the wheelchair, is sometimes available. Or a pole anchored to the ceiling and floor may be used by patients to support themselves as they move from the bed to the chair. Some treatment centers have hydraulic lifts that transport patients from the bed to a sitting position in the chair.

Wheelchairs. There are several different types of wheelchairs in use. The one most commonly utilized has two large wheels in the back and two smaller caster wheels that pivot freely in front. The large wheels have smaller rims set on the outside that are not in contact with the floor but are used by the patient to propel himself/herself. Most chairs have an adjustable footrest that can be moved to the side when the patient is getting out of the chair and also arm rests that can be removed to facilitate moving from the chair. Brakes that lock the big wheel are found on nearly all chairs. When the client is involved in recreational activity that requires a stationary position, the recreationist should continually check the wheel lock.

Wheelchairs are also propelled by motors or are pushed by another person. The motorized chairs are powered by a large battery; the controls are simple so that the slightest movement of the patient will control the chair. Chairs that are pushed are provided with handles projecting from the back of the chair, or if no handles are provided, the back of the chair itself is used. Some wheelchairs are collapsible; these are made with plastic seats and backs. It is possible with these chairs for individuals who may not be able to walk independently to take the portable chair with them in the car for use at their destination, thereby giving them a degree of independence that could not otherwise be achieved.

For clients in wheelchairs, curbs and stairs present problems that require assistance. Techniques that may be used by the recreationist to move the wheelchair up and down curbs and stairs of one or two steps (more should not be attempted) are presented in Table 12-1. Also given are techniques for moving the client to and from the wheelchair.

TABLE 12-1 ASSISTANCE TO WHEELCHAIR CLIENTS

TECHNIQUE FOR PUSHING WHEELCHAIR UP CURB OR STAIRS

Client in chair faces in direction of ascent.

Assistant at the rear:

1. Tilts chair backward and pushes forward.
2. Lowers front wheels to surface while lifting rear wheels
3. Pushes rear wheels onto surface

TECHNIQUE FOR MOVING CLIENT TO AND FROM CHAIR
(Use when client is able to stand)

One assistant:

1. Moves chair close to where client is to sit
2. Locks wheels of chair
3. Moves aside foot and arm rests
4. Stands in front to one side of the chair and lifts up under client's arms to raise client to standing position
5. Reaches down with one hand to release lock and swings chair away
6. Moves behind client to support torso while lowering client to another chair or to floor

Steps are reversed to move client back into wheelchair.

TECHNIQUE FOR MOVING WHEELCHAIR DOWN CURB OR STAIRS

Back of chair faces in direction of descent.

Assistant at the rear:

1. Draws chair backward until large wheels are off the surface but small wheels remain on the surface
2. Lowers back wheels slowly to surface.
3. Pulls backward while pressing down on handles to prevent front wheels from dropping when pulled off the surface
4. Lowers front wheels

TECHNIQUE FOR MOVING CLIENT TO AND FROM CHAIR
(Use when client is unable to stand)

Two assistants are required. Each stands on one side of the chair after removing the arm rests. Then each assistant:

1. Slides the hand nearer the front under client's thighs to grasp hand of other assistant
2. Pushes other hand gently behind client's back to clasp other assistant's hand
3. Lifts client up and forward from chair
4. Lowers client to another chair or floor

Steps are reversed to return client to wheelchair.

Scooter Boards. Scooter boards make an effective means of transportation for handicapped youngsters. They can be constructed in any dimensions desirable. Those sold commercially consist of a flat board approximately 14 × 18 inches to which four casters have been attached to permit the person on the scooter to roll freely in any direction. The youngster takes a position on the board by sitting or lying and then propels himself / himself by use of the hands pushing against the floor. A longer scooter can be made to accommodate the entire body while lying prone. The latter type of scooter was developed at Newington Children's Hospital and is used extensively there by children who are paraplegic.

Many different games can be played from the scooter, ranging from scooter basketball to tag games to relays. Some possibilities for scooter play are described in Chapter 14.

Outpatients

The involvement of outpatients in the recreational program varies from one treatment center to another. The clients who are returning periodically for treatment or diagnosis to general or rehabilitation hospitals in which they have previously been a long-term patient will generally welcome the opportunity to participate in the recreational offering during the day or days that they must remain there. Because they are already familiar with the routine of the program, they will fit in easily and can often be a real asset in assisting other patients who need help. This not only contributes to the program, it gives the clients a sense of responsibility and usefulness.

Clients can also be invited to return to the treatment center for the observation of special days and events conducted by the recreational service personnel. Clients who are elderly or not physically or mentally well enough to work often have few pleasures in life. Being invited back to take part in a party or celebration can mean a great deal to them.

One of the big responsibilities of the recreationist is leisure education of long-term patients, helping them acquire recreational skills during their hospitalization that they can utilize after they are released. Toward this end, the recreationist should become acquainted with the recreational offerings in the communities to which the patients will return. The program can then be planned to offer patients opportunities to become familiar with activities that they can continue in their home communities.

Before patients are released, they must have learned from their recreational experiences their tolerance level for activity so that they can judge the extent to which they should exert themselves when they are on their own. If they are restricted in movement, they should be taught how to compensate for their limitation and how to make the necessary adaptations to allow participation with others not so handicapped. Equally important, they must be given the self-confidence and assurance they need to take up their former life among members of the community.

Homebound

Homebound is a term applied to patients who, while they need not be hospitalized, are so disabled or ill that they are unable to leave their homes. Most of them are not bedridden, although some are able to leave their beds only for short periods of time. These patients are most often cared for by family or someone living in the home, a few receive care only from visiting public nurses, welfare workers, or personnel from other public agencies that provide home care services.

Home recreational service departments with sufficient financial resources have recreational services for the homebound in which adapted recreationists visit the home to develop an individualized program for the client and, if necessary, teach those who care for the client to aid the client in participation. The recreationist returns at intervals to refurbish supplies, check on progress, and offer encouragement. Often a corp of competent volunteers can be trained to conduct these individualized programs once the recreationist has initiated the program.

To develop a homebound program the first step is to locate those who are in need of such service. A search through community or hospital records will identify many homebound individuals. Once the program is in progress, news of it usually spreads by word of mouth, and others will call the recreation department to enroll. A second preliminary step is to research the community resources that may be utilized in the homebound program; among the possibilities are a traveling library, records of music and talking books, and clubs that will provide entertainment on special days.

TOLERANCE LEVEL

The prescription will indicate for the guidance of the therapeutic recreationist the physical tolerance level of the patient and also note the physical condition of different parts of the body. Parts of the body that are not affected by the disease or injury for which the patient is being treated can receive more strenuous workouts than the affected part or parts for which movement of any kind may be contraindicated. For example, a patient with a broken leg in traction is usually permitted to use his or her arms and upper body in vigorous movements but not allowed to move the injured leg. Such a patient could participate in throwing and catching games, darts, ring toss, and any number of similar gross motor activities that can be adapted to avoid movement of the leg.

Additionally, the emotional tolerance level of clients must be recognized, particularly in those who are mentally ill or mentally retarded. The near limit of tolerance is signalled by fatigue, boredom, and irritability. It is then necessary to terminate the activity, modify the performance, or change the activity entirely to revive interest and thwart an emotional outburst.

AGE AND INTERESTS

In addition to the physiologic and psychologic tolerance levels, consideration in programming must also be given to age and interests. Consequently, some knowledge of the general characteristics of different age groups and their common interests is useful. In the discussion of these characteristics and interests which follows, the patient population has been divided into three broad categories: younger children, older children, and young adults and adults.

Young Children

Young children have relatively little experience with social contacts outside the immediate family and do not usually participate eagerly in activities with unfamiliar people. They are self-centered, and their play is individual even though they enjoy having others play near them. Some children enjoy new experiences, but others are hesitant to deviate from that which is familiar. For the latter, the recreationist should, if possible, arrange for a few favorite toys to be brought from home. A favorite doll or stuffed animal can do much to ease the transition to the new environment because it provides a sense of security.

The majority of young children are developing a desire to please others and so are concerned about approval of their actions. Recognizing this, the recreationist should comment freely—but sincerely—on praiseworthy actions and efforts by the children. At a young age, children have keen interests and are generally easily motivated; they are usually eager to perform tasks within their ability.

Young children love to imitate not only people, but animals and inanimate objects that move. They enjoy simple songs and will attempt to join in singing them although not with great success. Listening to stories being read or told is another favorite activity.

During the early years, the imagination develops at a rapid rate. Consequently, most children are curious and enjoy new and strange objects and events if they feel sufficiently secure. The attention span is relatively short and interest shifts constantly. The recreationist must be alert to a child's shifting attention and be ready with a large reservoir of activities to capture the child's imagination.

Older Children

By the time they are 6 years old, most children find it easy to play and interact with others. As they acquire skill in reading and numbers, games and activities using these skills are increasingly appealing. Skill in the use of hands and fingers increases in older children to the point where throwing games of various kinds can be successfully performed. Arts and crafts, puzzles, and table games of various kinds are all activities enjoyed by older children. Because older children are gregarious, activities that involve others are greatly favored.

Since abilities and interests vary from child to child, opportunities for recreational participation should range from simple to complex activities. Both cooperative and competitive types of activities should be included, but special effort should be made by the recreationist to ensure that everyone experiences success in some way in competitive play.

Older children are frequently deeply involved in sports as participants, as spectators, or merely as fans of favorite sports personalities. This interest can be capitalized on to develop appealing recreational activities around the sports theme.

During pubescence, children often develop an antagonism toward members of the opposite sex. When there is evidence of this, the recreationist should provide segregated activities some of the time but should bring both sexes together frequently to encourage understanding.

Young Adults and Adults

Young adults often lack confidence and experience embarrassment in their attempts at new skills. The recreationist should be aware of this common characteristic and help the young adult gain self-confidence through successful, enjoyable experiences in recreational activities.

Sex antagonism disappears by young adulthood and is replaced by a growing interest in the other sex. Individual friendships grow rapidly among young adults and also among older adults. Group membership is important to many.

Young adults have, as a rule, developed a considerable body of knowledge that together with their skepticism of traditional concepts puts them at odds with the older generation. Indeed the ability of the young to deal with abstract ideas and to reason logically is often superior to older adults. For the young adult, an intelligent response to frustrating situations is more likely than an excessively emotional one. However, young adults often seek escape from unpleasant experiences through reading, viewing movies, and similar activities. If such an escape is used excessively, the recreationist must attempt to interest the patient in other activities.

As adults become older, they usually become less flexible mentally, as well as physically. They often do not welcome change and variation in the routines of life. The schedule of the hospital or nursing home, for example, may be difficult for them to adjust to. The older the client, the more difficult the adaptation, as a rule. The recreational program can ease the adjustment by offering activities that clients engage in routinely in everyday life. (Additional discussion of the characteristics of the aged is found in Chapter 10.)

With older mentally retarded clients and also some who are mentally ill, the attention span is so short and the range of interest so narrow that there is a temptation to offer these people recreational activities that are appropriate for young children. Usually this is a mistake: adults want to participate in adult activities. However, the activities may be modified to reduce their complexity or shorten the time required for their completion.

SIDE EFFECTS OF MEDICATION

Clients being treated with medication are not limited to treatment centers; many ill and disabled individuals among the general community populations are being treated with drugs of various kinds. Although neither the therapeutic nor adapted recreationist needs to have knowledge about drug treatment for curative purposes (type and dosage of medication is a medical decision), they both need to be aware of the possible side effects of drugs if these bear directly on the conduct of the recreational program for the clients taking the drugs.

In order for recreationists to be aware of the possible implications of a client's response in recreational activities, it is first necessary to obtain information about which drug is being taken and then to determine the side effects of that medication. In fact, the physician should routinely identify the important side effects when supplying the name of the medication to the recreationist. The practice of such routine reporting is more commonly established in treatment centers than in the community setting. However, it is just as important for the adapted recreationist to have the information as for the therapeutic recreationist. An excellent source on the side effects of drugs, other than the client's physician, is a reference book on prescription medication. Two of the best of such books are those by Stern and by Govoni and Hayes listed in the references at the end of the chapter.

The most frequently occurring side effects that have implications for recreational programming are: photosensitivity, overstimulation, depression, dizziness, drowsiness, hallucination, blurred vision, restlessness, nervousness, and motor dysfunction. (This is a representative, not a complete list.) Some examples will illustrate the importance of the recreationist knowing the side effects of drugs when selecting and conducting recreational activities for clients using those drugs:

- A client whose medication produces photosensitivity should not be involved in activities in the bright sunlight.

- When dizziness, drowsiness, or blurred vision is a possible side effect, recreational use of power tools or other dangerous equipment is contraindicated.

- Highly exciting activities are not suitable for those whose medications cause overstimulation or nervousness.

- If motor dysfunction is a side effect, intricate activities requiring high levels of motor skill are to be avoided.

If a particular drug treatment for a client is successful, in all probability the client will give evidence of benefitting from participation in the recreational program. However, if it appears that the medication being taken by the client effects successful participation, this information should be reported. In the treatment center, the reporting will be done to the rehabilitation team or the physician. In a community setting, the recreationist would discuss the matter with the client, if an adult, or with the parents of a client who is a child. In the situation of the recreationist working with school personnel to provide services for an ill or disabled student, the report on the effects of the medication should be made to school officials or the student's doctor.

Observations of the effects of the drugs on individuals by those in close contact with them is of vital importance to the prescribing physician. Sleator and Sprague feel that a drug treatment program for children will not be effective unless physicians routinely obtain information about their performance from those who work with and observe them.[2] It is undoubtedly useful to physicians to receive reports on adult individuals as well.

RIGHTS OF ILL AND DISABLED PEOPLE

Various federal legislative acts protect the rights of those who are handicapped by illness and disability by ensuring against discrimination and violation of their civil rights. All recreationists should be familiar with the general provisions of these laws in order not only to avoid transgression, but to actively promote adherence to them in the recreational setting. Handicapped clients deserve no less.

Rehabilitation Act of 1973

The rehabilitation act of 1973, known as the civil rights of the handicaped law, states that "No otherwise qualified handicapped individual in the United States . . . shall solely by reason of his handicap be excluded from participation in, be denied the benefits, or be subjected to discrimination. . . ."[3] The law further establishes that a handicapped person may require *different* treatment in order to be afforded equal access to programs and activities and that *identical* treatment in fact constitutes discrimination.

In terms of recreational services, the application of the law means that architectural barriers, such as steps that cannot be negotiated and restroom facilities that are impossible to use by those who are handicapped, must be adapted to ensure "access" to the benefits of the recreational services. Failure to make the necessary adjustments for accessibility denies the handicapped person an equal opportunity to obtain the same level of benefits from the recreational program as is available to the nonhandicapped, taking into account the nature of the particular handicapping condition.

Right of Privacy

The law also protects an ill or disabled person's right of privacy. Consequently, educational, recreational, and medical information cannot be released to other than the participating agency without the consent of the client or the client's parents. The law requires that each agency or physician "protect the confidentiality of personally identifiable information at collection, storage, disclosure, and destruction stages." When the collected information is no longer needed by an agency, the client or parents can require that the information be destroyed.

Other Rights

The right to education is also established by law, PL 94-142, and recreation is identified in the law as an educational provision to which the handicapped student is entitled. The ramifications of this provision are discussed in Chapter 6.

Those ill and disabled persons in a treatment center have the same rights as any other resident and citizen of a state in which they live and may, therefore, voice grievances to inside and outside representatives of their choice, free from all restraint.

States may pass additional laws for the protection of those with illnesses and disabilities. Laws by the states may increase the protection offered by federal laws but cannot diminish that protection by less stringent regulations. Many agencies and organizations treating and working with ill and disabled patients and clients have developed a bill of rights for the guidance of their personnel. The bill of rights is based on federal laws and any applicable state laws, and copies of it are made available by the organization to handicapped people to whom they provide services. An example of such a bill of rights, developed by the Iowa Health Care Association, is given in Appendix VIII.

REFERENCES

1. René Dubos, "Introduction" in *Anatomy of an Illness as Perceived by the Patient* by Norman Cousins (New York: W. W. Norton and Company, 1979), pp. 18-20.
2. Esther K. Sleator and Robert L. Sprague, "Pediatric Pharmacotherapy" in William G. Clark and Joseph del Guidice, eds., Principles of Psychopharmacology, 2nd ed. (New York: Academic Press, 1978) p. 35.
3. Department of Health, Education, and Welfare, "Federal Register, Part V, Monday May 17, 1976" (Washington, D.C.: Office of Education) p. 20296.

SELECTED REFERENCES

Ennis, Bruce and Emery, Richard, *The Rights of Mental Patients: The Revised Edition of The Basic ACLU Guide to a Mental Patient's Rights* (New York: Avon Books, 1978).
Friedman, Paul R., *The Rights of Mentally Retarded Persons: The Basic ACLU Guide for the Mentally Retarded Persons' Rights* (New York: Avon Books, 1976).
Goldberg, S. S., *Special Education Law: A Guide for Parents, Advocates and Educators* (New York: Plenum Publishing Corp., 1982).
Hull, Kent, *The Rights of Physically Handicapped People* (New York: Avon Books, 1979).
Robertson, John A., *The Rights of the Critically Ill* (New York: Bantam Books, 1983).

Chapter 13

Graphic and Performing Arts

The graphic arts of a recreational program include various forms of painting, drawing, and craft activities. The performing arts comprise dance, music, and drama. Together the graphic and performing arts constitute a large and important segment of the special recreational program in treatment centers and community settings. Because they are expressive media, outlets for personal statements of rage, frustration, and conflict, these activities provide many clients unparalleled therapeutic benefits. The performing arts are particularly beneficial to those with difficulty in verbalizing. The graphic art activities, on the other hand, are unique in the opportunities they offer for the redevelopment of lost fine motor skills. Both activities also promote symbolic or non-verbalized expression.

GRAPHIC ARTS

The environment, tools, and apparatus of the arts and crafts can all be modified to permit clients who are restricted in their movements to participate. Modification of the environment may require the construction of ramps, in-cut tables, and special chairs; use of mirrors and adjustable and demountable frames for holding canvases; and reducing or eliminating the vibration in certain activities that causes the client to tire more easily. With some ingenuity, the recreationist can overcome many environmental difficulties that tend to cause unnecessary exertion or present barriers to engaging in art or craft activities. Developing tools and apparatus to enable a client's participation requires a thorough analysis of the impairment or disability that reduces the range of motion, strength, and flexion or extension of extremities. Body posture must also be taken into account. The need to assume a supine, sitting, or other relatively fixed position will influence the way in which the activity may be performed.

Factors Which Determine Adaptation

A variety of factors require consideration whenever art or craft forms are to be employed within the special recreational program for those whose strength, posture, or motion are limited by virtue of disease, accident, or birth defect. In some motions, gravity is important in increasing or decreasing the effort involved. For example, several craft activities require lifting a weight (hammer, punch, drill, etc.) where the use of motion is aided by the pull of gravity on the tool or limb. However, the preparatory motion is inhibited by the same force. So it is often helpful to use an offset sling, a device which facilitates the striking movement for execution but does not require the individual to overcome inertia by counteracting gravitational pull. Gravity also will have an effect on body position if the individual must work at or above shoulder level.

The ability to grasp a tool may have some important influences on the client's use insofar as leverage is concerned. The closer the tool is gripped to the striking part (hammer, awl, maul), the less leverage and the greater the effort necessary to accomplish the task, but control is increased. The weight and shape of the tool may cause difficulty in accomplishing some craft objective if the tool is not appropriate for the particular disability. Such disparity may make the effort expended disproportionate to the activity's intended achievement. For example, a hammer too heavy for use in planishing might forestall important joint range activity, although this would be one reason for prescribing such an activity.

Ensuring Safety. Safety of the client is an important consideration in determining whether certain craft activities may be employed within the therapeutic situation. Activities that require many tools are contraindicated for the psychotic patient who may be suicidal. On the other hand, countless art and craft forms require no tools or implements other than the materials themselves. In a controlled and prescribed program clients, depending upon the nature and severity of their illness or impairment, may first participate only in activities that require no tools; and then, as they improve in ability to handle these activities, the clients are introduced to other activities that necessitate progressive use of more and more tools until the range of their accomplishment includes almost any device or implement.

Generally, kinetic or skill analysis of all craft or art activities should be made so the complete motion necessary for accomplishment of the activity is known. The cycle of a complete motion comprises a preparatory movement, executionary movement, and recovery movement. In certain cases more energy may be required for the preparatory movement than the executionary movement. When the preparatory movement can be made, there is no difficulty; however, in some circumstances muscular weakness prevents the preparatory movement necessitating either the use of some adapted device or the substitution of another activity. Only with a thorough analysis of the movements inherent in the activity can the recreationist determine whether or not the projected experience will be a safe and beneficial one.

In addition, the type of muscle contraction must be recognized. It must be known whether the muscles used contract statically, intermittently, rapidly, or slowly; whether there is passive contraction, extension, or stretching must also be understood. For example, in radial nerve palsy, the fingers have a tendency to curl despite the preventive appliances which are worn. There is great difficulty in contracting the extensor muscles voluntarily. Craft activities that utilize kneading motions of the fingers emphasize contraction of these muscles and so may effect improvement in extension as well as flexion of the fingers. Thus, clay modeling, dough kneading, and sawdust carving, which require a certain amount of kneading and finger extension, are beneficial recreational activities.

Joint range must also be noted because some activities require less flexion and extension so that little value is derived from the movement. Wherever joint movement will be required, the degree of the normal or practical range of movement in the joint to accomplish the activity should be noted. This is necessary so that over-exertion and possible damage to the joints will be prevented. The first position taken when an activity is begun will have a strong influence upon the joint range and effort necessary, depending upon the stance of the individual. Whether the patient is standing, sitting, bending, or reclining, the strength required, muscle use, as well as joint range involvement will vary depending on how the activity is to be performed insofar as position is concerned.

Finally, safety requires that tools should be scrutinized to determine the correct sizes and shapes for use by those who may have difficulty in grasping or who experience restriction due to limitation of joint range or capacity to move the instrument. Variations of tool sizes and shapes may require altered motions, new combinations of muscular contractions, and range of movement. When the analysis of mechanics and anatomy has been fulfilled, it is more likely that activities will be presented in realistic terms of what can be accomplished within the restrictions. Modifications of position, substitution of adapted tools, reliance upon healthy muscles to compensate for and assist weak or injured body parts, manipulation of the material to be worked upon, or changing the working space to accommodate the client and whatever appliances or contrivances must be used for support—all of these may effectively adapt a craft activity for the disabled person.

Selecting Arts and Crafts Activities

The selection of the craft activity, from which valuable consequences may be obtained, will rest upon several factors. Age, sex, and interest will be factors to be considered in motivating clients. Depending upon the prescription indicated insofar as orthopedic or surgical cases are concerned, a comprehensive range of crafts should be available with which clients can experiment. There are so many kinds of crafts that the recreationist who has analyzed the motions which are required will be able to offer stimulating projects as a means for initiating functional restoration. Patients who are forced to remain in bed for prolonged periods because of lower extremity fractures, pulmonary disease, or cardiopathic problems require therapeutic recreational activity which can satisfy their particular needs. In the absence of a rehabilitation team, physician and recreationist should ally themselves in the development of a plan which has for its objective the immediate improvement of the current condition and the eventual physical and mental betterment of the patient.

Where there is neural disorder, crafts may be utilized to train synergistic muscles (those that act in concert with another). When a muscle is partially paralyzed or recovering from paralysis, adapted craft forms should be introduced as soon as possible. Activity develops tolerance to fatigue and permits enhanced physical condition. Motions will probably be gross muscular movements initially but will progress to fine ones as strength and coordination are restored. The first goal in any sudden severe disability, such as occurs from peripheral nerve or spinal cord lesions, is the amelioration of depression which normally accompanies the impairment. Craft activities, provided at the level of the patient's capacity to perform in conjunction with kinetic analysis for optimum restoration, will do much to relieve the patient of anxiety.

A comprehensive array of activities capable of interesting both sexes and any age group can be performed in the prone position, for example, with the appropriate appliance. Perhaps the best activity for strengthening upper extremity muscles, for those clients who will use either wheelchair or crutches after leaving the hospital, is macrame. This art may be performed almost anywhere and is particularly useful for those in bed. Knotting various fibers requires exercise of flexors, triceps, and deltoids (muscles of the arms and shoulders) which need to be strengthened if the individual is ever to be able to gain the ambulatory independence that use of crutches makes possible. The end product is limited only by the imagination and creativity of the participant. Macrame is also utilitarian. When dense knots are made from woolen fibers, coverlets, throws, bedspreads, or ponchos may result. Or lovely wall hangings or tapestries may be created. In any case, this is the easiest bed exercise which forcefully contracts and, therefore, strengthens the muscle groups of the arms and shoulders.

Functional Considerations in Craft Activities

The most valuable activity is the one which carries out the intent of the treatment goal, i.e., forces the range of motion and effort expenditure. In most instances a single craft activity will be sufficient to accomplish what is desired; but there may be times when more than one activity is required to maintain the pace necessary to progress. As always, any prescribed activity will contain motions that are less useful to the patient; consequently, desirable motions should be stressed, or activities chosen which reinforce the more valuable patterns.

Adaptation of craft activities will necessarily mean devising tools, equipment, or apparatus which will enable patients to achieve more effective participation. Modification of apparatus, tools, body positions, stance, motion, or security may have to be undertaken if desirable objectives are to be achieved.

Apparatus Modification. Wherever a craft room utilizes power tools, large looms, or other such devices, platforms of various heights and sizes of solid construction will probably be needed. By use of variable height platforms clients can be placed at appropriate heights, relative to their activity, so that the desired range of motion can be either increased or changed. Special clamps, clips, or hooks may be devised for clients with little prehension in one or both hands. If a stabilizing holding device is provided, one hand may be able to do the work of two. For bed patients for whom postural traction is required, it may prove worthwhile to construct an easel which can be shifted for variable height and inclined plane demands. In some traction cases the patient's head is below the trunk of the body, thereby making an ordinary easel useless. The variable easel tips forward to permit art activities. The construction of an attached tray capable of holding paints, brushes, crayons, or pencils is an important aid. Slings, springs, adjustable lapboards, and overhead looms or reading boards are some of the other kinds of apparatus that must be devised to accommodate clients whose disability requires them to maintain supine positions or for whom the loss of muscular or joint range requires a stabilizing or assistive device.

Modification of Tools. The tools that are used in art or craft activities available for clients in well-organized special recreational programs are not generally valuable insofar as extending range of motion is concerned. Normally, tools are designed to minimize muscular effort. In order to benefit clients who need the desired exercise for increasing muscular conditioning and range of joint motions, a tool must be tailored to fit the individual and his or her disability. Handles may be modified to enable the client to grasp the handle or gripping part more easily. Among the alterations which are frequently employed are built-up handles that permit total contact with the hand. Tools frequently requiring adaptations are the hammer, mallet, knife, saw, plane, chisel, screw driver, hand drill, spoke shave, gouge, and rasp. Angled handles permit the client to reach and grasp the tool at the appropriate place. Stirrup attachments enable patients with restricted movements of rotation to grasp properly whatever levers are necessary for operation. Lengthening or shortening the handles can augment facility. in grasping.

Modification of Motion. Sometimes beneficial motion is available only in monotonous or unsatisfying drudgery. An example of this is the rotation movement of the forearm—best achieved with a screwdriver. But the constant use of a screwdriver can be boring and unrewarding for the patient. However, many woodworking procedures require elbow and shoulder flexion and extension. Motions in these planes can be redirected into rotation of the forearm by the adroit placement of cams, levers, pulleys, and right-angled gears.

Modification of Body Position. Almost all craft activities are accomplished in either a standing or sitting position. Those clients who, because of illness or disability, cannot either sit or stand must be accommodated by art or craft activities that can be performed while maintaining the required medically prescribed position. By utilizing the patient's bed as the rigid frame, weaving, macrame, painting, drawing, or clipping and pasting can be performed.

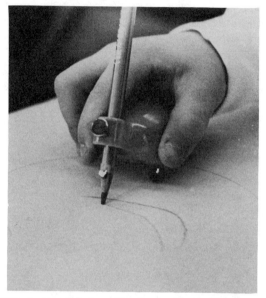

Fig. 13-1 A specially designed device with wheels allows a client with greatly reduced movement in the fingers and hands to draw or write. (Courtesy of the inventor, Takuma, Japan).

Art as a Therapeutic Adjunct

Art is an expressive medium which has been exploited in many of its forms from soap carving to sculpturing and painting. Art productions, both controlled and spontaneous, especially those by children and psychotics, have been studied for their personal-symbolic significance. Finger painting has been a medium for work with children as a therapeutic outlet, and as a means for understanding the child artist. Drawings and paintings as vehicles to interpreting unconscious processes have been a valued diagnostic instrument for more than half a century. One of the richest and most rewarding means of insight into the nature of human psychopathology is through the fine arts. The entire range of graphic and pictorial arts offers a source of experience and understanding of the disorganized personality. In painting, for example, artists are free to see the world as it appears to them. They may twist and distort the world of reality and use symbols and the images of the dream as a method for expressing themselves. Art activities have demonstrated their usefulness for achieving emotional catharsis, especially among patients who have difficulties in releasing tensions or in translating their ideas into words.[1]

Spontaneous art projects are more commonly performed in the treatment setting, where the patient can be observed during the process and where therapeutic discussions can follow on the heels of the completed work.

Therapeutic Values. Physically handicapped individuals may profit from graphic art work at least to the same extent as can the mentally ill. The therapeutic values to be derived from painting or drawing for one who has cerebral palsy or has lost the use of both hands and arms are significant; ability to express oneself through visual arts, particularly when the effort requires extreme discipline, can contribute to perseverance and eventual adjustment to a life with a physical disability.

The recreationist can gain considerable insight into the circumstances which influence the client by simply observing art activities. It can be significant to consider the implement with which the graphic or plastic art product has been created. Was the corporal self used as the medium for application or was there a surrogate body? Were thumbs, fingers, hands, or feet employed in the creation of the symbol? The feelings of the artist about the subject represented through sculpture, drawing, or painting may be inferred by the method of approach as well as the finished composition. The various forms of art enable clients to express their inner feelings and ideas. Just as drawings can be obliterated by smearing or scribbling, so too may feelings be covered over as though the individual were ashamed of the thought content.

The art works which clients perform are directly related to their life experiences and the feelings which they have about them. Individuals who have been rejected or who have failed in coping with social situations often symbolize these relationships in drawings or paintings that are indicative of their problems. Some clients compulsively paint scenes devoid of human beings; others depict a single lonely person being watched by apathetic crowds. Mentally ill persons often draw or paint in ways that can only be described as surreal and / or abstract. As the individual loses contact with reality there is a tendency to paint or draw with greater elaboration, filling in blank spaces compulsively, and creating forms which are magnifications of the bizarre.

Whatever the art form utilized, a great deal of therapeutic value exists in the process of creating and destroying. In finger painting, for example, the picture can be destroyed because the paint has to be smoothed out before another picture can be made. In the process much may be revealed about the client. What is smoothed away may be of greater significance in understanding the problems of the individual than what is finally completed. The kind of movements used, the relation of mood and color to the individual's feelings and the manner in which one subject in the picture can be, and is, changed to become something or someone else—all of these have a bearing on the client's way of looking at things and may represent deep-seated problems.

On occasion, art work helps the client to express hostility which is sublimated. Sometimes the art activity can be useful in alleviating pent-up emotions through catharsis. When individuals harbor aggressive tendencies, which cannot be worked out in direct release, they may become emotionally unstable or so preoccupied with hate that they are incapable of functioning. It is possible that art activity that permits release of emotional hostility through the use of colors that depict mood, strokes that symbolize violence, or an attack upon the drawing or painting surface that invites release becomes, in fact, the modality which permits the establishment of a therapeutic relationship between client and recreationist.

No one experience will resolve all of the difficulties which frustrated, hostile, or ill people have. However, a program which offers opportunities to display hostility in sublimated form or which is accepted by the recreationist without remonstrance can be the basis for helping the patient to express fantasies, fears, and anger. The full range of artistic expression may be employed to achieve specific therapeutic values. Clients may be enabled to overcome threats to their ego by the exposition of art. Concomitantly, such individuals might also be receiving psychiatric assistance. Whether for diagnosis, self-expression, insight, or satisfaction, art can reveal possible manifestations of difficulties which trouble the client. Finally, there is the possibility of complete emotional expression where verbalization fails to translate the real intent and meaning which the inarticulate individual wants to convey.

PERFORMING ARTS

Personal participation in any aspect of the performing arts offers direct therapeutic value to the client involved. There may be ancillary benefits also. Precisely what values will result from participation in the performing arts is not readily determined since reactions to music, dance, dramatics, and other similar activities evoke a range of emotional states which usually cannot be assessed. But there are some basic substantive effects which seem to occur as a consequence of engagement in performing art activities. These benefits can be enhanced by modifications of physical requirements that limit or prohibit participation by those who are ill or disabled.

Dance: Program Considerations and Adaptations

Dancing is a personal means of expression through physical movement. It combines the use of rhythmics, body motion, and control of extremities and torso for conveyance of ideas, emotions, or suppressed attitudes which are inappropriately transmitted through verbalization or which cannot be articulated. The use of hands and arms, head, torso, and legs in pauses, spins, leaps, and dramatic movements offer an emotional outlet which finds expression in no other form. Moreover, the vigorous dance movements provide total body exercise and thereby promote the benefits of physical fitness.

Dance may be performed at almost any age. It is useful in translating heritage and contemporary fads, for relaxation and fun, and as an expression of mood. It is an activity that helps to free the mind from depressing preoccupation and can be used to promote individuality, social contact, personal security, and identification. The dance provides a means for low-keyed explication of mood or dramatic signals which may reveal behavioral actions that could never be demonstrated in speech. It must be seen or participated in to be appreciated because, unlike other art forms, dance is not permanent. Some ritualistic pattern may be passed along from one generation to the next, but spontaneous movements which are not codified in some formalized sequence are lost.

The dance may be analyzed in terms of personal usage and specific value which may be obtained as a result of dance participation. Dances may be used to exhibit high skill or to diminish the possibility of anxiety through solo performance. Dance may be engaged in by couples or groups and such formations may be helpful in overcoming timidity, awkwardness, or lack of skill, depending upon the forms. Thus an individual who might be afraid to participate in a solo or couple formation could be assisted in a group formation. An individual who might be threatened by the close contact which couple dancing provides could be enabled to subordinate that fear when surrounded by or in line with many other persons.

Adaptations. The adaptation of conditions to meet needs arising from disability may be observed when wheelchair-bound individuals participate in square, round, or folk dances. In such atypical situations, the individual cannot dance because of disability. Nevertheless, by manipulation of wheelchairs, either by the individual or by having the chair propelled by ambulatory patients or volunteer workers, through the figures and formations, the clients in wheelchairs may actually participate. Dance activities can also contribute to therapeutic goals where disorganized personalities are concerned. The values to be gained by introducing maladjusted individuals to dance can be obtained through the utilization of spontaneous movement patterns, auditory reactions, spatial relationships, and optical sequences. Repetitive motions may have a soothing or stimulative effect on the dancer.

It has been observed that schizophrenic patients often display distur-bance by rotation of the body or spinning.[2] It is possible that other patterns may be introduced to such disturbed persons thereby blocking the char-acteristic movement and leading to the capacity to express distress in ways that have therapeutic value.

Perhaps no group of disabled people receives greater therapeutic value from dancing and rhythmic activities than those who are blind. Rhythmic movements and the physiologic reactions that accompany them are quite stimulating and motivating to blind clients. They are much more capable of achievement in dance because sound is of greater importance than vision in establishing muscular patterns. Unstructured dance offers greater assistance to the blind person insofar as spatial relationships are concerned. More significantly, it helps to teach poised movements and mobility for walking. Blind individuals can be taught to respond with ex-treme sensitivity to the sounds around them and can translate rhythms into dance patterns without much difficulty. In this way they may also appreciate time and space dimensions which provide a sense of security which might otherwise be missing.

The various forms of dance appeal in several ways to different indi-viduals with disabilities. For some the dance becomes a means of ex-pressing deep-seated feelings which cannot be expressed in any other way.[3] For others, the participation in a rhythmic movement offers an opportunity for learning kinesthetic sensitivity, balance, and spatial rela-tionships.[4] To still others it presents a social challenge and permits het-erosexual interaction. Basically, the various types of dance offer great appeal because of the patterned movements which motivate participants.

Music: Program Considerations and Adaptations

Music is universally recognized as an international medium. There has never been a culture which did not have some music by which it could create satisfying organized sound as a form of expression. Music, as a worldwide and instantly recognized language, promotes emotional dis-plays and stimulates mood changes in people. While it is difficult to be certain of which music can be tolerated by and used to benefit clients who are depressed, hostile, or disruptive, it is known that the playing of selected pieces of music can alter and modify moods. Not enough is known nor has there been sufficient experimentation to be able to state, with certainty, that a particular piece of music will always elicit a specific reaction from a given individual. Music appears to suggest certain emo-tions and this may be helpful when dealing with individuals who either need stimulation or relaxation.

Adaptations. Adaptation of music to meet disability needs may be possible through the use of any object that can be handled to produce sound. Thus, sandpaper blocks rubbed together produce a snare drum effect. Almost any sound can have some musical representation and literally anything can produce sound. Fabrication of so-called instruments is a question of ingenuity. The production of music does not require real instruments. Vocalizing, humming, whistling, clapping, drumming, strumming, blowing, and rubbing can all produce acceptable music, particularly if accompanied by at least one instrument which supports the melody.

Adaptation may also consist of developing prosthetic attachments so that instrumental music may be performed by clients who either want to learn or who already have the skill and knowledge to play. Peters has made several good suggestions for a school child that can also be utilized for clients in the recreational program:

> One way is to select an instrument for the child which can be handled without use of the disabled part. Another way is to adjust the instrument to the child. For instance, the piano pedals can be adjusted to the reach of a child with leg deformities, or an instrument ordinarily held can be placed in a fixed position.
>
> A third way is to adjust the child to the instrument. A variety of ingenious prosthetic appliances are possible to allow for the most discriminating motor movements. The teacher's knowledge of what movements are required in playing musical instruments, combined with the prosthetics expert's knowledge should result in a satisfactory adjustment for almost any disabled child.[5]

Recordings may provide the medium for appreciation, or accompaniment, for the kind of listening enjoyed by patients or clients. Recorded music may be used for stimulative or for sedative purposes. Background music intended to suppress noise has been found to have a calming effect.[6]

As with other therapeutic recreational activities, the patient may be encouraged to develop self-expression through the use of a specific musical instrument. The use of electronic devices, such as tape recorders and mixers, permits musical composition. One experiment performed with mental patients found that the application of music had definite value in strengthening group cohesion and interpersonal relationships, in facilitating emotional release, and in enabling the patient to experience better personality integration.[7]

Vocal Music. Singing is especially invaluable for expression of feelings, aspirations, or ideas. Vocal music offers the opportunity for individuals, who might otherwise remain inarticulate, to sing about what they cannot verbalize. The sense of cohesion in a group singing some well-known traditional folk songs or even popular songs can be sensed almost immediately. Losing oneself in the process of singing can cause some individuals to feel better physically. Some songs express themes of ambivalence, defiance, hostility, or action. All or some of these ideas may need expression by the individual who neither has the courage nor the capacity to discharge tension brought about by such feelings. Music making may become the avenue for indirect discharge of emotional feelings. Through music anti-social behavior or bizarre conduct may be sublimated and this has therapeutic value for the individual so involved.

Those who cannot sing may still gain emotional release by participating in rhythmic activities. Music accompaniment on rhythm band instruments of whatever homemade variety is produced, affords individuals a medium for making noise and demonstrating a full range of feelings which might otherwise be concealed. Pounding, clapping, blowing, or simply keeping time can be expressive and healthy for those who have no other way of legitimately giving vent to their emotions. Moreover, it provides an outlet for physical activity which may be highly beneficial for those who have a need for exercise of muscles and joints. The therapeutic values of music to both physically and emotionally ill persons can be seen in relieving the effects of boredom, in promoting a new or renewed interest which makes the client susceptible to treatment, and even in retaining whatever contact with reality the patient may have.

Carefully controlled musical experiences can assist in the general recreational program by creating an atmosphere more conducive to the therapeutic goals established by the rehabilitation team. Music need not be played or sung by patients themselves. Electronic devices may be the instrumentality for bringing music into the ward. In more fortuitous circumstances, musicians may give their time in voluntary efforts to bring live music to incapacitated patients. Regardless of the disability, clients can take some part in musical activity. The bedridden or wheelchair-bound person can participate by using modified instruments that are light enough to be supported on a stand, attached to a brace fitted to the bed or chair or by shaking or kicking a rhythm instrument that has been strapped to arm or leg. If the individual is unable to participate in these ways, peripheral participation may be possible by the simple expedient of nodding the head or shaking a finger or other body part that can be moved.

Drama: Program Considerations and Adaptations

Drama is a means of projecting specific ideas and emotions through action, verbalization, or both. It is a highly personalized form of expression where the focus of attention is on the individual performance. Drama provides a means for gaining attention and enhancing opportunities to be creative. More significantly, it often enables the participants to gain insight into their own problems as a consequence of playing a role or acting out a given situation.

"Psychodrama has been defined as a deep action method of dealing with interpersonal relations and private ideologies, and sociodrama as a deep action method of dealing with intergroup relations and collective ideologies."[8] In psychodrama, the patient is encouraged to enact on a stage a life situation or experiences relating to personal difficulties. The particular situation employed is suggested by the recreationist or by the patient. In the process of acting out, the patient reveals much of his or her underlying personality organization—motivations, conflicts, and usual ego defenses. Of even greater importance, however, is the cathartic effect upon the patient of the acting out of conflicts and traumatic experiences. Here may be expressed fears, resentments, jealousy, guilt, shame, or inner desires which cannot or may not actualize in everyday life. Learning to express oneself easily and spontaneously and to meet new situations as they arise in the dramatic reenactment usually proves advantageous to the individual because it offers freedom from inhibiting emotional frustrations and encourages greater resiliency and skill in interpersonal relations.

Dramatics permits the individual to play a unique role which differentiates the actor from all others. No one can play an identical role because there is always an interpretative aspect in attempting to create a character or in playing oneself. Of all the performing arts, drama best lends itself to adaptation. Regardless of handicap or disability, the individual who wishes to participate in dramatics is enabled to do so. Creative or spontaneous drama permits the widest range of adaptation to meet the needs of the individual performer. Here the individual is attempting to demonstrate some incident, idea, story, or role which suits the personality and immediate environment.

Drama has significant therapeutic values and has been utilized in the analysis and treatment of the mentally ill. Moreno developed the psychodrama as a medium for acting out repressed emotional fantasies.[9] Other dramatic forms have also been employed to release emotional tension. Bender and others tried puppetry as the medium through which children with emotional problems could express hostility, conflicts, and give vent to feelings which were otherwise denied.[10]

Spontaneous Drama. Pantomime, extemporization, and creative dramatics are spontaneous experiences typically based upon the experiences of the individual involved. Sometimes people find that they can express their feelings best through movement of the body or some of its parts. No words are required to convey what the person really wants to say. It assists the individual who finds verbalization too threatening. It may lead to the use of single words or phrases which gradually enable the individual to articulate some of the emotions which have been suppressed. Extemporizing is based upon cues or conditions with which the participating individuals are familiar. It may be a well-known theme, story, or situation which encourages a spontaneous development of characters and permits the outpouring of extremely personal feelings and attitudes that might otherwise be hidden. Because this form of drama poses no threat to the individual, since any untoward act or emotional expression may be cast off as "mere play acting," the participant may reveal feelings or attitudes of frustration, hostility, prejudice, or any negative emotion without guilt.

Adaptations. Dramatics may be adapted to meet the contingencies thrust upon any individual by illness or disability of almost any kind. For those who are fearful of performing before others, because such activity might prove embarrassing if lines were forgotten, dramatic readings can be substituted. Plays may be performed as though they were radio performances so that performers read the script without having to memorize lines. In this way fears will be alleviated and the individual enabled to participate in a beneficial experience. Other patients may be able to memorize lines but are afraid of the demands which a role may place upon them. Such roles can be rewritten—a favorite form of adaptation.

For clients who want to act, but cannot bring themselves to the point of exposure to an audience, simple activities can be devised. In some instances roles may be created for such clients in which they make entrances and exits without having to say anything. Sometimes they can be motivated to deliver "one-liners." As they find success in overcoming the basic fear of being on stage and as they develop confidence from whatever small speaking assignments are provided them, they may be encouraged to attempt more extensive performances. For patients who achieve security through reliance upon others, group or choral readings are possible adaptions of drama. Here the entire ensemble chants or recites a set piece, prose or poetry, in unison. The timing and tone are important to producing a pleasant effect, but for the performers, there is a certain freedom of expression since they may use normal speaking voices and do not have to "act." Choral speech provides a dramatic setting for performers, permits solo voice parts and group speaking parts, but is not as demanding as some of the other forms of drama. It does encourage some aspect of self-expression and offers security to the individual at the same time. A role is provided to those individuals unable to take a solo part or act in a play; they are encouraged to combine their voices with others, thereby contributing to the pleasure and satisfaction of the entire group.

Puppets and Marionettes. For patients who can only express themselves when there is no fear of personal exposure or for those who require complete anonymity before they can lose inhibitions, hand or rod puppets and marionettes on strings may be employed. Here the individual can remain concealed while manipulating the puppets and marionettes behind the scenes. Clients may forcefully express whatever feelings they may wish through the character and lines they give the puppet or marionette. In whatever way the patients project, showing love, hate, destructive tendencies, anti-social behavior, or other emotion, they will dare to express themselves because there is a substitute figure on which to heap any blame.[11] Of great significance is the identification which the clients make with the puppet or marionette. Whether the client is mentally ill or physically disabled, the use of puppets and marionettes may be adapted to meet specific needs. When a client is bedridden, it is possible to employ hand puppets or finger puppets which can be manipulated as the patient sees fit. Marionette theaters may be reduced in size and adjusted to fit on the client's bed or wheelchair so that manipulation can occur.

The therapeutic use of puppets has been explored by several researchers and the indications are that patients use puppets as a method for investigating and finding solutions to problems, for dramatizing fantasies, for expressing hostile or aggressive behaviors which otherwise could not be released, for ego-identification, and for a feeling of mastery.[12]

Puppets and marionettes may easily be adapted to conform to the level of skill which the client possesses. Many simplified puppet styles exist and these can be crafted quickly and used immediately. As patients develop a sense of the dramatic by using simple puppets, it is likely that greater expression will be evoked. Working with marionettes is much more complicated and requires skill and patience. When there is sufficient interest to carry the client along, and particularly where motivation is strong, the complicated procedures of puppetry and marionette manipulation offer an excellent therapeutic outlet for creative activity and catharsis.

Adaptation of drama and the utilization of substitutes which stand in for live actors require the ingenuity of the recreationist if these methods are to be successful. Depending upon the limitations of the clients, the recreationist will have to understand whether or not the individual is able to emote, needs the protection of a group before vocal expression is obtained, or requires the safety of a mask or doll to encourage true feelings to be displayed. Through these the client can gain either greater insight or be helped to achieve adjustment as a result of having revealed deep-seated conflicts or problems.[13]

REFERENCES

1. M. Naumberg, *Dynamically Oriented Art Therapy: Its Principles and Practices* (New York: Grune and Stratton, 1966).
2. Lauretta Bender, "Childhood Schizophrenia," *American Journal of Orthopsychiatry*, Vol. 17, No. 1 (1941) pp. 43-48.
3. Gertrude G. Bunzel, "Psychokinetics and Dance Therapy," *Journal of Health and Physical Education*, XIX (March, 1948) pp. 180-181.
4. S. R. Slavson, *Creative Group Education* (New York: The Association Press, 1948) p. 109.
5. Martha L. Peters, "Music and the Exceptional Child," *Therapeutic Recreation Journal*, Vol. II, No. 3 (Third Quarter, 1968) p. 6.
6. Donald Michel, "A Study of the Sedative Effects of Music for Acutely Disturbed Patients in a Mental Hospital," *Music Therapy* (1951) p. 183.
7. S. D. Mitchell and A. Zanker, "The Use of Music in Group Therapy," *Journal of Mental Science*, Vol. 44, (1948) pp. 737-738.
8. J. L. Moreno, *Sociodrama, A Method for the Analysis of Social Conflicts* (New York: Beacon House, 1944) p. 3.
9. J. L. Moreno, "Mental Carthasis and the Psychodrama," *Sociometry*, Vol. 3 (1940) pp. 209-244.
10. Lauretta Bender and R. G. Woltmann, "The Use of Puppet Shows as a Psychotherapeutic Method for Behavior Problems of Children," *American Journal of Orthopsychiatry*, Vol. 6 (1936) pp. 341-354.
11. Betty M. Lovelace, "The Use of Puppetry with the Hospitalized Child in Pediatric Recreation," *Therapeutic Recreation Journal*, Vol. VI, No. 1 (First Quarter, 1972) pp. 21, 38.

12. Jeanetta Lyle and Sophie Holly, "The Therapeutic Value of Puppets," *Menninger Clinic Bulletin,* Vol. 5, No. 6 (1941) pp. 223-226.
13. Dan Malatesta, "The Potential Role of Theatre Games in a Therapeutic Recreation Program for Psychiatric Patients," *Therapeutic Recreation Journal,* Vol. VI, No. 4 (Fourth Quarter, 1972) pp. 164, 166.

SELECTED REFERENCES

Anderson, E., *Crafts for the Disabled* (North Pomfret, Vermont: David and Charles, Inc., 1981).

Astel, Burt C., *Puppetry for the Mentally Handicapped* (New York: State Mutual Book and Periodical Service, 1981).

Atack, S. M., *Art Activities for the Handicapped: A Guide for Parents and Teachers* (Englewood Cliffs, New Jersey: Prentice-Hall, Inc., 1982).

Eddy, J., *The Music Came from Deep Inside: A Story of Artists and Severely Handicapped Children* (New York: McGraw-Hill Book Co., 1982).

Kay, J. G., *Crafts for the Very Disabled and Handicapped: For All Ages* (Springfield: Charles C Thomas, 1975).

Nordoff, P. and Robbins, C., *Therapy in Music for Handicapped Children* (New York: State Mutual Book and Periodical Service, 1981).

Robbins, C. and Robbins, C., *Music for the Hearing Impaired: Music, Special Education, Music Therapy* (St. Louis: Ragna music-Baton, Inc., 1980).

Shivers, Jay S. and Calder, Clarence R., *Recreational Crafts: Programming and Instructional Techniques* (New York: McGraw-Hill Book Co., 1974).

Walberg, F., *Dancing to Learn* (Novato, California: Academic Therapy Publications, 1979).

Chapter 14

Games, Sports, and Exercises

Games and sports have long been a popular feature of recreational programs. A more recent, but equally appealing, feature has been the exercise program, responding to the enormous public interest in physical fitness, athletic conditioning, and weight reduction. The fact of their widespread enthusiastic reception among the general populace identifies games, sports, and exercises as good program choices for ill and disabled clients, who take just as much pleasure in playing games and competing in sports as their nonhandicapped counterparts and are just as interested in being fit and slim. Suitable adaptations can enable clients with many kinds of disabling mental, physical, and emotional conditions to participate in a variety of games, to compete in sports, and to engage in exercise programs for fitness and weight reduction.

Competitive sports and games can be used to good advantage in the therapeutic and rehabilitative processes. For instance, the prescription for recreational activities may indicate a need for the client to develop assertiveness or self-confidence in physical performance, for which competitive sports and games provide suitable opportunities. Generally however, sports and games will be offered for their own sake, for the joy of participation and competition.

SPORT AND GAME ACTIVITIES

Selection of sport and game activities by the recreationist depends on the nature and severity of the disabling condition as well as the interests and needs of the client. Careful consideration must be given to the physical limitation and to the movements that are contra-indicated. Therapeutic recreationists will have to consider the specific requirements of the prescription and the need to supplement the exercises of the physical therapy program. The recreationist providing adapted recreational activities in the community must be concerned with choosing activities that can be engaged in with success and enjoyment.

251

With these considerations in mind, adaptations of the most popular sport and game activities are presented below for clients whose conditions range from bedridden to fully mobile but with certain physical restrictions or mental limitations.

Throwing and Catching Activities

A wide variety of catching and throwing activities is possible for both children and adults confined to bed as well as for those who are not. Among the possible items to be used are bean bags, assorted sizes of balls, balloons, and sponge rubber objects. With the exception of some types of balls, strings can be attached to the items to make retrieval easier. A simple target at which the objects can be thrown consists of concentric circles drawn on the floor with chalk; a more elaborate target can be constructed from a cardboard box divided into parts and decorated with pictures. A permanent standing target may be made from wood. Holes are made in the face of the target and each is given a designated number of points, depending upon the difficulty of throwing the object into the hole. To facilitate retrieval, cans with one open end are affixed behind each hole so that the ball or other object with attached spring can be pulled back through the hole. Another possibility consists of the use of nails instead of holes on the target face; the object in this case is to toss the bean bag at the target so that it hangs on a nail. Strings can be attached to the rings or the bean bags to make it possible for the patient to retrieve the rings; the target must be in an upright position for the rings to slip off successfully.

Various throwing and catching activities can be devised for bed play with balls. For the very young, a large soft ball should be used because it is easier to catch. Such a ball may also be necessary for weak or ill clients to avoid risk of injury in catching. Balls can be used for catching and throwing among several patients in bed, between two patients, and between bed patient and non-bed patients, recreationist, or volunteer. For individual play, a ball may be suspended from the ceiling with a rope so that it hangs at a suitable distance from the patient who is in bed or in a chair. The swinging rope will return the ball to a position within reach after each throw.

For basket shooting from the bed, a hoop may be attached to a stand and placed near the bed or improvised baskets made from wastepaper baskets or boxes may be set near the bed. For both of these activities, it will be necessary to have someone retrieve the ball for the client.

Balls may also be rolled at a target on the floor. Plastic bowling pins, Indian clubs, or improvised pins made of sand-filled milk cartons all make good targets. Possibilities for balls are plastic bowling balls, softballs, and soccer balls. Bed patients roll the ball in either prone or supine positions by swinging the arm over the side of the bed to release the ball along the floor in the direction of the target.

Blind clients can readily participate in catching and throwing. Whether the blind person is playing with a sighted person or a blind person, each player keeps the other one informed by indicating how and when the ball is tossed. The ball is thrown or rolled along the floor so that it bounces and can be heard by the blind person. In catching the ball in the air, the arms are held close together and extended forward, slightly bent at the elbow. As the ball comes in contact with the arms, they are brought to the chest trapping the ball. In catching a rolling ball the feet are spread and the hands are brought down between the feet with the palms facing the oncoming ball. The ball is trapped as it comes in contact with the hands or feet.

Young children enjoy throwing objects of different shapes; these may be made of sponge rubber cut into the shapes of animals or inanimate objects. Throwing handles on some of the objects adds further variety. A "frisbee" may also be cut from sponge rubber; this is an especially interesting throwing device since it can be thrown long distances. It glides at slow speed and is so soft that it will not injure the patient who is accidentally hit by it.

Disabled individuals with upper limb involvement may use the soccer skills of kicking and trapping for propelling and controlling the ball. Targets at which the ball is kicked may be set up. Bowling pins, milk cartons, or sticks driven into the ground are target possibilities. A soccer ball, volleyball, or playground ball may be used.

Yo-yo and Rope Spinning

Yo-yo tossing is a good activity for older children and also for interested adults. The yo-yo is played by dropping it over the side of the bed or chair, depending upon whether the patient is bedridden or able to sit in a chair.

Rope spinning is another activity for older children and adults which may be performed from the bed or chair. It is a difficult skill to learn but once mastered, it is easy to perform. A good stiff rope is needed. For spinning a rope from a chair or a bed, the slip loop must be made small enough so that the bed or the side of the chair will not interfere with its spin. To assist the beginner, the knot of the loop may be taped so the loop will not slip when the spin is begun.

Ring Tossing

Ring toss is another throwing game suitable for the bedridden patient as well as for other patients of limited mobility. The rings may be a commercial variety, but they can be easily improvised from stiff rope by braiding or taping the ends together to form a ring of suitable size. Jar rings or embroidery hoops may also be used. The target may be a nail driven through a board, which sits on the floor or table, or a triangular board with several nails or pegs affixed to it.

Dart Throwing

Dart throwing is suitable for all except the very young. The darts may be the standard type or may have suction cups at the ends replacing the more dangerous spikes. The latter, although safer, are more difficult to make stick on the target unless driven by great force such as release from a bow or gun.

Archery

Targets for archers in wheelchairs or on crutches will need to be placed on level ground without land elevation behind the target, as is generally desirable for stopping the arrows, because these patients will experience too much difficulty retrieving arrows from an elevated area.

Those in wheelchairs can most easily shoot the arrows by turning the side of the chair toward the target and then reaching over the side to draw the bow. Archers who use crutches can prop themselves with the crutches in such a way as to free their arms for shooting and still maintain balance. The usual method for doing this is to tilt the body toward the target, allowing the front crutch to take most of the body's weight. This action holds the front crutch firmly in place and frees the arm to hold the bow. The other arm must squeeze lightly on the other crutch during the drawing of the bowstring.

Clients with a missing or disabled arm will need to be supplied with some kind of device for anchoring the bow; a standard used to support a volleyball net is one possibility. The bow is fastened to the standard in a suitable position for the archer at the range at which he or she is shooting. The standard used for this purpose must have a heavy base or one of sufficient size to allow the archer to put a foot on it to hold it securely. In the case of a wheelchair patient with the use of only one arm, the bow is strapped securely to the chair. For those individuals who have difficulty in holding the bow in the hand as the string is released, a bow sling may be used. This is a device that is strapped around the bow and attached to the wrist.

The crossbow may be used effectively by those who are not strong enough to pull the string back. The bow can be used in a lying, sitting, or standing position. If the client cannot hold up the bow, it may be supported on a forked stick that has been driven into the ground.

To assist blind archers, a wire guideline may be strung from the shooting area to the target area; this enables them to go after the arrows and return to the shooting position. In addition, a stick about a foot in length can be anchored to the ground at the place from which the arrows are shot, pointing in the direction of the target. The blind archer can then feel the stick and make the alignment with the target accordingly. Two poles can be placed in the ground, aligned with the target and located at the points where the hand of the extended arm should be and where the back of the wrist of the drawing hand should be at the release of the arrow. In addition these poles may be wrapped with tape to assist the blind archer in sighting at the target. The placement of the tape is determined through trial and error with the assistance of a sighted person. With the tape in the correct place, the blind archer knows the sighting is correct when the backs of the hands touch the taped areas of the poles.

To enable blind clients to score with limited assistance, each section of the target may be outlined with a cord so that they are able to determine by feel what score to give the arrow retrieved from each section of the target.

Bowling

Bowling can be offered to almost every client who has the use of an arm. It can be played by all mobile patients, both ambulatory and in wheelchairs, and also in a modified form by bed patients. The game can be easily played by those who are blind with no modification of the skills; however, someone does need to tell them which pins remain standing and record the score. A guide rail is often used to teach bowling skills to the blind player. Holding onto the rail while the ball is released helps the blind bowler to keep in mind the location of the pins. However, seasoned blind players frequently find the use of the guide rail more hindrance than help. Clients with little strength and endurance or for whom strenuous activity is contraindicated can utilize the lighter weight polyethylene balls and pins, which can also be substituted for regular equipment when it is not available, for example, in correctional institutions. Play with this type of equipment is the same as with regular equipment with the exception of the grip, which is taken at the first joints of the fingers rather than the second joints as in bowling with a regulation ball. It should also be noted that the polyethylene ball is difficult to control in a spin so that only the straight ball should be thrown for successful results.

Clients who cannot take the necessary steps in delivering the ball may bowl from a chair or, if they are able to stand, may deliver the ball from the standing position at the foul line. To compensate for the lack of approach in the delivery, a preliminary swing is taken and the body leaned over as far as is necessary or possible to permit the ball to be released smoothly on the alley. In bowling from the bed, the arm is swung along the side of the bed and the ball released as smoothly as possible in the direction of the pins.

Wheelchair bowlers place their chairs facing the pins and lean over the side of the chair to deliver the ball. If the arm movements of such individuals are limited, it may be necessary to provide them with a trough-like device that is held in the lap and directed with the hands to send the ball in the desired direction down the alley toward the pins (Fig. 14-1). The device is made of lightweight metal and is used with a light polyethylene ball so that aiming and releasing are accomplished as easily as possible. If the bowlers in wheelchairs have use of their arms but cannot hold and release a ball, they may be able to bowl with use of a modified shuffleboard cue. The cue head is built up so that the head comes in contact with the center of the ball when the cue is pushed along the floor. In using this cue the ball is placed at the side of the chair on top of a jar ring to hold it in place. The player places the cue behind the ball and pushes it toward the pins. If both hands are needed to push the ball, it can be placed in front of the chair.

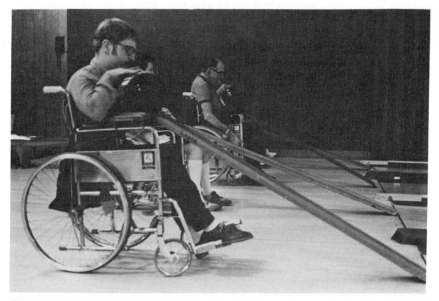

Fig. 14-1 Use of modified equipment while seated enables a client with restricted arm movement to enjoy bowling.

Golf

Golf can be readily adapted to the tolerance levels of those who lack endurance and strength: the number of holes to be played can be reduced, motorized golf carts can be utilized to reduce the amount of walking required, games of putting or of hitting into a net can be substituted for the game itself.

Clients with hand or arm disabilities will require adaptation only of the grip on the club. The most effective way to take the grip can best be determined through experimentation.

Those with limitations of mobility need to make adjustment in the stance to achieve the required balance for proper stroking. If a hip disability prevents bending forward at the hips, the golfer will need to stand closer to the ball or use longer than standard clubs. Lack of stability in the stance due to uneven weight distribution caused by leg impairment may be compensated for by spreading the feet apart to create a wider base. If a leg disability prevents the shifting of weight from one foot to the other, the length of the backswing must be reduced and the necessary force for the swing generated by the rotation of the hips rather than by the entire body.

Players on crutches can support themselves while stroking the ball, if they are right-handed, by bracing themselves with the left crutch only and, using a left-handed club, execute a back-handed swing with the right hand. Left-handed players must support themselves with the right crutch and use a right-handed club. In either case, some experimentation is necessary to find the best placement for the crutch; usually it is slightly behind and out away from the leg.

Those golfers who cannot balance themselves on one crutch and those who for other reasons cannot stand will be unable to play modified golf on a regulation course; however, they can engage in games that utilize golf skills such as driving balls into a golf cage or net and putting on the green while seated in chairs. Such chairs must have a wide base to prevent tipping. Wheelchair patients can also participate in these skill games. Players in chairs or wheelchairs must turn the chair to face the ball with their left side (for right-handed players) toward the direction of the intended flight of the ball. Extra long clubs may be needed by the wheelchair players in order to reach over the foot of the chair. There is a suction device on the market that slips over the handle of the golf club so that the ball can be picked up from the ground without stooping down.

Tennis

Play on the large area of a tennis court can, of course, be quite strenuous; therefore, adjustments in the size of the area to be covered in play may be made to reduce the amount of movement required and so make the game less demanding. In addition, regulation scoring can be dispensed with for those who have insufficient endurance and/or skill to keep the ball in play; one modified method of scoring is to count the number of times the ball is successfully returned during a given period of time. Reducing the size of the playing area is also a means of enabling those with restricted locomotion due to leg impairments to play tennis. If locomotion is not possible at all, the court may be reduced even more so that the player may remain stationary and make the necessary strokes by twisting the body.

The court size can be reduced to half of the singles court and chops and drop shots eliminated to accommodate players with restricted locomotion. A player in this case stands in the middle of the court about 2 feet behind the baseline. Another possibility is to increase the number of players to three or four on a side for a "doubles" game. If there are three players, one plays at the net and the other two play near the baseline on each side of the court; if there are four players, two play at the net.

Adaptations of the serving techniques are necessary for players who do not have sufficient strength or coordination to serve in the usual fashion or who have one or both arms missing. Those in the first category serve by bringing the racket in front of the body and tossing the ball into the air with the other hand; the ball is hit as it falls into range for stroking. One-armed players may make a similar adaptation except that they must toss the ball with the racket hand. To accomplish this, a regular grip is taken on the racket and the thumb and forefinger are projected beyond the handle to grasp the ball. The ball is tossed into the air and may be stroked as it descends or after it has bounced.

Double arm amputees, in order to play, will need to have the racket taped to the stump or prosthesis. The serve in this case is made by balancing the ball on the face of the racket and then tossing it into the air by means of a short quick upward movement and stroking it as it bounces off the ground.

Loose balls are retrieved with the racket. If the ball is stationary, the portion of the racket face near the handle is placed on the ball and it is drawn quickly toward the body to initiate a roll. The head of the racket is then slipped under the ball and it is brought to balance on the face of the racket. A loose rolling ball is retrieved by placing the racket face near the ball so it will roll onto the face, where it is brought under control by bouncing it gently. If the loose ball is bouncing, it is caught on the face of the racket and bounced lightly until under control.

Badminton

The easiest adaptation in badminton is reduction of the size of the court. Play may be limited to half the singles or half the doubles court, using the back serving line of the doubles court as the back line in either case. Players will not have to move to either side when playing half a singles court and will not need to move more than a step or two on a half doubles court. Elimination of the drop shot will remove the necessity for movement to and back from the net. Another modification that may be utilized to reduce locomotion on the court consists of working to keep the bird in the air for as long as possible by placing the bird close to rather than out of the range of the opponent.

Any player who has difficulty controlling the racket should modify the grip by taking hold higher on the handle than is customary. In serving, players with no wrist action may be allowed to serve in front of the service line in order to serve effectively to the back court. If it is not possible to take the correct position with the feet for serving, the player should manipulate the body by twisting at the hips.

Players with limited wrist action will not be able to smash as effectively as they can drop shot so they will have to use high clears and drop shots. Those with limited mobility playing on a half court with the drop shot made illegal will need to utilize smashes and high clears.

Badminton can be played successfully from wheelchairs. If there are several players in wheelchairs, they can be strategically placed to cover the entire court with minimum movement of the chairs. To increase court coverage from a chair, an extension can be taped onto the badminton racket. In addition, Velcro can be cemented around the top of a shuttle-cock and the top of a racket so that a player in a wheelchair can pick up the cock by touching the Velcro on the racket to the Velcro on the cock as the player is doing in Figure 14-2.

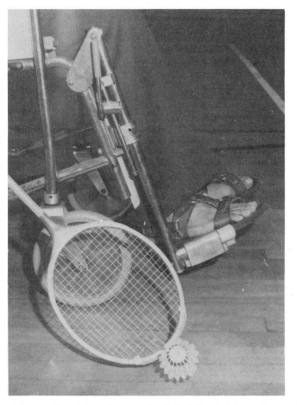

Fig. 14-2 A cock is easily retrieved by a wheelchair badminton player when Velcro is attached to the cock and to the racket rim.

Loop Badminton

Loop badminton is a game utilizing badminton skills that was especially developed for play by those who are unable to play regular or modified badminton. It is played with a badminton bird and table tennis paddles. The objective of the game is to hit the bird legally through a metal loop that is supported by an upright stand in the center of the playing court. It requires much less space than badminton and is more easily adapted to various limitations. Suggested size for the playing area is 10 feet by 5 feet. The loop, which may be constructed of heavy wire or of flexible strips of wood, is 24 inches in diameter and is secured to some type of upright stand such as a badminton or volleyball standard. The bottom of the loop is 46 inches from the floor. Restraining lines are drawn across the court 3 feet from the loop, which is located in the center of the court. Three dimensions for the court and loop may be adjusted as required by the disabilities of the players and the space available. Likewise, the playing regulations* may be freely adapted.

Table Tennis

Table tennis can be adapted for play by handicapped players in a number of ways. For wheelchair players, the table can be secured to the floor to provide support for holding onto the table to maneuver the chair. A further adaptation may be made by attaching a flexible steel rod to the side of the table beside the net. The ball is attached to the rod by a string which prevents the ball from rolling away when missed. This attachment works best on a portable table approximately 30 inches by 46 inches in size. The use of the rod is effective not only for players who are in wheelchairs, but for all those who have limited mobility.

Adapting the game for inexperienced blind players is done by limiting play to half of a regulation table on each side of the net. The other half of the table is covered with paper to produce a distinct sound when the ball lands on it, thereby enabling the player to differentiate between a good ball and an out-of-bounds one. Net of fine mesh, attached to standards, may be placed along the sides of the table to keep the ball on the table where it can be more easily retrieved, or thin boards may be permanently affixed along the edges to serve the same purpose. Another possibility is to substitute a string for the net; the player pushes the ball with the paddle so that it rolls beneath the string.

Modification of the paddle is also helpful to the blind or partially sighted table tennis player. One modification is a rectangular paddle made of a board $2\frac{1}{2}$ feet by $1\frac{1}{2}$ feet in area with handles attached to the two shorter sides. Another possibility is replacing the paddle with a space ball net which consists of a rectangular frame covered with netting, designed to be held in the hands.

The double handle paddle is gripped in both hands and held in front of the body. The ball is played by a pushing motion. Serving is accomplished by tossing the ball gently over the net to the opponent.

Those who must play from a chair usually find the pen holder grip more satisfactory than the handshake grip. In the pen holder grip the handle is held as if holding a pen in the hand with the head of the racket pointing down. Players in chairs and those on crutches who need to use the table for support may serve in front of the end line if this is necessary to maintain body balance.

---

*Regulation for scoring and playing are found in Fait & Dunn, *Special Physical Education: Adapted, Individualized, Developmental* (see selected references at the end of the chapter).

Players with only one hand can adapt the serve by holding the ball between the extended forefinger and thumb after taking the grip. The ball is tossed into the air and, depending upon the player's skill, is hit as it descends or after it bounces. Players without the use of either arm but with a functional stump can play with the paddle strapped to the stump. Serving in this case must be accomplished by tossing the ball into the air with an upward thrust of the paddle and hitting it before or after it bounces. In retrieving a loose ball, the player places the face of the paddle on the ball and draws the paddle quickly toward the body; simultaneously the paddle is slipped under the rolling ball to bring it onto the surface of the paddle, where it is brought under control by gentle movements of the paddle. If during play the ball comes to rest close to the edge of the table, it can be pushed with the paddle until it is near enough to reach with the head. The paddle is then placed flat on the table and the ball is pushed onto its face by nudging it with the forehead.

Shuffleboard

The shuffleboard court may be shortened for any disabled players who lack the strength or coordination to push the discs the total length of a regulation court. Blind players may be assisted in orienting themselves for proper aiming by placing strips of tape on the floor to be touched with the fingers.

The doubles game is in itself an effective adaptation for players with limited mobility since it does not require the changing of ends. The need to change ends may also be eliminated in singles by permitting one player to play from each end. The opponent counts the score and returns the discs by pushing them back to the other player for the next turn. Although this modification eliminates strategy to prevent an opponent from scoring, the game can still be an exciting one.

To push the discs, the wheelchair players should place the chair so that it faces the court and angles slightly to the side to permit the shot to be made from the side of the chair. A player in a straight chair may find it more effective to move the discs along the 10 off line to put them in the proper place for shooting than to move the chair into a satisfactory position. Bed patients who are able to lie on the front of the body or to sit in a semi-reclined position can play by extending the arm over the side of the bed to push the cue.

Simplified scoring may be desirable for young children or mentally retarded clients. To modify the scoring procedure, the number of discs that land within the scoring area can be counted, assigning each disc one point.

Tabletop shuffleboard makes an excellent game for those with limited movement. It may be played by bedridden patients by setting it on a table beside the bed. For those with limited movement of the arms, checkers may be substituted for the discs and the checker flicked with the finger, or the table may be placed upon the floor and the checkers pushed with a foot.

Basketball

To enable those with restricted arm movement and those confined to a chair to shoot baskets, the hoop may be lowered. If necessary to enable the player to retrieve the ball, a net may be strung from the chair to the backboard. Of great assistance to blind basket shooters in locating the basket is to hang a light string from the back side of the hoop above the head of the player but low enough to touch. In addition a small bell may be suspended inside the hoop so that a ball passing through the hoop will cause the bell to ring, informing the shooter that a basket was made.

A player with the use of only one hand, in order to catch the ball, will need to trap it between the lower arm and the body and then cradle the ball with the upper arm. Such players will make their passes with one arm, using the overhand for long passes and the underhand for short passes.

Players on crutches in receiving the ball are likely to find it easier to bring the ball to the side of the body instead of toward it because it is easier to maintain balance. They will have to utilize greater wrist snap than ordinary when making the two-handed chest pass. For most players on crutches, the one-hand pass will be the more easily and effectively executed, and one-hand shots will be more successful than two-hand shots. The maintenance of balance while receiving or passing the ball is facilitated by the use of the Canadian crutch (Loftstrand).

Blind players make the catch by extending both arms forward with the elbows slightly flexed. The ball is cradled in the arms as the fingers make contact with it to achieve effective control.

Basketball skill games and the game of basketball itself are played from wheelchairs with considerable success. Both one- and two-hand shots are possible. Power comes from the arms rather than the body.

Rules for playing wheelchair basketball have been standardized.* Samples of the rules follow. Players are forbidden to rise from the seat of the chair for the center jump or a jump after a tie-up. The ball may be advanced by passing or dribbling. A player dribbles by alternately moving the chair with a push on the wheels and tapping the ball on the floor. Making two or more successive pushes on the wheels without tapping the ball on the floor constitutes traveling. Contacts between players and wheelchairs are treated the same as contact between players in a regular game.

---

*Rules may be secured from the National Wheelchair Athletic Association, 40-24 62nd St., Woodside, New York 11377.

Softball

The strenuousness of the game can be modified by reducing the size of the diamond, decreasing the distance between the pitching mound and home plate, or by adding more fielders. Other suggested modifications include calling strikes only when the batter strikes and misses, not calling balls, and not permitting the batter to advance on calls. If a player is able to bat but cannot run, a teammate is designated to run for the batter.

Most disabled players will benefit from the use of a glove in catching, for it increases the efficiency of catching and, of course, reduces the risk of injury to the hand. Those with only one hand need to develop a special technique for catching with the glove and then throwing the ball. The technique, which is described below, can be used by anyone who has a functional shoulder joint and upper arm on the disabled limb. The technique consists of catching the ball with the hand of the functional arm and immediately placing the glove with the ball nestled in the pocket under the upper part of the disabled arm. The hand is removed from the glove without disturbing the ball and, in one continuous movement, the ball is grasped and thrown.

Players in wheelchairs or on crutches can master catching with a little practice. The crutches must be propped so that one arm bears most of the weight, freeing one arm so it is easier to catch the ball and throw it without losing balance. The upper portion of the body is utilized in throwing with the twist coming from the trunk rather than the hips. Anyone who is unable to twist or for whom twisting is contraindicated must make the throw completely with the arm.

Softball may be modified in several ways for blind and partially sighted players. Batting may be done from a tee. In running bases, a sighted runner may accompany the blind runner, making some kind of sound for guidance toward the base. The diamond is reduced in size and only one base is used. A run is scored when the player has run to the base and returned home safely. A large inflated ball is used. It is pitched by rolling it on the ground toward the hitter; the ball will make sufficient sound while bouncing to enable the batter to tell when and where to strike at it. The batter is out after three strikes; a foul ball is the same as a strike except on the last strike when another ball is rolled; three outs retire a side.

The ball is thrown underhand in every case so that it will roll and create a sound. Catching is accomplished by facing the direction of the ball with the feet spread to cover as great an area as possible. The hands with the fingers spread wide are placed between the feet ready to grasp the ball as it rolls toward the hands. In the case of partially sighted players, the ball may be thrown and aimed toward the extended hands of the catcher, who holds both hands with the palms up to form a basket for the ball to fall into.

To bat, blind players (if right-handed) stand with the left side to the pitcher. A kneeling position is taken on the left knee with the weight partially on the right foot; the left hand holds the bat near the end while the right hand is 4 or 5 inches above it. Batters notify the pitcher that they are ready and, when they hear the ball rolling forward, strike at it swinging parallel to the ground and a few inches above it.

Volleyball

Volleyball is another game that can be successfully modified for play by those in wheelchairs. The court may be enlarged or decreased, depending upon the number of players so that each player will not be required to cover an area larger than can be easily handled. For other handicapped players the area may be decreased or the number of players increased.

Those who have insufficient power to get the ball over the net in the serve may be permitted to move closer to it. A player with one arm will need to throw the ball high into the air and bat it with the same arm, using an overhand stroke.

Players who are unable to strike the ball to return it may be allowed to catch it and then throw it back over the net. If this is necessary for all or most of the players, the net should be placed somewhat higher. A score, when catching is permitted, is made when the ball is not caught or when it is thrown out of bounds or into the net. Throwing may also be substituted for the regulation serve. Blind players usually serve by throwing the ball. The ball is caught or trapped after it hits the floor. If it is not trapped or caught before it rolls out-of-bounds, the other side scores.

Wheelchair players will find the underhand serve the more practical. The serve is made by leaning to the side of the chair or by tossing the ball high into the air with one hand and hitting it with the other. The return is also made with one hand unless the player is skillful in maneuvering the chair into position to use both hands. The one-hand return is made by stretching the arm straight out to the side of the chair and, when the ball reaches shoulder height, striking it with the palm.

Players on crutches will utilize the same adaptations for serving and returning as the wheelchair player who plays with one hand. The player on crutches will need to develop skill at balancing with the crutches to free one arm for playing the ball.

Weight Lifting

Weight lifting is readily adapted to most handicapping conditions including some of those that require confinement to bed. However, for the majority of bedridden patients, weight lifting is a conditioning program for rehabilitation, rather than recreational activity, handled by the physical therapist or corrective therapist.

If a weight lifting machine is available, it is highly useful for those in wheelchairs and for the blind. Most machines are so constructed that a wheelchair can be rolled up to the machine to make the lifts; only for the bench press will the patient need to move from the chair. If moving is not possible or desirable, the muscles of the chest (pectoralis major), and shoulder (deltoid) and the triceps muscles of the arm can be conditioned by other exercises. The military press and spring exercises are good substitutes for the bench press.

The blind will find the weight lifting machine especially easy to use because it is not necessary to place on weights and fix collars as for barbells.

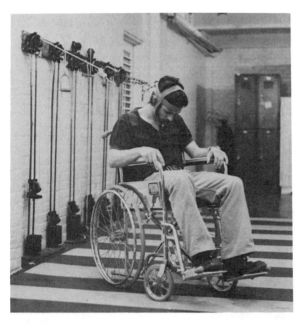

Fig. 14-3 A head harness can be attached to a wall pulley for exercising the neck muscles.

For those who are paraplegic or partially paralyzed in the upper limbs, wall pulleys are especially good. In a situation where the individual cannot grasp but is able to move the arms, the pulleys may be strapped to the wrists. For quadriplegics in wheelchairs, if it is not otherwise contraindicated, a head harness is attached to the wall pulley. The chair will need to be moved so as to allow the correct pull against the pulley weights. The neck can be extended, flexed, or moved laterally to exercise muscles.

Bag Punching

Bag punching is a suitable activity for perambulatory and ambulatory patients as well as for the blind. For those who must be seated the bag frame should be anchored on the wall low enough to be easily hit from the sitting position. If both standing and sitting participants are to use the bag, it will be necessary to have two different frames anchored on the wall at different heights. Although the height of the bag is adjustable in the frame, it is not possible to move it sufficiently to accommodate both sitting and standing participants.

Blind participants will need special instruction in bag punching. One of the most effective ways of introducing the blind client to bag punching is through the use of manual kinesthesis, i.e., leading the client's hands through the desired motion, making actual contact with the bag in good rhythm.

Track and Field Activities

Track and field events offer many opportunities for participation by the disabled. For convalescing patients the activities may need to be somewhat restricted, but for most others at least one type of track or field activity is possible with no or minimal modification. For example, individuals with lower limb disabilities are able to perform the throwing activities and those with upper limb involvement are able to engage in the running and jumping activities with no or slight adaptations. Even for wheelchair and blind participants the modifications are relatively simple.

For the long distance running events and jogging, blind runners are accompanied by someone with normal vision who either runs beside them or rides a bicycle just ahead of them to give the necessary auditory cues. For the shorter distance runs, it is preferable to string a guide wire along the track between supports at either end; no other supports should intervene so that the runner's hand can travel smoothly along the wire during the run down the track. If this arrangement is not feasible, someone can be stationed at the end of the course to guide the blind runner with continuous auditory cues.

Blind participants in the long jump or triple jump start from a stationary position at the takeoff point. To execute the high jump, they place themselves at the point of takeoff, swing the lead leg back and forth to achieve momentum, and then spring from the takeoff leg. The throwing events may not need any modification. In the javelin throw the distance of the preliminary run may be decreased to prevent the possibility of overrunning the foul line, or the throw may be made from a stationary position.

Running events for those in wheelchairs consist of the 50- and 100-yard dashes and a slalom race that tests the ability to maneuver the chair over an obstacle course. Throwing events can be performed from the chair with some adaptation of the style of throwing. If participants are able to use the trunk in throwing, they can develop a style utilizing a twist of the body to generate power. Otherwise, they must depend entirely upon the arm and shoulder for the necessary power.

Skiing

Many clients can participate in skiing with minor adaptations even though it is a relatively rugged sport. Use of outriggers enables those with lower leg involvement, including those with a leg amputation, to ski.

The outrigger is a short ski (16 inches) attached to a Canadian crutch by a hinge that allows the crutch to move forward or backward without tipping the ski. An outrigger is held by the hands on each side of the body to help the skier balance. The arm band is reinforced to stand the pressure exerted against it during the skiing.

Swimming

Special devices such as ramps and steps with hand rails may need to be installed to enable disabled clients to get in and out of the pool. A few may not be able to manage even with the assistance offered by these devices and so will need the aid of a helper. Whenever possible, it is desirable to have numerous helpers or volunteers present to assist with recreational swimming, particularly when instruction is being offered. Some, who have severe limitations in motor movement, will require support in the water. Such support can be provided by helpers and also by the use of flotation devices such as tubes, canisters, and water wings.

The disabled client can be taught the beginning and intermediate skills of swimming using the techniques commonly utilized in teaching non-handicapped people these skills. However, certain precautions must be observed.

Cardiac patients should not practice breath-holding; if necessitated by the severity of their condition, they should only float or swim without submerging the face.

Clients with ataxia may experience difficulty regaining their feet because of the poor sense of balance that is a symptom of the condition. Helpers should be ready to give assistance as needed.

Those with missing limbs will experience difficulty initially balancing the body in the water. They must be helped to find, through trial and error, the best adaptations of the conventional arm and leg strokes. The side stroke is usually the most easily mastered by those with a missing limb: the functional arm or leg is simply employed in the capacity of the missing member. Those with no legs will find that they can do the side stroke effectively in a partially prone position.

The back stroke is also usually easily accomplished by disabled swimmers since almost any type of movement will propel the body when it is supine in the water. In the crawl, the arm stroke may be modified by reducing it to less than a full stroke for any who have arm or shoulder impairments that prevent full movement. Those with weak shoulder joints subject to frequent dislocation should not perform the crawl stroke.

Floor Hockey

This game is a combination of ice hockey and field hockey, using indoor hockey sticks and a ball. The goals, which are placed at either end of an indoor playing floor, can be regulation hockey goals or simply large paper boxes anchored securely and cut so that the ball can enter. The game lends itself to play by various types of ambulatory and perambulatory players.

Tetherball

Nearly all types of handicapped clients can play tetherball with simple modifications. One-arm amputees have no difficulty in playing the game; double-arm amputees can play if it is possible to tape a paddle to a functional stump.

For playing from a wheelchair the rope holding the ball can be made longer to bring the ball within reach. However, with the longer rope the actual playing of the ball becomes more difficult. Therefore, it is more satisfactory to build an adjustable pole so the rope need not be made longer.

A table model of tetherball can also be constructed from a short pole anchored to a flat board. Table tennis paddles are used as paddles for the game.

Pool and Billiards

Pool and billiards are games that require a minimum amount of energy and are readily adapted to many different types of disabilities. Those who must stay in a reclining position can shoot pool or billiards from a cart that is approximately the same height as the table. If the client is right-handed, the cart is placed parallel to the table and the player grips the stick in standard fashion with the right arm. The stick lies across the chest. A regular bridge is required, but a sliding bridge attached to the cue stick may be substituted. A sliding bridge can be constructed from a smooth piece of wood rounded at the corners and taped to the cue.

The wheelchair patient playing on a standard pool table will need to grasp the cue with an underhand grip so that the cue can be brought over the shoulder. A bridge may or may not be used depending on the ability of the player.

Horseshoes

The game of horseshoes generally requires little adaptation for ambulatory or perambulatory players. It may be necessary to shorten the distance between the stakes or eliminate the preliminary steps for those unable to execute the steps. Those in chairs may throw the shoe by leaning to the side of the chair using regulation pitches. In cases where the player does not have sufficient strength to throw a regular iron horseshoe, a smaller lighter shoe may be substituted. The substitution may also be necessary for an ambulatory patient who is not able to take the preliminary steps in throwing or who lacks the strength to throw the standard horseshoe.

Box Hockey

Box hockey can be played with little modification by either perambulatory or ambulatory patients. The game is played on a court contained in a box that is about 18 inches by 60 inches in size. A partition in the center has holes in it through which a puck is knocked. Holes are also located at the ends of the court. Each player has a stick with which to attempt to knock the puck through the holes on the left. When the puck is knocked through the hole and out of the box, a score is made. The game may be played by two or four players.

Casting and Angling

No special adaptations need to be made in casting for either perambulatory or ambulatory clients if they are able to use both limbs. If there is a disability of one arm, a harness device that is strapped to the body may be used to anchor the pole. A holder attaches to the harness in which the end of the pole is placed after a cast is made, leaving the arm free to reel the line.

As a safety precaution for those fishing from wheelchairs, the chair's brakes should be set and/or rocks or logs placed in front and behind the wheels to hold the chair securely during the landing of a fish.

It is desirable that disabled nonswimmers who fish from a boat wear life jackets. Life jackets are also recommended for those who are blind regardless of their ability to swim if they are fishing in a body of water where it would be difficult for them to determine the location of the shore.

Canoeing and Boating

Canoeing and boating make excellent activities for clients with lower leg involvement because these activities do not require movement of the legs. The canoe or boat can be made more comfortable for the paraplegic client by the use of sponge rubber padding.

In a canoe without seats the pad is placed to cover the bottom of the stern and the gunwhale for protection of the legs and the back when the client sits in the stern. For seating in the center of the canoe, the pad is placed to the center and leaned up against the center thwart (brace) for a back support. The client sits on the pad with legs extended. In some canoes the thwarts are located so that it is not necessary to place the legs under them; this kind of canoe is recommended for use by paraplegic canoers. In canoes that have seats, the pad is draped over the back seat and up on the gunwhale to provide a back support if necessary. The client sits on the seat to paddle.

A paraplegic client can also row a rowboat. All rowboats have seats so it is not possible to utilize padding effectively. The rower sits on the seat. The J stroke is used if the boat is small, or strokes on both sides of the boat will keep it moving in a forward direction.

All disabled canoers and rowers should wear life jackets while they are in the craft.

Deck Tennis

Deck tennis makes an excellent mild activity for those with limited mobility. The size of the court can be reduced as needed to make it possible for the player to cover it easily. A more extreme modification is to change the objective from throwing the deck ring so that it cannot be caught by the opponent to throwing the ring so that it can be caught successfully. In this case, a score would be made by the thrower only when the opponent caught the ring.

Table Cricket

This game may be played either in a sitting or standing position. As many as four players may participate. Partners stand on the same side operating the sticks in an attempt to knock the ball through the goal on their left.

Scoop Ball

Scoop ball is played with a ball and a scooplike device, which is used to catch and throw the ball. The game is easily accommodated to play by bedridden and perambulatory clients. For those with limited mobility, a string may be attached to the ball to make retrieval easy when the ball is missed in catching. Targets similar to those described earlier for throwing and catching activities can be set up for throwing the ball at with the scoop. To increase the difficulty of throwing at a target, a moving target can be created by rolling a tire past the player. When several are playing, they can form a line and as the tire rolls by them, they attempt to throw the ball through the tire.

Scooter Play

The scooter, described in an earlier chapter as one of the pieces of equipment used to give mobility to those who have lower limb disabilities, can be used in recreational activities with great success. Players take lying or sitting positions as required by their conditions and propel themselves with their hands.

Any number of games can be readily adapted for play on scooters. Basketball may be played by substituting a wastebasket or similar container for the regular basketball hoop. The ball is advanced by passing and dribbling, depending upon the abilities of the players. To avoid the possibility of the fingers being rolled on by the scooters, players should maintain a distance of 3 feet from one another. A variation of soccer is played on the basketball floor with an Indian club set up at each end of the court. One player is assigned to guard the club against being knocked over by the ball, which is propelled by the hands or feet in any way that is possible for the players. Scooter hockey is played in much the same way except that the ball must be moved by bumping it with the front end of the scooter.

Parachute Play

Parachute play is suitable for many different types of disabling conditions with a minimum of adaptation. Mentally retarded clients in most cases, are able to perform the simple maneuvers of the activity, and often they can be involved in the more complex procedures such as changing places under the uplifted parachute or tossing a ball on top of the parachute. Blind children can perform readily in parachute play; however, they will be limited in the activity that requires change of place. If the participants are in wheelchairs, the edge of the parachute is held in their laps. Most of the activities performed in regular parachute play can be executed by those in wheelchairs.

Childhood Games

Disabled children should not be denied the joy of playing the familiar games of childhood like Pussy Wants a Corner, Drop the Handkerchief, Red Light, and Call Ball. Youngsters with physical and mental disabilities can, and should, be included wherever these games are played: on the playground, at camp, or at the community recreational center. The games should also be offered in therapeutic recreational and rehabilitation programs for children in treatment centers. Mainstreaming is usually fairly easily accomplished because the lack of complexity in play of the games makes extensive adaptation unnecessary. Modifications may include changing the usual procedures of playing the game, altering the playing space, and substituting a different kind of movement for the one routinely utilized.

The simple childhood games are played according to informal rather than strictly regulated procedures of play, so a change to accommodate the limitations of one or more players is relatively easy. One example will serve to illustrate the possibilities: The game requires that a player respond, upon hearing his or her name called, by catching a ball that is thrown by another player before the ball bounces more than once. For children whose mobility is impaired, the calling of the name can be made before, rather than at the same time, the ball is thrown to allow more time for the disabled player to make the catch. Additionally, the ball may be permitted to bounce 2 or 3 times before it must be caught.

Adjusting the area of the playing space that must be traveled through in a game generally consists of reducing the actual distance the disabled child must move. A child with crutches, for example, may be allowed to take a specified number of steps beyond the restraining line. Nearly all catching and throwing games can be reduced in distance to enable more successful participation by disabled children.

There are numerous possibilities for changing the manner of movement in which a game is ordinarily played. Walking, crawling, or moving on a scooter board can be substituted for running and skipping. Wheelchairs can be maneuvered in specific patterns to replace movements by the feet and body. The ideas suggested in the earlier discussion of sports and games for blind and deaf clients can be utilized also in games children play.

In the program of recreational activities of the treatment center there might be an insufficient number of children of an appropriate age to participate in the games. In these instances, modification to reduce the number of players needed is usually possible. Also, perhaps volunteers or visiting family members can be used to fill out the ranks. It may even be possible to bring children from the community into the treatment center on certain days to take part in the games.

COMPETITIVE SPORT TEAMS

Players with disabilities frequently become so skilled in playing sports with certain adaptations that they wish to join with other proficient handicapped athletes to form a team for competitive play with other teams of disabled players or with nonhandicapped teams. They certainly deserve to have such opportunities, and the recreational service staff in community settings should endeavor to provide the opportunities. In doing so there are several aspects of organizing the competitive sport team that require special attention.

Safety

Safety comprises provisions to ensure a safe environment for play and personal safety factors. A physical examination of the kind given to nonhandicapped athletes should be required of the disabled players prior to participation. A conditioning program is essential, as it is for all players of strenuous sports. Special attention must be given to keeping the court or field free of obstructions that, while easily avoided by others, would be a hazard to players with physical impairments. Wheelchairs and special equipment used in play of any sport must be carefully maintained.

Organization

Various problems of organization are often more difficult for disabled teams than for regular teams. Scheduling often poses a problem because there may be an insufficient number of teams in a given sport near enough to permit competition to be arranged. However, this can be partially overcome by soliciting nonhandicapped players to fill out the team or meet the roster. Also, in some situations teams of disabled players can successfully compete against teams of non-disabled players.

Obtaining equipment may pose a serious problem since much of it must be of special design. The serious athlete who uses a wheelchair needs a chair specially built for the various sports. Special wheelchairs range in construction from the heavy low-centered chair with spayed wheels for playing basketball to the extra-light chair appropriate for racing.

Financing sports for handicapped players may also be a problem. The cost per person to field teams of disabled participants is relatively high and, when the budget for recreational services is tight, justifying a significant portion of the funds to serve so few is difficult. However, because of the great interest of the players and their families and friends as well as certain community organizations, fund raising by them for the promotion of sport for the disabled is not an unusual undertaking. Many communities throughout the country have shown through their own successful fund drives that where interest and support can be generated, money is available to give disabled athletes the opportunity to compete in team sports.

Sports Associations for the Disabled

Various groups have formed to promote sports for participants with a specific disability, and more can be expected to organize in the future. To date there are about 18 different associations, which are listed in Table 14-1. Four of these actively promote national and international games for handicapped players: American Athletic Association of the Deaf, National Association of Sports for Cerebral Palsy, National Wheelchair Athletic Association, U.S. Association for Blind Athletes, and Special Olympics. Rules and regulations have been established by the organizations to govern competitive play; these and other information about fielding a team may be obtained by writing to the groups at their listed address.

EXERCISE AND CONDITIONING

It is well established that sedentary living has detrimental effects on well-being.[2] Hence attention has been focused on conditioning programs for ill and disabled individuals, who as a group are typically less active than other population groups due to a combination of factors including over-protectiveness of parents, lack of ability to perform motor skills, and fear of failure or injury in attempting to take part in vigorous activities.

Except for those who receive conditioning exercises as part of the treatment or rehabilitation program in the treatment center, most ill and disabled people can only receive the conditioning programs they need to achieve and maintain a desirable level of physical fitness from in-community recreational settings. The physical fitness programs now so common in community recreational programs can be readily adapted to provide the same service to disabled clients.

TABLE 14-1. ASSOCIATIONS FOR HANDICAPPED ATHLETES*

American Athletic Association of the Deaf
3916 Lantern Drive
Silver Springs, MD 20902

American Blind Bowling Association, Inc.
3500 Terry Drive
Norfolk, VA 23518

American Wheelchair Bowling Association, Inc.
N54 W15858 Larkspur Lane
Menomonee Falls, WI 53051

Amputee Sports Association
11705 Mercy Blvd.
Savannah, GA 31419

Canadian Wheelchair Sports Association
333 River Road
Ottawa, Ontario, Canada K1L 8H9

International Wheelchair Road Racers Club, Inc.
165-78th Avenue, NE
St. Petersburg, FL 33702

National Amputee Golf Association
5711 Yearling Ct.
Bonita, CA 92002

National Association for Disabled Athletes
80 Hugenot Avenue—Suite 11-B
Englewood, NJ 07631

National Association of Sports for Cerebral Palsy
66 East 34th Street
New York, NY 10016

National Foundation for Happy Horsemanship for the Handicapped
P.O. Box 462
Malvern, PA 19355

National Foundation of Wheelchair Tennis
3857 Birch St., #411
Newport Beach, CA 92660

National Handicapped Sports and Recreation Association
Capital Hill Station
P. O. Box 18664
Denver, CO 80218

National Wheelchair Athletic Association
2107 Templeton Gap Road, Suite C
Colorado Springs, CO 80907

National Wheelchair Basketball Association
110 Seaton Building
University of Kentucky
Lexington, KY 40506

National Wheelchair Softball Association
P.O. Box 737
Sioux Falls, SD 57101

North American Riding for the Handicapped Association, Inc.
P.O. Box 100, R.I.B. 218
Ashburn, VA 22011

Ski For Light
1455 West Lake Street
Minneapolis, Minn. 55408

Special Olympics, Inc.
1701 K Street, N.W., Suite 203
Washington, DC 20006

United States Association for Blind Athletes
55 West California Avenue
Beach Haven Park, NJ 08008

* These organizations can provide information about local, national, and international programs for handicapped athletes.

When developing a conditioning program for a client, the recreationist must first obtain a complete physical profile from the client's physician, indicating among other things the types of activities that are contraindicated. This is followed by administration of a physical fitness test to determine the current level of physical conditioning. Care must be taken to utilize a test that gives consideration to the contraindicated movements. The components of physical fitness that require improvement will be identified by the test results.

Nature of Physical Fitness

Although there is no complete agreement on the definition of physical fitness, exercise physiologists usually define the term by identifying the constituents that comprise physical fitness, i.e., its components.[3] The components are those qualities of physiologic capacities of the body that respond to progressive overload (a process discussed in Chapter 3). Components related to the learning of motor skills are not physical fitness factors, rather they are motor skill or motor fitness factors.

Components of Physical Fitness. There are four physical fitness components: strength, muscular endurance, cardiorespiratory endurance, and flexibility. A brief discussion of each follows; more complete information can be secured from the references listed at the end of this chapter.

Strength. The physical fitness component of strength, which is the amount of force that can be exerted by a muscle, responds readily to the progressive overload principle. Participation in such recreational activities as sports, games, and exercises is a good way of increasing strength if participation becomes increasingly more vigorous and/or of longer duration so that a progressive overload is attained. Only those muscles that receive the progressive overload will be affected and, if the work of the muscles levels off rather than becoming increasingly greater, the increase in strength will seek a plateau. Similarly, the muscles will decrease in strength if the workload becomes less.

Increasing and maintaining muscular strength have great importance to disabled clients, particularly those who use crutches, walkers, wheelchairs, and other assistive devices, because they are then able to move about more easily and with greater independence from help supplied by others. Moreover, with the increased strength to engage in physical work and play, the disability can more easily be accepted and desirable adjustment to it acquired.

Endurance. Like strength, endurance responds to the progressive overload principle. There are two types of endurance components: muscular and cardiorespiratory. Muscular endurance is the capability of the muscles to continue contracting or to sustain contraction over a period of time. Cardiorespiratory endurance, on the other hand, is the ability of the body (specifically the lungs, heart, and vascular system) to process and supply oxygen to the various parts of the body during work. When a greater amount of oxygen can be supplied, the body is able to sustain high levels of work over longer periods of time.

For disabled clients, endurance of the muscles and cardiorespiratory system is an asset in undertaking with greater efficiency and persistence the often arduous tasks imposed by the disability. Sustaining efforts to accomplish work or recreational activities is easier and therefore more pleasant; also recovery time from fatigue is reduced.

Flexibility. The component of flexibility can be defined as a condition of the muscles and joints that permits a wide range of motion. Greater flexibility is achieved by stretching the muscles that cross the joints, thereby increasing the distance through which the joints can be moved. Although it might appear that the progressive overload principle would not be applicable to stretching the muscles, since stretching is so different from contraction of the muscles, the principle does indeed apply. Exercises and activities that extend the joints beyond their accustomed range will increase flexibility. However, the extension must become increasingly greater to continue to achieve improvement.

Disabled clients who experience movement restrictions due to lack of flexibility benefit greatly from appropriate flexibility exercises. Greater range of movement in non-disabled limbs can compensate to some extent for loss of use elsewhere. Loss of movement-potential that is characteristic of some neuromuscular and joint diseases can be retarded to some extent by flexibility exercises. (Conditions for which flexibility exercises are contraindicated are discussed in a later section.)

Body Composition. Although it is not generally considered a component of physical fitness (because it does not respond to progressive overload), body composition is so closely related to achievement of physical fitness as to deserve discussion here. Body composition refers to the percentage of the total body weight that is fat.

Excessive body fat has been implicated in a variety of poor health conditions including heart disease, diabetes, and high blood pressure.[4] Overweight individuals have difficulty in moving with efficiency and so often experience limitations in vocational and recreational endeavors. Appearance may be so unattractive as to produce feelings of depression and rejection. When these problems are added to those caused by an incapacitating illness or disability, the handicapped client can be devastated. Improvement in body composition is possible for nearly everyone. A program of vigorous physical activity by reduction in caloric intake (the amount of calories in the food that is eaten) will reduce excessive body fat. Calories are burned during the activity and, if less calories are consumed than required by the body to produce energy during work, the fat stored in the body is utilized and weight reduction results.

Physical Fitness Testing

To determine the overall level of fitness, each component needs to be assessed. This assessment can be used as a reference point for determining improvement. In some situations test results may be used to make a comparison of fitness level to established norms.

Some clients may not be able to participate in physical fitness testing because of the nature of the illness or disability or because the condition may be aggravated by taking the test. It is generally recommended that those with muscular diseases such as muscular dystrophy and multiple sclerosis and bone diseases like osteoporosis and osteogenesis imperfecta not be tested by non-medical personnel. Usually, however, the test can be given to other ill and disabled clients if parts of it are modified or eliminated. In a situation where part of the test is omitted, the results of the test will indicate fitness in those parts of the body that were tested rather than overall body fitness.

In comparing test results of disabled clients, to the established norms, it is important to remember that such a comparison may not be meaningful. For example, a client with a missing thumb performing pull-ups will probably have a lower score than that indicated by the norms. The conclusion cannot be drawn from this comparison that the client has less than average arm strength and endurance since the score was likely influenced by grip weakness due to the missing thumb. While it is possible to make meaningful comparisons with norms that have been developed with non-handicapped populations, the best comparisons are made with norms established for use with specific disabling conditions.

Tests for Ill and Disabled Clients

There are few published validated tests of physical fitness currently in general use. Some of the more useful tests are: The American Alliance for Health, Physical Education, Recreation, and Dance (AAHPERD) modified test for mentally retarded subjects;[5] Winnick's test for use with youngsters with spinal neuromuscular conditions;[6] and Fait's test for use with mildly and mentally retarded persons.[7] All of these tests include motor fitness components as well as physical fitness components.

The AAHPERD test has three physical fitness items: flexed arm hang, sit-up, and 300-yard run and three motor fitness items: shuttle run, standing long jump, and softball throw for distance. The test booklet provides information about how the test is to be administered and norms. The AAHPERD test's health-related physical fitness items do include a body composition test but norms for ill and disabled clients are not given.

The test by Winnick includes a body composition test item and provides norms for disabled clients. Other physical fitness items in his test include right and left grip strength, arm hang, pull-up, and long distance run. Norms are provided.

The items on the Fait test that measure physical fitness are (1) the bent arm hand that measures static muscular endurance and shoulder girdle, (2) leg lift that determines the dynamic muscular endurance of the flexors of the leg and of the abdominal muscles, and (3) 300-yard run-walk that measures cardiorespiratory endurance. The other two items on the test, static balance and thrust, are measurements of motor fitness. The complete test and directions for administering it are in Appendix IV. Norms are provided for all test items (see Appendix V).

Tests of Muscular Strength

Muscular strength can be measured in two ways: by use of weights or with a scale or similar type mechanism. In the former measurement, a weight is selected that approximates the strength of the muscle group to be tested. This weight is lifted with care being taken that the lift involves the muscle group for which the measure is desired. If the weight is too heavy or too light to adequately measure the maximum strength, adjustments are made until the right weight is secured. Sufficient rest between trials must be provided to ensure that fatigue does not limit the expression of actual strength.

Of the scale type mechanisms used in measuring strength, the dynamometer is the most common. This device records in pounds or kilograms the amount of force exerted against the dynamometer. The hand dynamometer (manuometer) measures grip strength. One of the most useful of this kind of mechanism has a rubber bulb for a grip (see Fig. 14-4 A and B) which enables a more effective grasp by those who have a physical condition limiting the ability to grip. The grip measurement can be used to predict general body strength of normal muscles if sets of muscles have not received specific strengthening exercise, since there is a relatively high relationship between grip and total body strength.[8]

If dynamometers are not available, heavy spring scales can be substituted for most parts of the body. The end of the scale is attached to the appropriate part of the body to measure a given set of muscles and the other end is attached to an immovable object. A complete contraction of the muscle will produce a reading on the scale that represents the strength of the muscle.

Tests of Muscular Endurance

Since muscular endurance is the ability of the muscle to continue contracting or to sustain contraction over a period of time, muscular endurance is tested by determining how many times the muscle can contract or sustain a contraction given a specific weight load. The most commonly used weight for the testing is one that is held or secured to the appropriate part of the body for testing the desired muscle; the subject then moves the weight by contracting the muscles as long as possible.

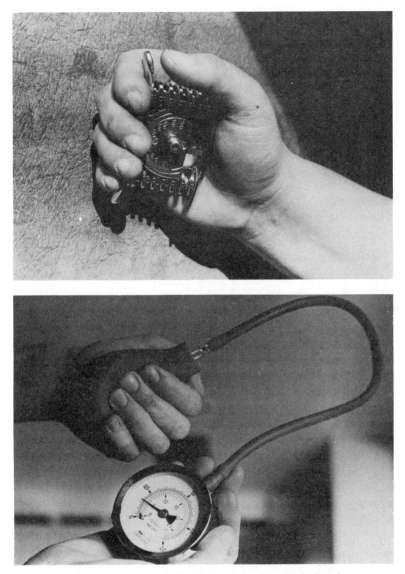

Fig. 14-4 A, Hand dynamometer. B, Hand dynamometer with bulb grip.

The number of times the movement is made is the score for the endurance test.

This test may not produce a valid measurement because contracting a muscle until it can no longer contract produces pain that many individuals cannot tolerate; therefore, they cease movement before the muscle has been fully exhausted. Also, working a muscle to exhaustion may be contraindicated for some ill or disabled clients. To overcome these limitations, Fait's Endurance Ratio may be utilized: A weight is selected that is judged to be one the specific subject will be able to lift many times before the muscle being tested becomes exhausted. The weight is held or attached to the appropriate part of the body and the subject is instructed to move the weight a given distance for 10 seconds. The number of times the weight is lifted for the first 5 seconds is counted and recorded, followed by count and recording of the number of times in the last 5 seconds. The two scores are used to determine a ratio representing the endurance level of the tested muscle. For example, if the score in the first 5 seconds is 6 times and the score for the last 5-second period is 3, the resulting ratio can be expressed as $3/6$ or $3 - 6 = .5$. The closer the dividend is to 1, the more endurance the subject has. A score of 1 or more is an indication that the test is measuring muscular speed rather than muscular endurance and that either the weight or the time needs to be increased to obtain a true measurement.

Tests of Cardiorespiratory Endurance

Measurements of cardiorespiratory endurance are obtained by three types of evaluation tools: oxygen consumption tests, heart rate tests, and performance tests. Oxygen consumption tests are performed in a laboratory situation by highly trained specialists using equipment designed for the purpose. The test determines how much oxygen can be delivered to the muscle cells in a given time, thus indicating the efficiency of the heart.

Heart rate tests of cardiorespiratory endurance are accomplished by having the subject do a given amount of work that taxes the cardiorespiratory system. This can be achieved by continuous stepping up on and down from a bench or by riding a bicycle ergometer at a selected speed and resistance. The more capable cardiorespiratory system will demonstrate less increase in heart rate (measured by taking pulse count) per given work load than a less efficient heart. To make the comparison the pulse rate is taken before the exercise and *immediately* after the exercise and the two scores compared.

The most frequently utilized performance test is the distance run; distances of 300 yards to $1\frac{1}{2}$ miles have been suggested by authorities. The longer the distance of the run, the more accurate will be the measurement of cardiorespiratory efficiency, assuming the client remains motivated to run to or close to the point of exhaustion. Since these tests do require maximal effort, they can be dangerous for those who are aged or extremely sedentary and those with health problems.

To eliminate the need for all-out effort in testing cardiorespiratory endurance, Fait's Endurance Ratio, described in the section on muscular endurance testing, can be utilized here as well. The run for the client is set at somewhere between 60 and 170 yards, depending on the client's cardiorespiratory fitness. The run is made at full speed for the entire distance. The first half is timed, and then the second half. As for the muscular endurance test, the two scores become a ratio. Consequently, if for example, the first half of a 60-yard run was covered in 10 seconds and the final half in 17 seconds, the ratio may be expressed as 10/17 or .58. Interpretation of the score is the same as for muscular endurance.

Cardiorespiratory endurance tests should not be given to those with cardiorespiratory problems.

Tests of Flexibility

The most familiar measurement of flexibility is the toe touch while holding the knees straight. This, of course, measures the flexibility of the hamstring muscles (back of the upper leg) since tightness of these muscles restricts the toe-touch movement; hence, the test is limited to measurement in one area of the body.

As indicated in the earlier discussion of it as a component of physical fitness, flexibility is highly specific, so each muscle set must be tested separately. Procedures for testing various sets of muscles are given below.

Trunk Extension:	From a prone position on a mat the subject, whose hips are held down, raises the chest and chin as far off the mat as possible, and a measurement is made from the mat to the top of the sternum.
Shoulder Elevation:	Lying prone on a mat with the chin touching the mat, the subject raises a wand held at shoulder width and arms' length in both hands as high as possible. Measurement is made from the mat to the bottom of the wand.
Shoulder Extension:	In a similar position to the shoulder elevation except with the wand held at shoulder width behind the back so that the wand rests across the hips, the subject elevates the wand as high as possible. Measurement is from the bottom of the wand to the floor.
Hip Abduction-Rotation:	The subject is seated on a mat and the soles of the feet are placed together, knees to the side. The subject spreads the knees as far as possible. Measurement is from the bottom of the knee to the mat.[9]

Flexibility exercises should be performed by some individuals only under the supervision of a physician. Cerebral palsy is one example of conditions that require stretching or other flexibility exercises to be done in strict compliance with the medical prescription because of the importance that only certain specified muscles be stretched.

Test of Body Composition

Measurement of body composition differs from the use of comparison with height and weight charts that have been developed to show norms for males and females. Such charts or tables indicate total body weight and do not distinguish between actual fat and the rest of the body weight.

Body composition measurement is obtained by measuring the subcutaneous (beneath the skin) fat with fat calipers (Fig. 14-5). This mea-

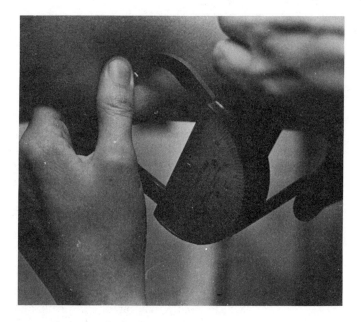

Fig. 14-5 Calipers used in measuring body fat.

surement is called the skin fold measurement. The two most common sites for measurement are the triceps (back of the upper arm) and the subscapular area (below the shoulder blade) because they are easily measured and are highly correlated with total body fat. For a complete description of the method of measurement and established norms for nonhandicapped children, see the AAHPERD publication given in the reference list at the end of the chapter.

Developing Muscular Strength and Endurance

Muscular strength and endurance are most rapidly improved by the use of some type of resisting exercises. The resistance or weight may be created by springs, elastic cable, barbells, or the body itself. Examples of the body becoming the resistance in exercise are the push-up, sit-up and pull-up. Many gymnastic activities such as stunts on the parallel bars and rings and, for younger age groups, the wheel-barrow race, seal walk, one-leg hopping, and medicine ball passing can provide sufficient overload to increase muscular strength and endurance through use of the body as the resistance. The number of muscle groups that can be exercised in this way is somewhat limited, however.

In using resistance exercises to develop strength a relatively heavy load should be used. The weight should be sufficiently heavy so that the lifter can only perform the lift about 10 times. As the lifter becomes stronger, the weight is progressively increased.

In developing muscular endurance it is recommended that the weight be light enough to permit 30 or 40 repetitions of the lift at a rapid rate.

All ill and disabled clients who are going to participate in muscular strength and endurance exercises should obtain approval from their doctor. Most physicians do not recommend resistance exercises for those with muscular disorders such as muscular dystrophy or bone diseases such as osteoporosis.

Exercises that may involve diseased or disabled parts of the body require approval by the client's physician. When exercising other parts of the body, care must be taken that muscles in the protected area are not brought into action in the movements required by the exercise. To guard against any possibility of this occurring, an all-out effort should not be made in lifting.

Clients in wheelchairs, including those with leg paralysis, can do many of the arm exercises. For example, pull-ups can be done using an overhead bar while push-ups can be made by pushing against the arms of the wheelchair while in the sitting position. The wheels must be checked to ensure the brake is tightly secured any time the clients are engaged in activities of this kind.

If clients in wheelchairs experience minor back difficulties, they may be allowed to lift with the arms if the back is held straight so that the weight is taken evenly on all parts of the spinal column. Since lifts from a prone position do not place undue strain on the back, lifts can be made from this position if the back is held flat against the floor. Participants with weak or injured shoulder muscles should usually avoid lifting weights that require lifting above the head. In almost all cases individuals with heart disorders are not permitted to participate in weight lifting.

Development of Cardiorespiratory Endurance

Any exercise that requires a large amount of oxygen and hence places an overload on the cardiorespiratory system will increase cardiorespiratory endurance. An estimate of the intensity can be obtained by counting the pulse rate *immediately* after cessation of the exercise. The pulse rate should be taken for 10 seconds and multiplied by 6 to secure an accurate estimate of the work done since the heart rate (pulse) decreases quickly after exercise is stopped.

For an exercise to increase the efficiency of the heart it has to be sufficiently strenuous to increase the heart rate 40 to 60% of the maximum heart rate. The 60% rate is for the young person with no disability that would affect heart function; the 40% rate applies to aged or extremely disabled individuals with low cardiorespiratory efficiency.

To determine the maximum heart rate, a target rate is arrived at either by estimation of the maximum ability of the heart to beat or by an actual measurement of the heart's maximum rate. The heart is only able to beat at a specific rate at its maximum. (The workload may be increased but the heartbeat has reached its maximum and cannot beat any faster.) In actual measurement the client is given an increasingly greater workload, usually on a treadmill, while the heart beat is monitored to determine its maximum rate. This procedure is called a stress test. Only those who have extensive training should give the stress test and then only in the presence of a physician.

In estimating the maximum heartbeat for an individual it is assumed that a maximum heart beat is 220 minus the age of the client. In either estimating or measuring the maximum rate, a percentage of the difference between maximum rate and resting heart beat is calculated to obtain the target rate. In the case of individuals without cardiac problems, it is recommended that the percentage be 60. For example, estimating the target rate for a person 60 years old with a resting pulse rate of 80, using a percentage of 60, produces a target rate of 128, that is $(220 - 60) - 80(.60) + 80 = 128$. This formula should not be applied by recreationists for individuals with cardiac problems without the recommendation of the client's physician. For these persons, the doctor will use a different percentage based on the severity of the condition in arriving at a suitable target rate.

Evidence would indicate that to improve cardiorespiratory endurance the duration of training must be between 20 and 40 minutes.[10] It is recommended that the lower figure be used for disabled clients who are not in good condition. Thus, for the previous example, the heart rate of approximately 128 should be maintained in exercise for 20 minutes at least 3 times a week for improvement to be achieved.

Any type of activity that will produce a heart beat of desired target rate is appropriate for obtaining the cardiorespiratory conditioning effect. Especially good are jogging, swimming, and dancing; also any vigorous exercises while sitting may be utilized.

Developing Flexibility

Flexibility is achieved by placing a progressive overload on the muscles involved, i.e., the muscles are stretched more than they are accustomed to being stretched. All flexibility exercises should be performed slowly, never using bouncing movements. When the muscle is stretched and the body part has reached the end of the range in that position, the position is held for 15 to 30 seconds. Each exercise should be repeated at least 3 times a day. Specific stretching exercises are described in the books by Adams given in the reference list at the end of the chapter. The same precaution to be exercised in giving flexibility tests should be observed in offering flexibility exercises.

Decreasing Body Fat

Losing weight by decreasing the amount of fat content of the body is dependent on the amount of energy in the form of food that is ingested compared to the amount of energy expended by the body. If more energy is taken in than is used by the body, the body will put on fat. When the opposite occurs, fat is decreased.

Any diet and exercise program to be effective must be based on a recognition of these facts. The greatest problem in weight reduction is the difficulty for many people to decrease their food intake or increase the energy output.

Disabled individuals have a greater difficulty in maintaining appropriate weight than nonhandicapped people do. The chief reason is the lack of sufficient amounts of exercise to burn the required number of calories to effect reduction. The recreationist can assist these people in increasing their work output by engaging them in active games and specific exercises. Both should be analyzed for compatibility with the assessment of client's capabilities. The activity selected should be one that uses a maximum of energy within the realm of the clients' ability to participate in exercise. For example, to provide an energy-consuming activity for a client who is a complete quadriplegic, the recreationist must consider that the only response the client is able to make is movement of the head. Resistance exercises which utilize a head harness attached to wall weights is one possibility for a suitable workout.

In most cases to affect body composition, both diet and exercise must be regulated. The first step is planning an exercise and diet program in which the caloric intake and expenditure are calculated. By keeping a daily record of the caloric content of the food consumed and the amount used in exercise, it can be determined if the body fat is going to increase, decrease, or remain the same. If the caloric intake and output are equal, the fat content of the body remains constant. To decrease the fat, either the caloric intake must be reduced or the caloric output must be increased by longer, more strenuous exercise. (Tables showing the number of calories contained in various foods and the amount of caloric consumption that occurs in various types of exercise are given in Appendices VI and VII.)

When decreasing the caloric intake, care must be exercised that the nutritional content of the food not be reduced to an extent that becomes detrimental to health. Any diet should include the Basic Four Food Groups:

(1) the milk group, (2) meat group, (3) vegetable and fruit group, and (4) bread and cereal group.

In developing a weight reduction diet, it is wiser not to follow any of the various highly publicized diet plans that gain great popularity from time to time. While they may reduce weight, they tend to be medically risky for some individuals, especially those who have illnesses and disabilities, because the nutrients supplied by the diets are insufficient. The assistance of the client's physician should be enlisted in planning the diet and exercise program.

REFERENCES

1. M. Sherril Moon and Adelle Renzaglia, "Physical Fitness and the Mentally Retarded: A Critical Review of the Literature", *Journal of Special Education,* 16, November 3, 1982, p. 1.
2. Joseph Winnick, *Early Movement Experiences and Development Habilitation and Remediation:* (Philadelphia, W. B. Saunders Co., 1979), p. 12.
3. Harold Falls, *et al,* Essentials of Fitness: (Philadelphia, Saunders College Publishing, 1980), p. 4.
4. W. B. Kannel and Tavia Gordon, Physiological and Medical Concomitants of Obesity: "The Framingham Study" in *Obesity in America,* George Bray, editor: (Washington, D. C., U.S. Department of Health Education and Welfare, 1980), p. 125.
5. American Alliance for Health, Physical Education, Recreation and Dance, *Special Fitness Test Manual for Mildly Mentally Retarded Persons,* (Washington, D.C., AAHPER, 1968) passim.
6. Joseph Winnick and Francis Short, "The Fitness of Youngsters with Spinal Neuromuscular Conditions," *Adapted Physical Activity Quarterly,* 1, November 1, 1984, p. 37.
7. Hollis Fait, "Physical Fitness Test for Mildly and Moderately Retarded Students," in *Special Physical Education: Adapted, Individualized, Developmental* by Fait and Dunn (Philadelphia, Saunders College Publishing, 1984) p. 544.
8. Charles McCloy and Norma Young, *Tests and Measurements in Health and Physical Education,* 3rd ed.: (New York, Appleton-Century-Crofts, Inc., 1954) p. 128.
9. Hollis Fait and John Dunn, *Special Physical Education: Adapted, Individualized, Developmental:* (Philadelphia, Saunders College Publishing, 1984), p. 461.
10. Harold Falls, *op cit,* p. 152.

SELECTED REFERENCES

Adams, R. C., *et al., Games, Sports and Exercises for the Physically Handicapped,* 3rd. ed. (Philadelphia: Lea & Febiger, 1982).
Allen, A., *Sports for the Handicapped* (New York: Walker & Co., 1981).
Arnheim, D.D., *et al., Principles and Methods of Adapted Physical Education and Recreation* (St. Louis: C. V. Mosby Co., 1977).
Hedley, E., *Boating for the Handicapped: Guidelines for the Physically Handicapped* (Albertson, New York: Human Resources Center, 1979).
Lane, J. and Schlaef, R., *Wheelchair Bowling: A Complete Guide to Bowling for the Handicapped* (Huntington Beach, California: Wheelchair Bowlers of Southern California, 1980).
Price, R. J., *Physical Education and the Physically Handicapped Child* (New York: State Mutual Books and Periodical Service, 1980).

Chapter 15

Horticulture, Animal Husbandry, and Culinary Arts

The participation of ill and disabled clients in activities that require the kinds of skills needed for horticulture, animal husbandry, and the culinary arts may at first appear incongruous. However, with proper modifications participation is possible by most clients in a variety of gardening, animal care, and cooking activities. Some of the activities are particularly good choices for those clients who are institutionalized or homebound and often difficult to interest in recreational pursuits.

The nature of both horticulture and animal husbandry suggests a need for outdoor space of considerable dimensions in which to carry out the activity. Actually a modified garden need be no larger than a window box or flower pot. Animal husbandry can be adapted to indoor areas no larger than that required for a bird cage or fish aquarium. Although not as adaptable as gardening and animal care, the culinary arts can be offered on a modified scale: by choosing dishes that need only a few ingredients and have a limited number of steps in preparation, cooking can be adapted to the limitations of even severely disabled clients.

In addition to offering scaled-down versions of the activities of horticulture, animal husbandry, and the culinary arts, adaptations are possible in the skills used to perform the activities. Ways in which to modify skills to enhance participation by handicapped clients are described in the sections of this chapter.

When planning the suggested activities, recreationists should keep in mind that many disabled persons may never before have had any involvement with plants and animals. Perhaps their environments precluded such experiences. For example, it is not unusual to find that many urban dwellers have never seen farm animals of any kind and have no idea how food is grown, transported, and prepared for sale in markets. Some people have never owned pets much less fed an animal or learned how to care for one. They have never grown garden vegetables or cared for a house plant and so have no appreciation of the joy and wonder inherent in such activities. Hence, considerable motivation may be required to stimulate clients' interest in plants and animals.

Introductory activities may serve to provide that stimulation. Photos, films, books, exhibits, demonstrations, and hands-on activities can be offered so that the client gains enough exposure to the delights of the world of plants and animals to wish participation in it. Once the desire is kindled, the client's own sensory apparatus will likely continue a restimulation of interest in growing plants and caring for animals.

HORTICULTURE

"How does your garden grow?" is not merely a line from a nursery rhyme. As a question put by one ill or disabled client to another, it is a clue to the importance of horticulture as a therapeutic modality. There is something comforting and satisfying about being able to cultivate plants and see them grow. As a plant flourishes, there seems to be a positive transfer of psychic strength to the handicapped person whose active participation in other activities is limited. There is great pleasure to be obtained from preparing the soil, planting bulbs or seeds, nurturing the plants, and watching their progress toward fruition. The enjoyment extends to talking with other gardeners about the problems and pleasures of making a garden grow.

Unique Therapeutic Benefits

Clients who feel that the severity of their physical illness or disability prevents any possibility of participation in normalized recreational activities derive great psychologic support from their ability to care for plants. The psychologic benefit is evident in an increased perception of personal usefulness, i.e., recognition by the client that despite incapacity there still remains an ability to perform activities necessary to the support and maintenance of another living organism. Horticulture also offers a degree of independence to mentally ill individuals who are being treated in a controlled environment and to those who, like severely mentally retarded persons, are largely dependent on others for almost every aspect of survival. Feelings of helplessness common to any handicapped person tend to diminish as the client learns to control the plant's environment for successful growth. Participating in the planting and nurturing of plants produces a sense of mastery that is psychologically beneficial to one who is no longer able to exert full autonomy because of restrictions imposed by aging, illness, or disability. As a consequence of a commitment to plant care, greater alertness, acceptance of responsibility, physical movement, and a sense of personal accomplishment are often evident.[1]

Moreover, many clients need to develop resiliency to frustration and to acquire the ability to adjust to stress produced by personal incapacity and societal barriers that tend to discriminate against the disabled. In caring for plants, they confront such problems as plant blight, insect infestations, aridity, soil compaction, and other conditions that endanger plant life. Whether the plant is on a window sill or in an outside garden, the ability to cope with the unanticipated upsets or sudden changes that produce ill effects on the plant may help the client to develop the greater capacity to deal with the frustration and stress that appear to be a part of everyday living.

Among the therapeutic values that may be associated with plants is their use as purely decorative forms within the treatment setting. In one study, it was reported that the arrangement of flowering plants in the dining room used by chronic mental patients was followed by a significant rise in verbalization, time spent in the dining area, and the quantity of consumed food. The positive effect on severely withdrawn patients was specifically noted and statistically significant, although no explanation was given for this response.[2] While there may be a number of causes for such reactions among patients, it appears that the only difference was the introduction of flowers. Such experiences, if replicated, could be indicative of the importance that plants have within the environment and the influence that they have upon human behavior.

Horticultural Therapy

While the therapeutic value of horticulture has long been understood, the current recognition of "horticultural therapy" as a special modality began with its use at the Menninger Foundation in 1919. Later the New York University Institute of Rehabilitation Medicine became actively involved with recreational activities centered around plant care and gardening. It may be obvious why horticultural activities have gained popularity as one aspect of a recreational program, but still unclear is the therapeutic value which is claimed for horticulture beyond its benefits as a recreational activity.

Although a number of therapeutic benefits are alleged for horticulture, little has been done to substantiate such claims on a systematic basis. Most of the articles written about the values intrinsic to the experience have been more inspirational and observational than scientifically or experimentally based. Nevertheless, the therapeutic value of horticulture continues to be proclaimed by those who have some expertise in this specialization. As horticulture is increasingly used in various treatment centers, a better appreciation of its benefits and the way it influences behavior will, presumably, result. Such new insights will undoubtedly promote scientific research into the mechanisms by which horticultural activities bring about desired changes. When the importance of its contributions is fully understood, horticulture should become an important element in therapeutic programming.

Adapting Activities

Various gardening projects are possible indoors as well as outdoors. Clients who are able to move about and to perform the movements necessary to cultivation of the soil can be provided with plots of ground outside the treatment center or in community gardens, if the client is in an adapted community recreational program. Indoors, planting boxes, dishes, or flower pots can be supplied for window gardens in which seeds, seedlings, bulbs, or tubers may be planted and nourished.

For those patients whose ego needs are diminished or whose attention spans are relatively short, the need for instant success or gratification can be sustained through the introduction of flowering plants. Here the patient obtains satisfaction from possession of mature plants as well as the pleasure of seeing them at their flowering peak. Caring for such plants, in pots or window sill planters, requires little effort. The reward of seeing the plants each day should be sufficient. A plant that is full of buds and only just opening its first flower is infinitely preferred to those in full bloom because there is only a remote chance that the flower will not bloom and success is practically assured. As the plant begins to blossom, gratification will be obtained. Moreover, the enjoyment of the patient will be prolonged through the added days required for the buds to open.

For those patients whose ego strength is resilient or who have learned to defer instant gratification without becoming obsessed with failure, depression, or inability to cope with disappointment, the science and art of horticulture can be a delightful experience. The recreationist utilizing horticulture as an activity should be knowledgeable about the kinds of plants to be grown in the treatment center environment, what plants will, in fact, flourish in an indoor situation, and which will have the most striking floral effect. Plants should be chosen for their ease of handling, need for light without full exposure to the sun, and temperature necessary for sturdy growth. Moreover, the care of plants should be well within the ability of the client to tend to them.

Outdoor gardening by clients who must use wheelchairs, crutches, or walkers but have reasonably good movement of the arms can be facilitated by elongating the handles of the tools they use. This can be done by replacing the regular handle with a specially made longer handle, or the regular handle can be extended with pieces of wood approximately the same diameter as the handle which are taped or bolted to the original handle.

It is essential for the wheelchair gardeners and helpful for those using crutches and walkers if the surface alongside the plants is sufficiently hardened to permit easy access and maneuverability. Packing the earth with a lawn roller is one way of achieving a hard surface; surfacing the paths with clay is another possibility.

Indoor gardening may be done in planters or flower pots placed on the window sill. If the window can be easily opened by the client, window

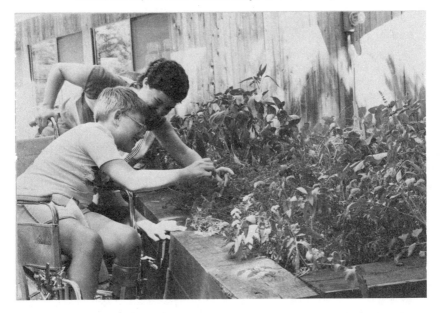

Fig. 15-1 Elevating the garden bed is one way of adapting horticulture for clients who must remain seated while caring for plants. (Hemlocks Outdoor Education Center.)

boxes can be attached outside the window for gardening in appropriate weather. The containers for growing plants can also be set directly on the floor, or placed on platforms with casters that will roll across the floor to where the client is located. For bedridden clients, the plant containers can be placed on a movable bed stand and placed directly over the bed in front of the client, who is then raised to a sitting or semi-reclining position to garden.

Much of the planting and cultivating of container-grown gardens can be performed with the hands alone. However, if the client needs or wants to use tools, small trowels and hand hoes may be provided; even large sturdy spoons may be pressed into service. Lightweight watering cans with long spouts are desirable for supplying water to the plants. A tote bag or a handmade bag of similar material and design can be used to hold the tools within easy reach during gardening, possibly attached to the bed or bed stand. The same type of bag is useful for small tools used by gardeners with assistive devices.

For those whose limitations are so severe as to permit little or no movement at all, gardening activity may be pursued with the help of a volunteer, or horticultural experiences related to plant design and decoration may be offered. Adaptation may also take the form of the client's acting as a plant advisor to other patients with greater physical ability but who lack knowledge about plant cultivation.

ANIMAL HUSBANDRY

Animal husbandry is the careful management and protection of domestic or other animals so that they are secure within their natural habitats or enabled to survive and procreate. Animal husbandry may also imply the care and feeding of a variety of small or large animals who live in enclosures, pens, or zoos. This latter aspect permits the exhibition of animals to those who might not ordinarily get to see such creatures because their mental or physical limitations are such that normal access is denied. For the most part animal tending in institutional settings is restricted only by accommodating space, administrative policy, and the knowledge that the recreationist has concerning the handling of the types of animals which would be most helpful in meeting the needs of patients.

Unique Therapeutic Benefits

For some time, there has been recognition of the fact that certain animals, serving as pets, can have a comforting and calming effect on individuals in a disturbed emotional state. Holding, petting, talking to, and attending to the needs of the animals can be especially profitable to those whose confinement tends to strip them of identity or to restrict their independence. The care of animals places clients in a role where another creature is dependent on them and responsive to their attention. Thus, cats and dogs, which take on almost human characteristics, are popular pets.

Laboratory animals, such as rats, mice, gerbils, hamsters, and the like may also be enjoyed and cared for by clients. Well known psychologic experiments indicate that these animals can be taught to perform or otherwise demonstrate responsiveness to the human guardian. The same holds true for a variety of birds, which may be kept as pets. Not an animal, in the technical sense of the word, but nevertheless rewarding in their own way are tropical fish. Swimming fish seem to have a soothing effect on those who observe them. The same care that nurtures other animals must be provided to fish: feeding, changing of water, and maintaining proper balance of aquatic plant and animal life.

The single greatest argument for the use of animals in the special recreational program is the fact that they seem to reduce isolation, loneliness, and anxiety within the individual who has access to them. Small animals, such as dogs, cats, hamsters, gerbils, birds, and fish elicit responses from patients who otherwise show no reaction to social overtures made by people. Animals, which become pets, are non-threatening even to those whose mental conditions make a threat of the most innocuous objects. Animals of many types have a calming effect on clients and make them more receptive to other therapeutic modalities.

Animals really ask for nothing except care, and in return offer complete trust and "friendship." The companionship of animals often helps to reduce tension in clients. Furthermore, animals respond to training, some more so than others, but even fish gather for feeding. The client is thus given the opportunity to control the life and security of another organism which can share the feelings, but never makes excessive demands, of the client.

Pet Therapy

Although scientific studies concerning "pet therapy" have not been carried out with any rigor, there are some reports by interested observers that support the belief in the efficacy of animals upon the behavior, attitude, and temperament of pet owners, especially those who are institutionalized for emotional instability. Of course, the use of animals for therapeutic purposes is not solely directed toward the mentally ill clients. Many kinds of patients may profit from close contact with animals, whether the benefit comes from an entertainment and fun orientation, as in seeing animals, holding, petting or feeding them, or from the sense of comfort and tranquility induced by the animal's response to the care it is given. Clients achieve the needed love, security, and a sense of responsibility provided by animal husbandry activities.

Adapting Activities

Although bird feeders and bird and animal cages may be purchased commercially, they may also be constructed in the crafts shop if the treatment center has such a facility. Patients who have the ability to construct their own animal feeders or enclosures should be encouraged to do so, since this is another recreational activity that might have some therapeutic benefit for the individual. Where it is deemed necessary to acquire commercial items, these may be purchased with allocations from the department budget, or perhaps donated by individuals or by business establishments that sell such items.

Feeders and cages have to be emplaced and stocked with the proper food and water before an animal is housed there. In the case of a bird feeder, whatever bird feed is used is certain to attract the local bird population and probably squirrels, also. The only prerequisite is that the feeder be placed so that the patient can observe it easily. This, of course, applies also to cages housing small animals and birds, and fish bowls and aquariums.

When young animals are brought into the treatment center or community setting for clients' observation or care, the only equipment necessary may be baby bottles with nipples so that milk may be given to the animals. If animals cannot be brought into the facility, it may be possible to transport clients to a nearby zoo or other kind of animal shelter for observation purposes. Visits can also be made to nearby farms and local pet shops.

The likelihood of keeping live animals in the treatment center will be subject to administrative policy, but if it can be shown that such animals do not contribute to unsanitary conditions, may be cared for easily, and contribute to the stabilization of patients' emotions or even to the rehabilitation of the patients, it is not beyond the realm of reality that an enlightened administrator may permit fish and birds, at least, in appropriate places in the treatment setting.

If animals, as pets, are kept within the treatment center, then such activities involved with them are routinized, i.e., performed by the client each day, and are nonscheduled or performed at will. Casual observation by recreationists may be advisable to make sure that the care and feeding of the creatures is without difficulties for the client and that the animal is not neglected.

Where aquariums and fish bowls have been placed in the patient's room, the activity of feeding and care of fish may be adapted by the use of curved or bent implements which assist the client with limited movement in feeding the fish. Of course, access to the aquarium must be easily obtained. The same holds true for bird and animal cages. Whether set on legs or supported by a stand, the cage must be easy to open and clean by an individual who cannot stand. Movable platforms and bed tables can be used to bring the cage or aquarium to clients in beds or chairs.

It may be possible to bring small or young animals to visit clients. Even those who cannot sit up, but are forced to remain prone or supine, may take part in feeding, petting, or grooming animals if a volunteer is available to make sure that the animals are securely confined or docile enough to take food from a hand-held container which the client proffers.

Bird feeders, placed outside of a patient's window, simply require filling when the food supply is exhausted. This means that the patient will have to have access to bird feed, be able to open the window, and place the feed in the feeder. If possible, therefore, the feeder should be placed outside windows designed to open without exerting great force, that is, ones operated by a crank. A pole with a cup attachment may be used to extend the reach to fill the feeder.

CULINARY ARTS

The culinary arts include all aspects of food preparation and service: not only cooking and baking but all the activities of acquiring the food, making the menus, putting the food on the table, and cleaning-up after the meal can be considered elements of the arts. The wide appeal of the culinary arts has made them a popular activity in community recreational programs for special populations. It is not unusual to find some aspect of cooking and baking being performed by clients as an integral part of therapeutic recreational service. If eating the prepared dishes is not contraindicated by dietary restrictions or if the preparation can be performed with the knowledge and guidance of dietetic personnel in the treatment center, the various forms of the culinary arts afford a pleasant change of pace in the recreational program as well as enjoyment by the clients both of the process and the end product.

Unique Therapeutic Benefits

Everything associated with eating should, theoretically, be of positive benefit to clients. After all, without the proper nutrition health becomes precarious and the human body is unable to function properly. Appropriate and nourishing food is a main sustainer of life, and as such, all of those arts and crafts related to the preparation and serving of food may have positive value to the individual. However, there are victims of self-starvation who cannot bring themselves to eat and, if they do, eat such minuscule portions as to place them in imminent danger of progressive malnutrition and eventual starvation. These individuals, preponderantly females, suffer from anorexia nervosa. Another manifestation of the same illness is bulimia. In this instance the individual usually resorts to auto-regurgitation. Other than such persons, almost everyone who is able to eat, looks forward to well-cooked and attractively served meals as one of the pleasures of the day.

Cooking skills assume significance for an individual who is otherwise limited in terms of movement or is without interpersonal relationships so vital to social intercourse. Demonstration of ability in the culinary arts may do much to remove the blight of unsocial behavior or arouse a level of peer admiration and praise that produces a responsive note in the individual. The psychologic support thus engendered may be the trigger that permits greater social contact and increases desire to gain group affiliation.

Many individuals do not know how to prepare food for themselves much less for anyone else. They are relatively helpless when it comes to reading and following recipes. Therefore, although often taken for granted, achievement of cooking skills indicates a unique level of mastery by the client. This knowledge may serve that person in situations where the ability to control a variety of environmental elements may have disappeared.

Participation in the culinary arts can be therapeutically beneficial to clients. However, there is little in the way of experimental evidence to support this contention. Once again, observation by practitioners must be substituted for replicated procedures. Where culinary arts have been introduced to the treatment center recreational program, there appear to be positive outcomes in terms of patients' cooperation among themselves and with staff, greater socialization, an attempt at more decorous conduct at the table, and even manifestation of neater dress. Such improvement may be the forerunner of other activities of greater assistance in the process of rehabilitation. Where rehabilitation is not possible, participation in the culinary arts may make life a little more bearable within the institutional setting. For disabled clients in the community adapted recreational program perhaps the greatest benefit is the encouragement to undertake daily tasks, once viewed as beyond their reduced capacity. Success in preparing food in the recreational setting goes far in convincing clients that they can do the same at home—and perhaps accomplish other housekeeping tasks as well.

Adapting Activities

Cooking as a recreational activity is informal, fun, and contains something for nearly everybody to do. Cooking offers many opportunities for leadership to occur among the patients. There is the need for group planning and participation, for cooperating with others, and for becoming self-sufficient. Cooking develops many qualities that will prove necessary after rehabilitation or useful to the individual if rehabilitation is not being considered. Participation in the culinary arts promotes learning about different foods; comparison shopping for quantity, quality, and value; culinary skills; planning menus; estimating food needs; reading recipes; special ways for preparing dishes; and, of course, cleaning up afterwards.

Cooking provides for the display of skill, knowledge, and immediate gratification of successful performance. Almost every patient likes to eat. Of course, there will be some patients for whom food is anathema because of phobic reactions or other mental aberrations. However, for the most part, eating is an enjoyable activity and both the sight and smell of good cooking should be stimulating enough to cause participation; especially if the activity is undertaken at appropriate meal times. Some aspects of cooking may be engaged in between meals; for example, snacks in the late afternoon before the dinner meal and in the late evening after dinner or in preparation for serving later at meals. Naturally, in treatment centers all such activity must be coordinated with the dietary department so that cooking activities neither conflict with proper patient treatment nor contribute to excessive calories.

Cooking may be programmed indoors or outdoors, as a special occasion or as a routine activity. However it is scheduled, there should never be a burden placed upon any one individual. The chores of cooking must be evenly distributed so that each person can contribute whatever knowledge or skill is possessed as well as learn new skills or hone old ones.

Cooking classes, rather than cooking per se, are another form of the culinary arts that may be offered to clients. They are usually presented under the supervision of a qualified recreationist or a volunteer. Cooking classes are in effect demonstrations with individualized instruction or group instruction being given before an assemblage of clients. At the conclusion the products of the class may be distributed among the group.

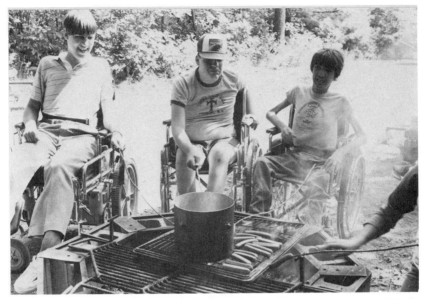

Fig. 15-2 Recreational culinary activities for disabled clients should, if possible, include cooking in the out-of-doors. (Hemlocks Outdoor Education Center.)

If the food preparation has been performed well, the outcome may be an enthusiastic response of clients to the activity and the wish to participate in such classes or in personal food preparation more frequently.

Ideally, the kitchen facilities in which the culinary art activities are conducted are designed for accessibility to clients with physical disabilities. Tables, counters, and work surfaces are lower than average height so that those who must remain seated during food preparation can work at a comfortable level. Space is provided under the sink and some counters to allow a wheelchair to be moved beneath them bringing the occupant of the chair right up to the space where work is to be performed. Large handles are placed on cupboards and appliances, which are located within easy reach, to facilitate opening and closing. Electrical switches and outlets, also, are located at appropriate heights in places of ready accessibility; additionally, they are color-coded for mentally retarded clients who have difficulty remembering which ones serve which purpose. The kitchen is painted in colors of an intensity and hue that enables vision impaired clients to discern objects more clearly. Special lightweight pots and pans with over-sized handles are provided for those who have difficulty handling cookware due to lack of strength or disabilities of the fingers or arms.

Most kitchens, however, are less than the described ideal; they may lack some or all of the desirable accommodations for disabled clients. The recreationist must then make adaptations of the existing facilities and equipment. Even when remodeling to create lower work surfaces and space for wheelchairs is not possible, there are still several modifications that can be accomplished at small cost. A circular rotating shelf, known as a lazy-Susan, can be placed on a low shelf or counter top to hold needed food supplies or cooking utensils. Then instead of clients in chairs having to stretch dangerously to reach items, a shift of the turntable brings the items to the client. Handles on appliances, cookware, and cooking and eating utensils can be enlarged for improved gripping with large wooden handles bolted or taped to the existing handles.

There is also a commercially available gadget that looks like elongated tongs which extends the reach of clients who must remain in chairs or whose body movements are greatly restricted. The gadget can be manipulated with one hand to clasp an item in its grip while picking the item off the floor or lifting it down from a shelf. The grip on the item is released mechanically to deposit the item where desired. This useful gadget has many applications in the kitchen and elsewhere.

The use of volunteers is helpful in the kitchen, particularly in assisting severely physically disabled clients in facilities that have not been designed for their use. Volunteers can make certain preparations before the culinary activity begins to facilitate use by clients with limited mobility and also by mentally retarded individuals. For example, prior to the time the client comes into the kitchen, for a cake baking project, bowls, pans, utensils, and ingredients can be assembled in one spot that is readily accessible to the client. Care must be taken, however, not to do things that the clients can do for themselves as this tends to thwart the development of independence and self-reliance.

REFERENCES

1. Langer, E. J. and J. Rodin, "The Effects of Choice and Enhanced Personal Responsibility for the Aged: A Field Experiment in an Institutional Setting," *J. Personality and Social Psychology,* Vol. 34, No. 2 (1976), pp. 191-198.
2. Talbot, John A. "Flowering Plants as a Therapeutic Environmental Agent in a Psychiatric Hospital," *HortScience,* Vol. 11, No. 4, (1976), pp. 365-366.

SELECTED REFERENCES

Amary, I.B., *Effective Meal Planning and Food Preparation for the Mentally Retarded— Developmentally Disabled: Comprehensive and Innovative Teaching Methods* (Springfield: Charles C Thomas, 1979).
Bienz, D. R., *The Why and How of Home Horticulture* (New York: W. H. Freeman and Company, 1980).
Blakeslee, M. E., *The Wheelchair Gourmet: A Cookbook for the Disabled* (Bloufort, South Carolina: Bloufort Book Co., 1981).
Browne, J., *Growing from Cuttings* (New York: State Mutual Book and Periodical Services, 1981).
Cooper, G., *Animal People* (Boston: Houghton Mifflin, 1983).
Daubert, J. R. and Rotfert, E. A., Jr., *Horticultural Therapy at a Psychiatric Hospital* (Glenacre, Illinois: Chicago Horticultural Society, 1981).
Daubert, J. R. and Rothfert, E. A., Jr., *Horticultural Therapy for the Mentally Handicapped* (Glenacre, Illinois: Chicago Horticultural Society, 1981).
Fisher, T. R., *Workbook and Manual Introduction to Horticulture* (Bloomington, Indiana: TIS, Inc., 1982).

Read, R., *When the Cook Can't Look: A Cooking Handbook for the Blind and Visually Impaired* (New York: Continuum Publishing Company, 1981).

Reiley, H. E. and Shry, C. L., Jr., *Introductory Horticulture,* 2nd ed. (Albany, New York: Delmar Publications, 1983).

Rothert, E. and Danbert, J. R., *Horticultural Therapy at a Physical Rehabilitation Facility* (Glencoe, Illinois: Chicago Horticultural Society, 1981).

Chapter 16

Social and Service Activities and Passive Entertainment

Certain recreational activities have come to be of considerable significance to the development of both therapeutic and adapted recreational programs, whether organized in the treatment center or in the community center. These activities are those of a social and of a service nature and those that require only passive participation.

Among the social activities are some that may be classified as formal and others as informal. Examples of formal activities include parties, banquets, ceremonials, concerts, balls, teas, and festivals. Informal activities range from pot-luck suppers and community singing to coffee klatches and spontaneous get-togethers.

Service activities are that broad range of services which client volunteers may provide. They include those services concerned with (1) organization and planning, e.g., membership on councils, committees, and interest groups; (2) direct activity leadership or instruction in any aspect of the recreational program; and (3) support of technical endeavors, e.g., clerical work, decorating trays and tables, delivering mail to patients, and other non-personal but necessary services.

Passive entertainment activities include those in which clients watch or listen to others perform, and do not become directly involved, physically or mentally, with the presentation. Examples are movies, plays, musical concerts, television productions, sports events, etc. Another type of passive entertainment encompasses activities that require minimal physical response by clients. Included are card games, board games (checkers, monopoly, etc.), games with little equipment (dominoes, pick-up-sticks, etc.), and electronic games.

SOCIAL ACTIVITIES

While all experiences of a recreational nature have social overtones, only those which bring together two or more people in close contact where some direct relationship and communication exist may be considered social. Communication, in this sense, does not have to be verbal. It is sufficient if people can satisfy their need to belong to a group by merely being present at an activity in which the group is involved. Close proximity to other people and coincidental participation or sharing of common interests with them often open up avenues of receptivity and acceptance so essential to sociability.

Social recreational activities sometimes seem to occur without any planning or development. There is no game, team activity, play, dinner, picnic, or performance-viewing activity that is not social. Hence, it is often assumed by recreationists that social activity is inherent in all recreational experiences and nothing needs to be done to encourage its occurrence. This is a grave error. Institutionalized persons in particular, but nearly everyone generally, require social contacts. Social activities of a recreational type have a place in any comprehensively drawn program where improvement in social interaction is desired and where good mental health is an objective.

Interestingly enough, the most common social activities are ignored while other esoteric forms are promoted—sometimes to the detriment of those for whom the activity is being planned. Thus, simple conversation between two or more persons may be more vital in the rehabilitation of the individual than some highly organized formal social activity. Often, those who are not aware of the profound effect that verbalization can have on the mental health of an individual dismiss conversation as not meaningful. However, it may be one of the most important social activities in a recreational program.

Value of Social Activities as a Therapeutic Tool

Social interaction is necessary for normal development. Whether the need to be with other people is learned or naturally discharged through certain essential stimuli, it is obvious that affiliation is an extremely powerful social motive among many people. Among the reasons for affiliation is the need to fulfill a gregarious impulse. The presence of other people provides an individual the opportunity to assess a personal emotional state by comparing it with others. Affiliation tends to reduce the anxiety of being alone. People need contact with others for the sense of love or affection that all human beings require at some time. People need others to share experiences, to give and receive information, to reduce feelings of anxiety and loneliness, and to relieve boredom.

Social isolation intensifies feelings of deprivation, heightens fears, delays the ability to make decisions that may have to be determined by obtaining information from others, and increases feelings of stress. This is particularly true when individuals sustain traumas associated with unavoidable losses or personal catastrophes; where there is little or no support from one's environment; a personal sense of inadequacy; a lack of social skills; or as a result of the need to compete with others. All of these factors are innately bound up with feelings of insecurity and lay the individual open to whatever vicissitudes are likely to accumulate in the daily confrontations of living. How much more vulnerable the individual is as a consequence of some pathologic condition may only be conjectured. However, to offset such negative experiences, specific social interactions may be introduced into the individual's environment by the recreational program.

Individuals may need to be introduced into group situations so that they can learn to function in ways which are enhancing of their self-perception while simultaneously participating in the give and take of group life. When several people are working together on the same task at the same time, especially when they are not in competition with each other, their performance may be better than when each person works alone. The presence of others, particularly when such persons offer emotional support tends to have a calming effect and permits the recipient of such support to learn to perform at a more efficient level. That outcomes which produce greater self-esteem, reduce anxiety levels, or encourage the development of interactional skills are therapeutically valuable cannot be denied. The significance of selecting the appropriate group, milieu, and situation so that these effects are more likely to be generated is part of the therapeutic recreationist's arsenal of counseling and programming knowledge. An assessment of each patient or client's needs must be made to determine how the socialization factor may best be put to use and then the individual must be introduced to social activities under optimum circumstances. How this is performed is the subject of the following paragraphs.

Selecting Social Activities

Not all contacts will be beneficial to patients or clientele suffering from some personal failure or trauma. If social groups are formed, they must be of a kind that will produce positive outcomes for all concerned. Groups should be formed with particular qualifications. Group membership should be predicated on common interest, background, and values. The activities undertaken by the group should be so arranged that there is little or no internal competition among the membership as competition only serves to strengthen feelings of anxiety. It may be that a dyad, that is, a two-person group, should be attempted at first. The recreationist will be in the best position to estimate the probability of success within any group situation as patients or clients act, react, and interact during group sessions.

Of extreme importance, in terms of facilitating desired performance, attitude, or appreciation, is the need to select group activities that require cooperative effort to succeed. Until diminished ego strengths can be reinforced and built up, the competitive aspects that predominate in many social forms should be controlled and eliminated. The emphasis should be upon mutual support, understanding, and assistance if the therapeutic value is to be obtained.

Developing Social Activity Prescription

A basic reason for the initiation of recreational activities for those who are institutionalized or those whose disability tends to limit their participation is to provide socialization. Clients who exhibit symptoms of withdrawal from reality are prime candidates for a social prescription. Of course, many individuals who are afflicted with disabilities that limit their mental or physical growth and outreach are similarly restricted by the lack of social stimulation and involvement with other people—either by choice or the lack of it.

Recreationists must have the resources at their disposal which will permit the planning and development of social activities that have as their outcome the promotion and stimulation of encounters designed to compensate for or counteract those prominent effects of disability—especially social isolation. The kind and degree of a client's involvement in social interaction is a function of the client's attitude, intellect, emotional stability, interest, and previous experience. But also involved are the recreationist's understanding, knowledge, and skill in dealing with recreational fundamentals, outcomes, and values. There must be continuous awareness of the need of the individual—in terms of any existing disorder—and the requirement for individualized assistance. To this end the prescription is fashioned.

If the disorder warrants, the prescription may be written to include specialization. This means that members of the treatment team recognize that a variety of intrinsic and extrinsic limitations are imposed upon the individual as a consequence of the disorder and that such impact may be reduced through activities that facilitate contacts and connections with reality. Frequently, catastrophic damage to the person results in withdrawal and isolation from others. To offset this negative behavior, social association may be recommended as the activity of primary choice. Then it is up to the recreationist to suggest and produce those activities of a social character that will most benefit the client's needs. An individualized prescription may be worked out, but it does not omit small group, large group, or even mass activities from the socialization process.

Other Considerations. Developing social activity prescriptions will depend upon the degree of impact of the affiliation on the client's emotional control and ability to perform physically. Certain activities will suggest themselves with regard to the client's previous experiences, skills, interest, intelligence, and capacity to be with others for any length of time. To a significant extent, many essential human functions are created from and satisfied through group experiences. The way these groups are established, scheduled, defined, and led constitutes part of the recreationist's methodology. Activities must be chosen for the positive effects assumed to be generated from the associations implemented through group contact.

Almost every recreational activity has a group base. The group becomes the setting in which members meet others who either share or want to share common ideas which are familiar and acceptable. Recreationists must make sure that all such group activities depend upon a certain amount of cooperative effort toward a shared goal. This makes the likelihood of ego-identification between individual and group more cohesive and thereby elicits a protective and supportive environment in which the members experience a collective feeling. The experience of an identifiable consciousness enables each group member to recognize personal expectations realistically and makes that person better able to understand and, perhaps, cope with anxieties with greater objectivity.

SERVICE ACTIVITIES

Activities which are voluntarily engaged in by people who wish to assist others in learning skills and developing appreciation, or in making the community or institution a better place as a result of their interest, talent, and sense of responsibility may be termed service activities. Such activities are typified by selfless donation of time, energy, and sometimes money, purely for the personal satisfaction derived from assisting another person, institution, or the entire community. Perhaps more than any other activity, service to others may be considered as the most rewarding. It is as enjoyable as any of the other recreational activity categories, requires the same sense of personal expression, and may result in an even greater or more intense emotional response of well-being and warmth. Watching an individual develop skill, knowledge, emotional maturity, or an appreciation as a direct outcome of one's personal help gives the donor a feeling of achievement and a sense of self-esteem.

Service activity is as broad as the entire field of recreational service. More importantly, services can be offered by anyone. Nothing prevents a disabled individual from helping others. There are many instances where physically impaired persons volunteer to perform vital services for those who require assistance. Nor is it unusual for patients in treatment centers, especially in long-term institutions, to undertake voluntary activities within the recreational program thereby broadening activity possibilities for other patients while, at the same time, reaping the benefit of personal satisfaction and peer recognition for giving their time and skill.

Value of Service Activities As a Therapeutic Tool

Donation of their services to the recreational program or some other phase of the treatment center's operations can be as helpful to the volunteer clients as to the recipients of the services. In committing themselves to assisting others, clients subordinate their personal problems to the work at hand. The knowledge that this work has importance and that they are making a contribution is immeasurably satisfying and reassuring to disabled clients. Prestige accorded by peers in the treatment center in recognition of the client's having been accepted as a volunteer has much positive influence on the way the client views him or herself. As a therapeutic tool, use of clients as volunteers has great potential for promoting acceptance of limitations and adjustment to the changed circumstances caused by the illness or disability.

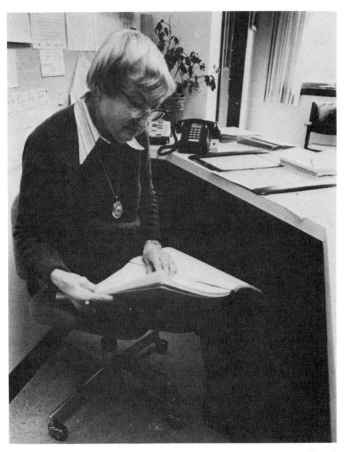

Fig. 16-1 The donation of time and assistance by clients to the recreational program is a service activity that benefits both the client and the program.

There may be vocational carry-over, as well as therapeutic benefits. The skill developed in assisting with the preparations for or instruction of an activity, in performing clerical duties, or in providing almost any other types of vocational service may be utilized in a job after release from the treatment program. The experience gained as a successful volunteer can be an important asset when the client's qualifications are being considered by an employer.

Identifying Service Possibilities

It is the responsibility of the recreationist to ensure a balanced program by investigating the possibility of incorporating the service phase of recreational experience into the program. To whatever extent an individual possesses some talent or ability, it may be useful to others and therefore a viable contribution to the program. There is no phase of the program that may not be made more valuable to participants because someone wanted to take the time, expend the energy, or be of service to someone in need.

It is not unusual for some especially talented, skilled, or knowledgeable person who has experienced some severe or limiting disability to volunteer to share his or her interests with others who are in the same disability predicament. There are many examples of disabled persons with art, craft, musical, sport, dance, dramatic, and other recreational skills coming forward to lend their time and efforts as instructors, guides, or advisors to those who are even more disabled or less able to be accommodated within the mainstream of program activities. Sometimes these volunteers are motivated to give help because they can empathize with the recipient or because of the chance to expiate guilt feelings or other emotional tensions. Regardless of motivation, opportunities for volunteer participation by disabled persons in the community or treatment center are almost unlimited. There is a place for both the skilled and unskilled. There are all kinds of activities and assistance which can be rendered directly to people and also in the provision of resources and technical aid that do not require face-to-face work.

Service possibilities can include, but are not limited to, sighted individuals or blind readers of braille reading to blind persons; older adults becoming foster grandparents to mentally retarded children; highly skilled sports instructors teaching amputees to ski, swim, handle archery equipment, sail, and similar activities. In one remarkable instance, a blind music teacher took a group of profoundly retarded persons and taught them how to chord music. Over a period of time this group became a well-trained chorus capable of singing in four-part harmony and performing before audiences.

The dedicated volunteer can perform the most useful of service activities by supplying the personnel necessary to accommodate disabled persons in a variety of typical recreational activities. Disabled clients usually require additional support and encouragement, not to mention adaptation of activities, which may be of a magnitude far beyond that which can be delivered by the recreational service staff due to personnel and budgetary constraints. With volunteers many activities in all categories may be offered because the ratio of membership to leadership is augmented.

PASSIVE ENTERTAINMENT ACTIVITIES

For obvious reasons, passive entertainment, wherein the individual simply sits and watches a performance, may appear to be ineffectual or non-inspirational, but for those individuals whose attention spans are fleeting or whose condition leads to hyperactivity, the ability to sit and watch the performance of others may, indeed, be a sign of marked improvement. Any show, dramatic presentation, movie, concert, circus, or some other form of entertainment can be so enjoyable and mind-riveting that individuals are actually caught up in the excitement of the performance or involved in the projected imagery to such an extent that they are thoroughly absorbed. Aside from some physical response as a result of an outstanding performance, the observers may be able to empathize with the characters being represented by a stage presentation or feel themselves fulfilled in listening to or watching an artist in concert.

Some individuals, whose self-image is of such negligible quantity that they think they are unable to do anything, may be stimulated by being able to observe the skilled performance of another. There are individuals who do not have the interest, skill, or knowledge to participate in a wide variety of recreational activities and, therefore, insist that they cannot learn anything or will not take the time to try to learn. These are the very people for whom passive entertainment may be beneficial. Sometimes, all that it takes to generate a real desire to emulate a spectacular performance is to be present at one. Whether the stimulation arises from a movie, dancing, art, gymnastics, swimming, or any other kind of performance the possibility exists that the proximity, excitement, enthusiasm, and pure pleasure derived from the experience may elicit either curiosity or a desire to try the skill that has been observed.

Value of Passive Entertainment as a Therapeutic Tool

Entertainment may be therapeutic, in the broadest sense of the term, by permitting the disabled individual to escape from the mill-run miseries, psychologic problems, or physiologic limitations which are imposed by a disability. Sitting passively within an audience and being carried away by the performance, free for a time from all pressures and problems, can prove extremely satisfying. The entire concept of entertainment consists of diversion. It should be an occasion for pleasurable feelings, happy moods, displacement of fears, and a sense of being a part of a larger collection of people who are doing exactly the same thing—enjoying themselves.

Escape from the reality of pain, frustration, insecurity, misplaced or misdirected sympathy, and other emotional burdens may be offered within the context of passive entertainment. The individual does not have to do anything but be the receiver of stimuli that are designed to arouse positive feelings. Surely, there is a place for escape within the therapeutic milieu. However, too much dependency upon escapism becomes a defense mechanism and may lead the individual down a trail to fantasy—that is, the inability to distinguish between what is real and what is wish or dream.

The therapeutic value of entertainment comes in terms of reducing boredom, generating enthusiasm, providing fun, and generally brightening attitudes and outlooks. Moreover, passive recreational activities allow the individual to be a part of a collection of people and diminish loneliness. Such is the real function of entertainment: To produce positive behaviors and offer refreshment without requiring any commitment or effort on the part of the person receiving the benefit.

Structuring Passive Entertainment Events

Too much reliance upon passive entertainment, where the patient simply observes without any attempt at participation or motivation to eventually perform in some activity, is not conducive to rehabilitation. Therefore, passive entertainment should be utilized sparingly within the organized structure of the overall program. Entertainment may be injected into the series of activities in which patients or clientele are exposed on a once-each-week basis so that they do not become unnecessarily addicted to passive amusement.

Passive entertainment forms can be offered as a change of pace, as

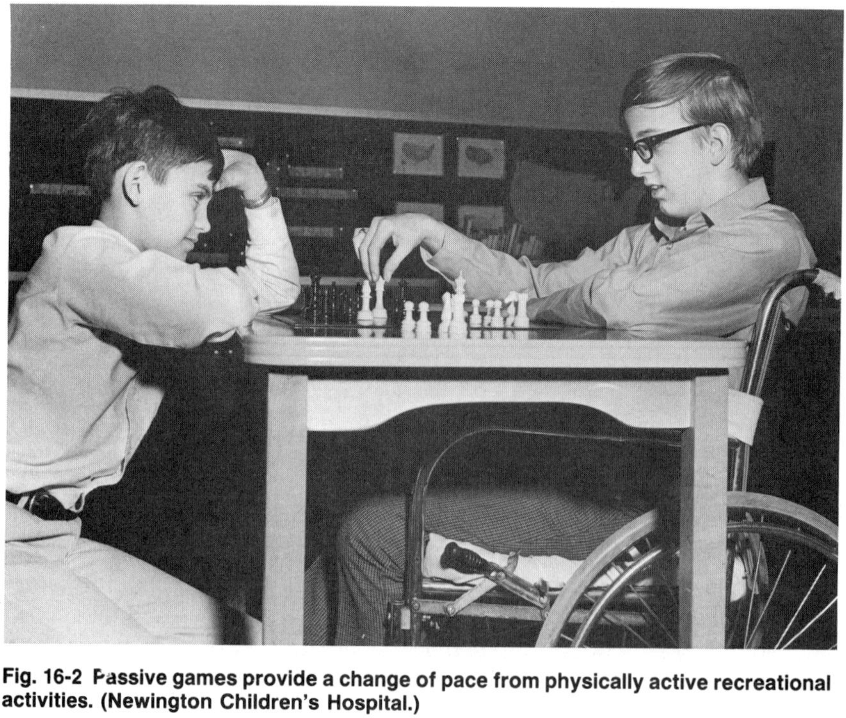

Fig. 16-2 Passive games provide a change of pace from physically active recreational activities. (Newington Children's Hospital.)

it were, from the typical routine of active recreational interests which ordinarily comprises the comprehensive therapeutic recreational program. There are certain passive entertainments which may be considered in the category of special events, despite the fact that client in-put to the planning and execution of such events is negligible or nothing. These events may consist of out-of-institution activities where clients are taken to see shows of various kinds, sporting events, or to visit some site where the operation is considered to be entertainment, e.g., a fashion show. In these instances, the logistics of support necessary for activities of this type require planning and coordination of transportation procedures, dietary and medical arrangements where necessary, the use of supplementary personnel and / or volunteers to assist patients or clients taking the excursion, and the time factor involved.

Passive entertainment should be introduced into the program as a complement to the other program activities. If there is a general theme toward which the program is moving, passive entertainment should emphasize that theme. If the recreationist is attempting to stimulate patient or client participation in specific activities, passive entertainment can be used to focus attention on the particular experiences so that there is some carry-over value and reinforcement of the stimuli that may assist in motivating the patient to try.

Although some aspects of passive entertainment need not have client in-put, much of the program should be assisted by client planning. Therefore, the development of entertainment events can become a part of the client involvement in program development. In whatever way clients are encouraged to take part in planning activities for themselves and others, the procedure must be enjoyable. With guidance and counseling supplied by the therapeutic recreationist, patient activity planning committees can be directed toward those passive entertainments which may be most valuable in meeting client needs.

Preparing Patients and Clients for Entertainment Events

In many instances, depending upon the patient's condition or the client's attitude, individuals have to be prepared for entertainment. This may mean a series of messages or reminders developed to publicize the event. It may involve training to increase an individual's attention span, to sharpen the person's focus of attention, or to inhibit some of a client's more bizarre manifestations of hyperactivity or emotional noncontrol. In the case of the last example, a longer period of preparation may be required during which the patient or client undergoes rehabilitative treatment which may utilize operant conditioning.

For the most part, however, preparations will consist only of determining what entertainment forms are attractive and interesting and then scheduling them at a time and place that will be convenient, accessible, and comfortable for enjoyment of the experience. Sometimes a passive entertainment possibility occurs on the spur-of-the-moment: a visit by a celebrity, a circus passing through town, or a politician on the campaign trail. If it is felt that the appearance of any of these would benefit the patients, then by all means expedient plans should be made to exploit the situation. For such impromptu entertainment, client preparation is necessarily limited and may involve nothing more than finding the most comfortable position for clients to sit, stand, or recline while watching the performance, or trying to elicit from a client a response to the activity so that desired outcomes will be realized.

Preparation may also have to be thought of in terms of the client's condition and the time necessary to feed, dress, and transport the individual to the place where the entertainment will occur. If the performance takes place within the institution, there will be the necessity for assuring that all clients are in their places, whether seated or lying, prior to the time of the show. If a trip outside the treatment center is planned, then the logistics of getting the clients properly washed, fed, dressed, and into vehicles for conveyance to the site of the performance must be undertaken.

Passive Games

The various passive games are widely included as diversionary activities in recreational programs offered in treatment centers and correctional institutions and for homebound clients. They have many advantages: the equipment (except for the electronic games) is inexpensive and easily stored; space needs are no problem; instruction is simple; skill requirements are minimal; and adaptations are usually easily made. The games are absorbing and enjoyable, and most of them offer opportunities for socializations with one or more partners and with those who stop to observe the progress of the activity. Because of these advantages, there is a temptation to use them excessively in the recreational program for ill and disabled clients. Recreationists must resist, however, and attempt instead to provide a balanced program.

One other concern must be mentioned. Some players tend to make even the simplest of the passive games highly competitive. Because clients in special recreational programs have greater anxiety and lower tolerance to frustration, emotional outbreaks are likely to occur unless the recreationist guards against the games becoming overly competitive.

Special Events in Treatment Centers

Special events are unique recreational activities presented occasionally to add extra spice and life to the routine program. The event may present entertainment of a passive nature to the clients, but it may also involve the clients in the planning and presentation.

Special events require so much time, energy, personal commitment, and resources that they are scheduled infrequently. Naturally, the incidence of special events will depend upon the kind of treatment center or recreational setting. Where clientele remain institutionalized for long periods, only one or two special events may occur. Where patient turnover is rapid, special events will be offered more frequently. High patient turnover means that relatively few patients will have extended hospital stays and so would be exposed only to the routine types of activities used for therapeutic gains if special events were not programmed at least once every 3 months. In long-term institutions, the too-frequent advent of special events is likely to cause loss of interest in the speciality and to become too great an energy drain upon clients who would normally be participating.

Most special events are projects that attempt to combine the activities of all into one culminating activity. This often takes the form of a festival, pageant, or similar production that can make use of all of the diverse activities which form the therapeutic recreational program. Typically, a central theme is chosen to give unity of presentation and rally all potential participants so that ego-identification with the theme is achieved.

The adaptation of special events only requires modification of mobility, the development of easily accessible entrances for central stage productions, and the use of a variety of prosthetic attachments and appliances which make the participants more capable of achieving satisfactory performance in their own eyes. Ramps, coverings, and the adaptation of material which conforms to the theme of the event will be necessary.

An example of such adaptations may be illustrated by the following occurrence at one of the larger metropolitan New York hospitals for long-term patients. A theme of carnival had been selected for the summer special event. It would take place during the week of July 4th. A major consideration for the carnival was the production of a masquerade ball to which patients from every unit were invited. Each unit, through its recreational council, decided to be represented in the event by an appropriate tableau or amusing skit. One unit, essentially composed of rheumatoid arthritics, decided to prepare an entry that was based upon the excavation of Tutankhamen's tomb in ancient Egypt. Since there were to be 10 participants in all, the unit decided to have one central figure representing the pharaoh and 9 attendants. The patient who was selected as the pharaoh was a man who could not sit up. His attendants, some of whom were paraplegics or arthritics, were ambulatory in wheelchairs. The contingent appeared in suitable costumes, apparently carrying the reclining figure of the pharaoh—in reality lying upon a stretcher covered with a plain sheet, and decked out in the royal regalia. Broom and mop handles had been attached to the stretcher and camouflaged so as to seem to be the support for a litter. Four attendants on each side of the litter wheeled themselves toward the stage, while a fifth attendant waved a simulated palm frond over the recumbent figure. The palm frond was attached to the chair and could be waved by a wire held in the patient's hands.

The use of ramps effectively enabled all the patients in this part of the event to gain access to the stage and parade across it without any difficulty. From the spectator's point of view, it would have been hard to tell which physical disabilities were being covered because, with few exceptions, the costumes were draped so that they concealed withered limbs, distorted bodies, and the seat supports of spastic patients from the gaze of the viewers. In each instance, ward contingents propelled themselves onto the stage. The pharaoh's entourage was assisted only to the extent that a volunteer pushed the stretcher up the incline to the stage. The members of the party then took their accustomed places and carried off their roles without difficulty.

Thus are adaptations made to compensate for any physical limitations which disease, accident, or birth place upon the institutionalized person. In countless other ways recreationists must extend their ingenuity so that whatever the idea for a special event, the client may be facilitated in its performance. Whether by camouflage, construction of ramps, platforms, or guide rails, or the attachment of equipment or prosthetic devices for ease of use, the recreationist must be aware of the physical capacity of the individual and the kind of movements required to carry out the intent of the performance while still maintaining the integrity and therapeutic benefit which such activity can have for the individual involved.

Special events, like any other recreational modality utilized by recreationists within the therapeutic recreational program, have features which are of value to the patient. The hours spent in the design and creation of a costume, head dress, mask, or other artistic endeavor may mean as much to the individual as will participation in the activity itself. Whatever lends itself to participation and self-expression may, with skilled observation and analysis of the client's behavior prior to, during, and after the event, be reflected in gained insight on the part of both client and recreationist. In turn there occurs a more intense degree of involvement by and with the therapists in other disciplines. To the extent that some aspect of recreational participation, under prescription, results in greater cooperation with other therapists or greater susceptibility to psychologic assistance and/or therapy, the special event may be considered one more advantageous technique in the arsenal of modalities employed by the therapeutic recreationist.

SELECTED REFERENCES

Erickson, M., *Hospital Volunteers Handbook* (Jamaica, New York: Learned Publishing, Inc., 1980).

Raumer, J. A., *Helping People Volunteer* (Morganville, New Jersey: Marlborough Press, 1980).

Chapter 17

Camping and Nature-Oriented Activities

Group living in the natural environment, as in camping, or involvement with flora and fauna through nature-oriented activities can only enhance the life of the ill or disabled person. Camping offers a chance to live in and appreciate the outdoors as a member within the freedom of an essentially democratically controlled group. Nature-oriented activities foster learning and appreciation through hands-on study of natural objects in both indoor and outdoor environments. There is room for both kinds of experiences in the recreational program of the treatment setting and, more particularly, in the community program where adaptation rather than therapeutic assistance is offered. No client need be denied the therapeutic benefits associated with closeness to nature. Adaptations of the environment to produce or reproduce the effects of outdoor experience is possible even for those who are institutionalized or homebound.

There are a number of possibilities for bringing nature-oriented activities to those who cannot go out into the natural environment. Where appropriate space can be set aside, an almost infinite variety of natural objects and specimens may be collected, exhibited, and worked upon. For example, exhibits may be arranged of organic and inorganic specimens such as insects and pebbles; mineral collections may be started from near and far places; growing flowers and plants can be displayed; and insects and small animals can be kept for observation in terrariums, bowls, cages, or cases. Such activities bring elements of the outdoors to those who otherwise would never be able to observe the myriad colorations, geometric configurations, or differentiated sizes and shapes which abound in the natural world.

In addition, other studies of natural science may be introduced to institutionalized clients. Astronomic observations may be made by those who are confined to bed, stretcher, or wheelchair if the proper instruments and views can be provided; observation of the outdoors through hospital windows can be highly enjoyable when binoculars or telescopes are made

313

available. Meteorologic calculations and weather stations may be as easily improvised within the confines of a hospital ward, as they are at camp. Clients may not be able to go out to the woods, hills, and lakes of the countryside, but there are facets of the outdoors that can be brought directly to those who must remain within the hospital or home.

For those who can be transported to camp, the recreationist has the mandatory responsibility to see that camping is made available. It is one phase of a balanced recreational program which can have significant therapeutic value to those for whom it is prescribed. It is of equal importance that those individuals with disabilities, who reside in the community be enabled to participate in adapted camping activities. Such experiences can be modified to accommodate whatever atypicality is encountered.

Camping As a Therapeutic Adjunct

Camping contributes a supportive atmosphere in the treatment milieu. By its residential nature, camping provides for control of the client without the visible restrictions imposed by institutional walls and wards. Camping permits maximum life and group situations without the forced formations usually encountered within the treatment center. There are opportunities for the demonstration of emotions, knowledge, skill, and attitudes in ways that may promote the reduction of tension and heighten individual actualization.

Note must be made, however, that camping may not be the optimum prescribed activity for some clients whose emotional problems are of such magnitude that deep depression results, and, in some instances, suicide or attempts at suicide follow as an aftermath of institutional return.[1] It should be understood that the freedom engendered through camping and the release which accompanies activity away from any institutionalized setting may evoke depressive responses upon return to the confinement of a hospital. This will be felt particularly by those who are emotionally disturbed. To forestall such occurrences of self-destruction, it will probably be necessary to prepare the client for a return to the institutionalized setting by intensive counseling techniques. Such counseling is analogous to the decompression necessary for deep-sea divers to prevent nitrogen bubbles from forming in the bloodstream and causing much pain and sometimes death. Preinstitutional return counseling provides the "decompression" that guards against the client's resort to suicidal gestures as a means of expressing dissatisfaction with institutionalization.[2]

Despite problems that may arise when camping with those who are emotionally disturbed, there is a therapeutic factor in camping which cannot be denied. The value of the camping environment offers a therapeutic milieu which, because of real living situations and the close relationships that can be established between recreationists and clients, should prove eminently satisfying insofar as treatment goals are concerned. If therapeutic recreational activities are designed to intervene in the pathologic behavior exhibited by the patient or to arrange conditions where recuperation is speeded up, then camping is an ideal experience.

One of the objectives of the recreationist is to be able to empathize with the client. By this is meant a sensitivity for and awareness of the needs of individuals within the group. Empathy permits a knowledge of the individual and his or her needs so that they can be satisfied. By satisfying the needs of others and resolving problems or conflicts as they arise, the client may be enabled to employ his or her own cognitive powers in situations that call for making decisions. This can also break the cycle of dependence and the mold of pathologic behavior.

As with all recreational situations, camping offers an uninhibited view of the client in a 24-hour-a-day living situation. This extended and intensive association provides a great deal of information about how clients regard themselves and relate to others. Any untoward behavior is readily seen and steps may be taken to stop it. On the other hand, behavior that is acceptable is easily reinforced. All of the recreational activities which have value to the client/patient may be offered in the camp setting. Values which accrue from facilitating self-expression, creativity, group interaction, or physical exercise are available at camp.

Camping also offers therapeutic values in the sense that activities which are performed can lead to mastery of skills, appreciation of the natural sciences, self-actualization, and achievement of personal goals. The give-and-take of camp life permits the individual to associate freely with others and begin to behave in ways that are socially acceptable. Many of the activities are exciting and in themselves may facilitate catharsis or relieve anxiety and tension. As always, camping activities and the camp experience itself are selected and prescribed because of the therapeutic value that they have for a particular patient in accordance with a specific rehabilitation or treatment objective.

Role of the Recreationist. Many clients cannot tolerate camping, regardless of their health. In some instances the camping environment offers nothing but frustration, loneliness, anxiety, and a time of total misery for the individual involved.[3] This is so because personnel have not fulfilled the assignment for which they were employed. It is the task of recreationists, employed within the treatment center, to make the environment a therapeutic medium. This is best performed by working closely with the incapacitated person, being sensitive toward and anticipating needs, resolving problems before they become calamities, and making the camp atmosphere enjoyable. The recreationist has a key role to play in this process when camping is the method utilized to promote phases of the client's rehabilitation.

To create social situations within a beneficial physical setting where patients can sense their significance as human beings, where their in-

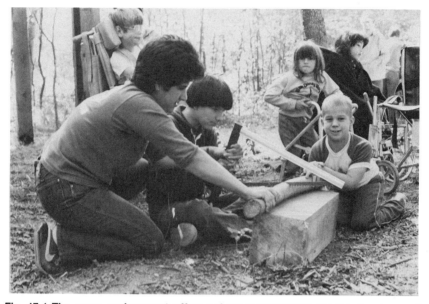

Fig. 17-1 The camp environment offers unique opportunities for the development of skills and achievement of personal satisfaction. (Hemlocks Outdoor Education Center.)

dividuality and personal worth are respected is one method by which the camping environment may be used therapeutically. The camp becomes the environment in which helping relationships are established. The various nature-oriented activities become the media by which assistance can be given and received. Activities are opportunities for the development of personal growth, skill, and self-expression. Further, they provide the basis for discovering capacities which might have been overlooked in a less open situation. Activities which are properly structured and presented can be personally satisfying and enjoyable. Under such circumstances, it is only natural to believe that helping relationships will be formed and that these will enable the client to behave in ways that are personally beneficial. Intervention in undesirable behavior may result in those changes which are necessary for the treatment or rehabilitation goal to be achieved.

The Recreationist as a Listener. The recreationist may perform a much needed function as a listener. In the camp situation, a tendency toward verbal communication, which may sometimes be inhibited in the more formal surroundings of the treatment center, is seen. The recreationist will realize that listening to others, not simply for understanding, but for the therapeutic value obtained when one is permitted to articulate personal problems, can facilitate insight or personal growth. Even the most inarticulate person will be helped when a sympathetic listener is available. The opportunity to speak, without interruption, is seldom offered in a culture where conversation is really self-expression rather than listening to another person or attempting to gain new knowledge. Individuals who have never been able to express themselves or have been denied opportunities for verbal self-expression may well become voluble when confronted with an appreciative listener. Camping activities may be the medium which stimulates a desire for speech. The recreationist can serve a most important therapeutic aim and establish rapport with any patient if prepared to be a readily available receiver.

Providing Opportunity for Independence. The chief impact which camping will have upon the client will be the heady atmosphere of permissiveness. This does not mean anarchy or abandoned behavior which cannot be condoned. Rather it suggests circumstances which are not restricted by complex institutional rules and regulations. Individuals are not restrained from trying to accomplish projects or activities—unless contraindicated by medical necessity. The range of possible outdoor experiences is so extensive that individuals can find something which is achievable that might have been overlooked in more routinized treatment settings. No one fully understands the potential which people can attain if they are given the proper environment to try. It is conceivable that with empathetic recreationists as counselors the personal associations established can lead to the development of skills, knowledge, or latent talent that promotes healthier psychologic outlooks and modified behavior conforming to optimum treatment objectives.

In discussing the need for establishing helping relationships so that individuals are enabled to search effectively for new meanings in their lives, Combs has this to say about changing the environment:

> To bring about change in behavior requires changing personal meanings. But this is no simple task, for perceptions lie inside people and are, consequently, not open to direct manipulation. To change behavior it is necessary, somehow, to involve the behavior in the process. In one way or another, he must be induced to explore and discover new meanings with respect to himself and his world. A person's self, however, is precious. It cannot be heedlessly placed in jeopardy. The turtle cannot go anywhere until he sticks his neck out. He will not stick his neck out unless there is something out there he wants and he feels it is safe outside. In similar fashion the self can only be committed when there seems some likelihood that commitment will result in a measure of fulfillment and that the self will not be damaged in the process. This is true for everyone, especially for the sick and inadequate persons whose selves are so threatened that they must be continually maintaining and protecting themselves from further destruction.[4]

Perhaps at camp the environment for change will enhance opportunities where self-perception, expression, and involvement can occur. To effect modification in meanings, the recreationist must be adept at producing the kind of climate in which self-actualization flourishes. This requires a condition in which the individual realizes that any attempt that he or she makes to assist recuperation or rehabilitation will be greeted enthusiastically, that such attempts will receive support and be positively reinforced, that protection is provided against ego diminishment, and finally that satisfaction will be obtained in consequence of the attempt. How adequately this happens will rest with the recreationist's understanding of individual needs and the behavior which needs encouragement so that the patient profits from the situation created.

Recreationists must be enablers. They should know when to be active and when to be passive. They must know when to listen and when to offer response. They must be knowledgeable about possible activities and understand and accept the client as an individual, and they must have the ability to use relationships in such a constructive manner that the client is able to achieve therapeutically desirable goals.

TYPES OF CAMPS

Whether the program of the camp is developed around therapeutic prescription or is adapted to the clients' abilities depends on the purpose of the camp and the way it is organized. In the former, medical personnel are chiefly responsible for setting program goals that are harmonious with the overall treatment plan. In the latter, goals are established by the camp recreationists and administrators. Camps may be organized to care for and treat those with some disease entity or those who are multiply handicapped. If the number of clients is small enough, a variety of disabilities may be included within one camp. However, special camps have been developed to accommodate particular problems.

Where special camps are in operation, clients can be given initial camping experiences that enable them to develop skills to a sufficient degree to function well in similar environments. In some instances, clients who have been in a special camp have transferred to camp programs that are not specialized. The primary experience has been beneficial and enjoyable enough to encourage those with a lesser handicap to participate in organized residential or day camp programs for those without disabilities.

For others, whose disabilities are too severe to permit camping in other than closely supervised and therapeutically operated environments, the special camping experience offers unique choices to participate in nature-oriented situations that cannot be obtained elsewhere.

Clientele. *Orthopedic, Neurologic, and Cardiac Clients.* Individuals with orthopedic, neurologic, and cardiac problems may benefit enormously from the relaxed atmosphere which a camp can offer. Activities can range from absolute passivity, e.g., watching clouds, to participation in swimming, boating, or other strenuous physical activity. All such activity is carefully supervised in terms of the individual's capacity to perform. To the extent that emotional problems manifest themselves as a direct consequence of the disability, the client may be introduced to graded activities which progress toward mastery; this may induce a more optimistic and stable outlook on life.

Epileptic Clients. As with those who are neurologically impaired or disabled, the epileptic client can benefit greatly from exposure to nature-oriented activities and camping practices. Where special camps are organized to care for and administer to those with epilepsy, it is probable that the individual can participate in all or nearly all of the activities which normal persons would undertake without restriction. In many instances the individual who receives regular medication is enabled to reside and completely adapt to the exigencies of camp life. As with all disability, the reaction of others to the person afflicted has much to do with the individual's ability to withstand emotional disturbance and cope with everyday life. Psychologic problems are minimized when others have a favorable reaction to the epileptic client and do not treat him or her as someone who is different and needs to be watched for bizarre behavior. Specialized camps are often best for those with more developed personality maladjustments.

Diabetic Clients. Camping is thought to be a basic necessity for the rehabilitation of those who are diabetic. Children with diabetes have greater opportunities for participating in the camping experience than do adults, but there is a growing number of camps which specialize in the treatment and care of the older age group. Obviously medical supervision is essential for the diabetic camper. The need for dietary control, activity prescription, and medical observation makes camping a ready therapeutic adjunct. Although the treatment and costs per camper are almost identical to those of the patient in a hospital setting, the relaxed atmosphere of the camp and the desired effects in terms of emotional stability and self-realization are much greater.

Mentally Retarded Clients. Camping for mentally retarded individuals is considered quite routine these days. Under proper supervision, those retarded individuals without other incapacitating disabilities may actively engage in an infinite variety of recreational activities appropriate to a camp setting. The enriched experiences received in out-of-door situations are particularly stimulating to those whose participation in so many activities is rather limited. Retarded clients can probably engage in the full range of camping activities, limited, of course, by their mental ability to appreciate and recognize hazardous undertakings. With competent supervision, however, dangerous explorations can be vetoed.

Blind Clients. Camping for blind individuals is well established in the United States. Blindness does not really prevent the individual from participation in nearly every kind of outdoor experience. With well-planned facilities and the removal of barriers or hazards that might become nuisances, blind campers can move about without escort and are capable of participating in every kind of camp activity.

Deaf Clients. Like blindness, deafness is no obstacle to camping. The only restriction upon deaf clients may occur as a result of personality maladjustment and, perhaps, a lack of communication between camp authorities and the deaf camper. Regular camps accept deaf children; when emotional problems are of such proportion that regular camps do not wish to take responsibility, special camps have been organized for the purpose.

Alcoholic, Drug Abusing, and Obese Clients. Camps may be organized around special medical needs of individuals who would otherwise find themselves confined to an institution or voluntarily commit themselves to some treatment regimen. In these cases, specialized camps are organized by hospitals, schools, or nationally recognized agencies involved with the treatment of these problems. All activities are carried on under medical supervision and camping activities are prescribed for therapeutic purposes. The avowed aim of such programs is to maintain emotional stability, reduce patient anxiety, and eliminate dependence upon the agent which is both cause and effect of the problem. In the camping environment, the resolution of emotional issues, which often are the underlying basis of the addiction, may be enhanced.

Aged Clients. Camping for older adults is neither new nor confined to those who are residing in nursing homes or geriatric facilities. Camping is as rewarding to the older adult as to the younger counterpart. Whether the outdoor experience is provided by a residential day camp or is a simple outing to a nearby park, the change from four walls to the pleasant aspect of comfortable outdoor situations necessarily offers a heightened sense of awareness to one's surroundings and adds zest to living. Much in the outdoors promotes a thirst for living. Older adults whose health is good are reportedly good campers and can withstand the rigors of inclement weather or changed surroundings. The regularity of camp life, nourishing food, stimulating activities, and opportunities to socialize permit life to flourish and reduce morbidity.

The Program

Camping and nature-oriented programs can have great symbolic meaning to the client and may leave a lasting good impression because individual experiences are interrelated and complement or supplement one another. Ideally, each activity draws upon the contributions of others because of the associations that are made as the camping program unfolds. Almost every form of recreational activity can be offered with or without adaptation in a camp setting or an artificially created nature environment.

Among the activities which should be a part of any nature-oriented program will be:

- aquatics
- astronomy
- agriculture
- archery
- games
- conversation
- lapidary work
- geology

- art
- crafts
- ceremonials
- scouting
- exploring
- hiking
- boating
- tripping
- dances

- ecology
- hobbies
- dramatics
- tournaments
- music
- reading
- meteorology
- pomology
- entomology

This listing is neither exhaustive nor impossible to schedule. It merely relies upon the ingenuity and skill which all recreationists must have if they are going to work with the ill, disabled, or handicapped.

Adaptation of Camping and Nature-Oriented Activities

When clients are so sick, either emotionally or physically, that they cannot be permitted to undertake a camping experience, then nature should be brought to them. Individuals who have never been exposed to nature-oriented activities should be given that opportunity under medical supervision. The experience of working with, handling, smelling, hearing, or seeing flora and fauna within simulated typical habitats might bring associated benefits which other recreational participation cannot fulfill. The following adaptations can be made to provide satisfying experiences.

Bed-bound patients may learn about various leaves, bark, berries, pods, weeds, grasses, grains, and roots by smelling, touching, tasting, or using them in a planned series of nature activities. Berries may be used for dyes, and seeds, twigs, pine cones, pods, and fungi can be used for decorations, ornamentation, and art work. Natural clay may be brought to the hospital for manipulation and the production of objects and utensils.

Patients who must remain in bed, particularly children, may be transferred to stretchers, or beds which can be rolled to appropriate locations on the hospital grounds. Such adaptations are readily available where the hospital is either surrounded by lawns or is situated in an open space or rural environment. When weather permits, patients may be transferred to the grounds for a day camping program. Any number of typical day-camping activities may be incorporated into the experience. Bed or table height stretchers may be utilized for nature craft activities, cooking fires may be a part of the program with participants permitted to grill their own food with long-handled forks. For young children, water activities may be included by creating specially constructed shallow pools in which a certain amount of free splashing is permitted and/or encouraged. In addition, model boats may be sailed.

Even where an urban hospital cannot provide lawns, trees, or bushes to offer a sense of nature, adaptations can still be made. Almost every hospital has a flat roof which can be constructed to present a natural appearance. A variety of planters with numerous types of flora may be placed at appropriate points on the roof, perhaps to give the appearance of a forest glade. Recycled water can be employed to provide a running stream or a small waterfall, the water being collected into a shallow pool and then used over and over again. Careful supervision is necessary to make sure that those children who want to can benefit from water play. Adjustable tables or rests can be provided to enable patients to participate in musical, craft, art, game, or dramatic activities. Some type of recreational activity may be possible all during the year if patients can be sheltered from extremes of temperature or direct exposure for too long a period to sun or wind.

Other adaptations should include the modification of any possible space that can be provided to accommodate some aspect of outdoor activity. Thus, if there is a lawn in the vicinity of the hospital and patients are capable of some movement, then some nature study can still be offered. Ant colonies may be viewed and flying insects can be trapped without a great deal of movement. With the assistance of microscopes, it is likely that water droplets and grains of earth can be examined. This is not camping, but it is another aspect of exploring the physical universe. It enables the natural phenomena to be observed, learned about, and appreciated. All that is necessary is time and the patient's attention to discern the infinite variety of organic matter in the natural environment.

Where camps are neither accessible nor available, the use of nearby parks and forests for short outings, picnics, explorations, or excursions is a completely satisfactory substitute.

Adapting Conditions to Meet Community Needs

Camping activities may be offered to disabled residents of a community if areas are planned to accommodate those who might ordinarily be prevented from using park and forest spaces. While every effort should be made to offer handicapped individuals recreational activities that can be enjoyed in the outdoors, i.e., camping and similar activities, some modificatons are necessary due to disability. Many textured surfaces, which blind persons can feel and translate into their own experiences, may need to be developed. A variety of trails can be laid out for use by blind as well as wheelchair restricted persons. Trails may be arranged so that a blind person has a guide rope or wire to contact and maintain direction. The trail should be arranged so that it cuts across many different kinds of terrain, particularly containing varied sounds and smells.

Safety precautions must be recognized and followed. Rest periods are necessary—fatigue factors are powerful deterrents for the disabled. The supervised program should contain diverse activities, although not necessarily competitive or anxiety-producing ones.

Modified primitive camping is possible for many who suffer from physical disability. Essentially, primitive camping practice requires improvisation—

that is, doing things in a simple way with whatever objects are at hand. This means that modification and adjustment of the environment are not only practical but challenging. Activities such as campfire cooking, sleeping out overnight, shelter building, food caching, and fire-making all require adapted materials, utensils, beds, or the development of a camping site. Even severely disabled persons can assist with cooking meals and arranging materials for outdoor sleeping. Outdoor activities such as fishing, archery, stalking, or field observation can be performed by physically impaired persons without much adaptation.

Hiking or field trips can be modified so that a group of persons with varied disabilities can participate. While a hike is generally intended to cover a specified distance, presumably through picturesque areas, field trips do not have any specified points to cover. Hiking can be designed so that even heterogeneous handicaps can be accommodated. For example, those with moderate impairment can begin the hike at a later time so that more severely disabled individuals may start earlier and rest more frequently; both will reach a given destination simultaneously if the hike is correctly planned. Transportation may also be provided to those whose fatigue or lack of endurance prevents them from completing the walk. Any combination of these factors can be used to facilitate hiking. Field trips on the other hand are often designed without any destination in view. The objective is more exploratory, taking much time and focusing on observations, specimen collecting, or discovering materials with which to fabricate articles or nature crafts.

REFERENCES

1. David J. Muller, "Post-Camping Depression: A Lethal Possibility," *American Journal of Psychiatry,* Vol. 212, No. 1 (July, 1971) p. 141.
2. James L. Ryan and Dale T. Johnson, "Therapeutic Camping: A Comparative Study," *Therapeutic Recreation Journal,* Vol. IV, No. 4 (Fourth Quarter 1972) p. 180.
3. Jay S. Shivers, *Camping: Administration, Counseling, Programming* (Englewood Cliffs, New Jersey: Prentice-Hall Inc., 1971).
4. A. W. Combs *et al, Helping Relationships: Basic Concepts for the Helping Professions* (Boston: Allyn and Bacon, Inc., 1971) p. 220.

SELECTED REFERENCES

Boy Scouts of America, *Exploring Division, Exploring for the Handicapped* (New Brunswick, New Jersey: BSA, 1975).
Croucher, N., *Outdoor Pursuits for Disabled People* (Mystic, Connecticut: Lawrence, Verry, Inc., 1981).
Kraus, Richard G. and Scanlin, Margery M., *Introduction to Camp Counseling,* (Englewood Cliffs, New Jersey: Prentice-Hall, Inc., 1983).
Mitchell, A. Viola and Meier, Joel F., *Camp Counseling: Leadership and Programming for the Organized Camp,* 6th. ed., (Philadelphia: Saunders College Publishing, 1983).
Shea, Thomas M., *Camping for Special Children* (St. Louis: C. V. Mosby Co., 1977).
Shivers, Jay S., *Camping: Administration, Counseling, Programming* (Englewood Cliffs, New Jersey: Prentice-Hall, Inc., 1971).

Appendices

Appendix I

Standards for Certification
National Council for Therapeutic
Recreation Certification*

Professional Level—Therapeutic Recreation Specialist
(minimum requirements)

A. Baccalaureate degree or higher from an accredited college or university with a major in therapeutic recreation or a major in recreation and option* in therapeutic recreation. Degree must be verified by an official transcript from the registrar. A student's copy is not acceptable.

OR

B. Baccalaureate degree or higher from an accredited college or university with a major in recreation *and* 2 years of full-time paid experience in a clinical, residential, or community-based therapeutic recreation program. Degree must be verified by an official transcript from the registrar. A student's copy is not acceptable.

Professional Provisional—Therapeutic Recreation Specialist (Non-Renewable)
(minimum requirements)

C. Baccalaureate degree or higher from an accredited college or university with a major in recreation. Degree must be verified by an official transcript from the registrar. A student's copy is not acceptable.

This alternative permits temporary certification while a person acquires the 2 years of full-time paid experience in a clinical, residential, or community-based therapeutic recreation program necessary for renewal of certification as a professional.

Professional Equivalency Process—Therapeutic Recreation Specialist
(minimum requirements)

---

*National Council for Therapeutic Recreation Certification. Current Revision: February 1983, p. 3.

327

D. Baccalaureate degree or higher from an accredited college or university in one of the related or allied health fields *plus* 5 years of full-time paid experience in a clinical, residential, or community-based therapeutic recreation program *plus* 18 semester or 27 quarter hours of upper division credits in recreation/therapeutic recreation competencies. Degree must be verified by an official transcript from the registrar. A student's copy is not acceptable.

Para-Professional—Therapeutic Recreation Assistant
(minimum requirements)

A. Associate of Arts degree from an accredited educational institution with a major in therapeutic recreation or a major in recreation and an option** in therapeutic recreation. Degree must be verified by an official transcript from the registrar. A student's copy is not acceptable.

OR

B. Associate of Arts degree from an accredited educational institution with a major in recreation *plus* one year of full-time paid experience in a clinical, residential, or community-based therapeutic recreation program. Degree must be verified by an official transcript from the registrar. A student's copy is not acceptable.

OR

C. Associate of Arts degree or higher from an accredited educational institution with a major in one of the skill areas (arts, crafts, dance, drama, music, physical education) and one year of full-time paid experience in a clinical, residential, or community-based therapeutic recreation program. Degree must be verified by an official transcript from the registrar. A student's copy is not acceptable.

OR

D. Completion of the NTRS 750-Hour Training Program for therapeutic recreation personnel, with verification by an official certificate of completion.

OR

E. Four years of full-time paid experience in a clinical, residential, or community-based therapeutic recreation program.

*PROFESSIONAL OPTION

The *professional option* includes:

a. A minimum of three courses dealing exclusively with therapeutic recreation content, and

b. Completion of a 360-hour field placement experience in a clinical, residential, or community-based therapeutic recreation program, and

c. Completion of supportive coursework to include a minimum of 18 semester or 27 quarter units from 4 of these 6 areas:

psychology
sociology
physical / biological science
special education
human services
adapted physical education

**PARA-PROFESSIONAL OPTION

The *paraprofessional option* includes:

a. A minimum of two courses dealing exclusively with therapeutic recreation content, and

b. Completion of a 360-hour field placement experience in a clinical, residential, or community-based therapeutic recreation program, and

c. Completion of supportive coursework to include a minimum of 12 semester or 18 quarter units selected from psychology, sociology, physical / biological sciences, human services, and physical education activity classes.

Appendix II

Philosophical Position Statement of the National Therapeutic Recreation Society
(A Branch of the National Recreation and Park Association)
(Adopted, May 1982)

Leisure, including recreation and play, are inherent aspects of the human experience. The importance of appropriate leisure involvement has been documented throughout history. More recently, research has addressed the value of leisure involvement in human development, in social and family relationships, and, in general, as an important aspect of the quality of life. Some human beings have disabilities, illnesses, or social conditions which limit their full participation in the normative social structure of society. These individuals with limitations have the same human rights to, and needs for, leisure involvement.

The purpose of therapeutic recreation is to facilitate the development, maintenance, and expression of an appropriate leisure lifestyle for individuals with physical, mental, emotional, or social limitations. Accordingly, this purpose is accomplished through the provision of professional programs and services which assist the client in eliminating barriers to leisure, developing leisure skills and attitudes, and optimizing leisure involvement. Therapeutic recreation professionals use these principles to enhance clients' leisure ability in recognition of the importance and value of leisure in the human experience.

Three specific areas of professional services are employed to provide this comprehensive leisure ability approach toward enabling appropriate leisure lifestyles: therapy, leisure education, and recreation participation. While these three areas of service have unique purposes in relation to client need, they each employ similar delivery processes using assessment or identification of client need, development of a related program strategy, and monitoring and evaluating client outcomes. The decision as to where and when each of the three service areas would be provided is based on the assessment of client needs and the service mandate of the sponsoring agency. The selection of appropriate service areas is contingent on a recognition that different clients have differing needs related to leisure involvement in view of their personal life situation.

The purpose of the *therapy* service area within therapeutic recreation is to improve functional behaviors. Some clients may require treatment or remediation of a functional behavior as a necessary prerequisite to enable their involvement in meaningful leisure experiences. *Therapy,* therefore, is viewed as most appropriate when clients have functional limitations that relate to, or inhibit, their potential leisure involvement. This distinction enables the therapeutic recreator to decide when *therapy* service is appropriate, as well as to identify the types of behaviors that are most appropriate to address within the therapeutic recreation domain of expertise and authority. In settings where a comprehensive treatment team approach is used, *therapy* focuses on team identified treatment goals, as well as addressing unique aspects of leisure related functional behaviors. This approach places therapeutic recreation as an integral and cooperative member of the comprehensive treatment team, while linking its primary focus to eventual leisure ability.

The purpose of the *leisure education* service area is to provide opportunities for the acquisition of skills, knowledge, and attitudes related to leisure involvement. For some clients, acquiring leisure skills, knowledge, and attitudes are priority needs. It appears that the majority of clients in residential, treatment, and community settings need *leisure education* services in order to initiate and engage in leisure experiences. It is the absence of leisure learning opportunities and socialization into leisure that blocks or inhibits these individuals from participation in leisure experiences. Here, *leisure education* services would be employed to provide the client with leisure skills, enhance the client's attitudes concerning the value and importance of leisure, as well as learning about opportunities and resources for leisure involvement. Thus, *leisure education* programs provide the opportunity for the development of leisure behaviors and skills.

The purpose of the *recreation participation* area of therapeutic recreation services is to provide opportunities which allow voluntary client involvement in recreation interests and activities. Human beings, despite disability, illness, or other limiting conditions, and, regardless of place of residence, are entitled to recreation opportunities. The justification for specialized *recreation participation* programs is based on the clients' need for assistance and/or adapted recreation equipment, limitations imposed by restrictive treatment or residential environments, or the absence of appropriate community recreation opportunities. In therapeutic recreation services, the need for *recreation participation* is acknowledged and given appropriate emphasis in recognition of the intent of the leisure ability concept.

These three service areas of therapeutic recreation represent a continuum of care, including *therapy, leisure education,* and the provision of special *recreation participation* opportunities. This comprehensive leisure ability approach uses the need of the client to give direction to program service selection. In some situations, the client may need programs from all three service areas. In other situations, the client may require only one or two of the service areas.

Equally important is the concern of generalizing therapeutic recreation service across diverse service delivery settings. The leisure ability approach of therapeutic recreation provides appropriate program direction regardless of type of setting or type of client served. A professional working in a treatment setting can see the extension of the leisure ability approach toward client needs within the community environment. Likewise, those within the community can view therapeutic recreation services within a perspective of previous services received or possible future needs.

All human beings, including those individuals with disabilities, illnesses or limiting conditions, have a right to, and a need for, leisure involvement as a necessary aspect of the human experience. The purpose of therapeutic recreation services is to facilitate the development, maintenance, and expression of an appropriate leisure lifestyle for individuals with limitations through the provision of *therapy, leisure education,* and *recreation participation* services.

The National Therapeutic Recreation Society is the acknowledged professional organization representing the field of therapeutic recreation. The National Therapeutic Recreation Society exists to foster the development and advancement of this field in order to ensure quality professional services and to protect the rights of consumers of therapeutic recreation services. In order to provide consistent and identifiable services throughout the field, the National Therapeutic Recreation Society endorses the leisure ability philosophy described herein as the official position statement regarding therapeutic recreation.

Appendix III

Texas Revision of Fait's Basic Motor Skills Test*
Basic Movement Performance Profile

1. Walking
   - 0—makes no attempt at walking
   - 1—walks while being pulled
   - 3—walks with toe-heel placement
   - 3—walks with shuffle
   - 4—walks with heel-toe placement and opposite arm-foot swing

2. Pushing (wheelchair)
   - 0—makes no attempt to push wheelchair
   - 1—makes some attempt to push wheelchair
   - 2—pushes wheelchair once with arms only
   - 3—pushes wheelchair with continuous motion for 10 ft.
   - 4—pushes wheelchair carrying adult occupant continuously for 10 ft.

3. Ascending Stairs (up 4 stair steps)
   - 0—makes no attempt to walk up stairs
   - 1—steps up one step with assistance
   - 2—walks up 4 steps with assistance
   - 3—walks up 4 steps; two feet on each step
   - 4—walks up 4 steps; alternating one foot on each step

4. Descending Stairs (down 4 stair steps)
   - 0—makes no attempt to walk down stairs
   - 1—steps down one step with assistance
   - 2—walks down 4 steps with assistance
   - 3—walks down 4 steps, two feet on each step
   - 4—walks down 4 steps, alternating one foot on each step

5. Climbing (4 rungs; 1st choice, ladder of slide, 2nd choice, step ladder)
   - 0—makes no attempt to climb ladder
   - 1—climbs at least one rung with assistance
   - 2—climbs 4 rungs with assistance
   - 3—climbs 4 rungs, two feet on each rung
   - 4—climbs 4 rungs, alternating one foot on each rung

6. Carrying (folded folding chair)
   - 0—makes no attempt to lift chair from floor
   - 1—attempts but not able to lift chair from floor
   - 2—lifts chair from floor
   - 3—carries chair by dragging on the floor
   - 4—carries chair 10 ft.

7. Pulling (wheelchair)
   - 0—makes no attempt to pull wheelchair

*Test development financed by the Joseph P. Kennedy, Jr. Foundation.

1—makes some attempt to pull wheelchair
2—pulls wheelchair once with arms only
3—pulls wheelchair with continuous motion for 10 ft.
4—pulls wheelchair carrying adult occupant continuously for 10 ft.

8. Running
0—makes no attempt to run
1—takes long walking steps while being pulled
2—takes running steps while being pulled
3—jogs (using toe or flat of foot)
4—runs for 25 yds., with both feet off the ground when body weight shifts from the rear to front foot

9. Catching (bean bag tossed from 5 ft. away)
0—makes no attempt to catch bean bag
1—holds both arms out to catch bean bag
2—catches bean bag fewer than 5 of 10 attempts
3—catches bean bag at least 5 of 10 attempts
4—catches bean bag at least 8 of 10 attempts

10. Creeping
0—makes no attempt to creep
1—will assume hands and knees position
2—creeps with a shuffle
3—creeps alternating hands and knees
4—creeps in a crosslateral pattern with head up

11. Jumping Down (two foot take-off and landing from 18 in. folding chair)
0—makes no attempt
1—steps down from chair with assistance
2—steps down from chair
3—jumps off chair with two foot take-off and landing with assistance
4—jumps off chair with two foot take-off and landing while maintaining balance

12. Throwing (overhand softball, 3 attempts)
0—makes no attempt to throw
1—grasps ball and releases in attempt to throw
2—throws or tosses ball a few feet in any direction
3—throws ball at least 15 ft. in air in intended direction
4—throws ball at least 30 ft. in the air in intended direction

13. Hitting (volleyball with plastic bat)
0—makes no attempt to hit ball
1—hits stationary ball fewer than 3 of 5 attempts
2—hits stationary ball at least 3 of 5 attempts
3—hits ball rolled from 15 ft. away fewer than 3 of 5 attempts
4—hits ball rolled from 15 ft. away at least 3 of 5 attempts.

14. Forward Roll
0—makes no attempt to do forward roll
1—puts hands and head on mat
2—puts hands and head on mat and pushes with feet and/or knees in an attempt to do roll

Appendix IV

Fait Physical Fitness Test for Mildly and Moderately Mentally Retarded Individuals*

Twenty-Five Yard Run. (Measures the speed of running short distances.) The subject places either foot against the wall (or block) with the foot parallel to it. He or she then takes a semi-crouch position with the hands resting lightly on the knees. The forward foot and trunk are turned in the direction he or she is to run. The head is held up so that he or she is looking toward the finish line. At the command of "Ready: go!" the subject begins the run. The watch is started on the "Go" and is stopped as the subject passes the finish line. However, the subject is directed to run to a second line, which is about 5 feet beyond the finish line to prevent slowing down during the approach to the true finish line. The time of the run is recorded to the nearest one-tenth of a second.

Bent Arm Hang. (Measures static muscular endurance of the arm and shoulder girdle.) A horizontal bar or doorway bar may be used for this test. A stool approximately 12 inches high is placed under the bar. The subject steps onto the stool and takes hold of the bar with both hands, using a reverse grip (palms toward the face). The hands are shoulders' width apart. The subject brings his or her head to the bar, presses the bridge of the nose to the bar, and steps off the stool. This position is held as long as possible. The timer starts the watch as the subject's nose presses to bar and the body weight is taken on the arms. The watch is stopped when the subject drops away from the bar. The tester should be ready to catch the subject in the event of a fall. The number of seconds the subject held the position is recorded on the score card.

Leg Lift. (Measures dynamic muscular endurance of the flexor muscles of the leg and of the abdominal muscles.) The subject lies flat on the back with hands clasped behind the neck. A helper should hold the subject's elbows to the mat. The subject raises his or her legs, keeping

*Test development financed by the Joseph P. Kennedy, Jr. Foundation.

335

the knees straight until they are at a 90-degree angle. Another helper, who stands to the side of the subject, extends one hand over the subject's abdomen at the height of the ankles when the legs are fully lifted. This serves as a guide to the subject in achieving the desired angle and encourages the subject to keep the legs straight. He or she should be instructed to touch the shins against the helper's arm. The subject is to do as many leg lifts as possible in the 20-second time limit. The test begins on the command of "Go" and ceases on the command of "Stop." The score is the number of leg lifts performed during the 20 seconds.

Static Balance Test. (Measures ability to maintain balance on one leg.) The subject places hands on hips, lifts one leg, and places the foot on the inside of the knee of the other leg. The subject then closes his or her eyes and maintains balance in this position as long as possible. The watch is started the moment the eyes close. As soon as the subject loses balance, the watch is stopped. The score is the number of seconds to the nearest one tenth of a second.

Thrusts. (Measures the specific type of agility that is measured by the Squat Thrust or Burpee.) The subject takes a squatting position with the feet and hands flat on the floor. The knees should make contact with the arms. At the command "Go," the stop watch is started. The subject takes the weight upon the hands so that he or she may thrust the legs straight out behind. The legs are returned to the original position. The score is the number of complete thrusts the subject is able to perform in 20 seconds. One-half point is awarded for completing half of the thrust.

300-Yard Run-Walk. (Measures cardiorespiratory endurance.) If the run is to be given outside on a track, it can be administered to large numbers at one time by placing the runners in one long straight row or in two rows with one behind the other. The runners in taking a starting position should place one foot comfortably ahead of the other. A semi-crouch position with the hands resting lightly on the knees is taken. At the command to go, the stop watch is started. The subjects run the prescribed course. They are allowed to walk part of the distance if they are unable to run the total distance. As each runner crosses the finish line, the timer calls off the time to a recorder who makes a check beside the corresponding time on a prepared sheet. As the timer continues to call off the times as the runners pass the finish line, the recorder goes down the line of times and checks the times called. If two runners cross the line at the same time, two checks are placed beside the appropriate time on the sheet. As the runners finish, they line up according to the order in which they finished. One person will be needed to help the runners stay in correct order. When the runners are all in line, the name of the runner and the time it took to complete the race can be matched and placed on the score card by comparing the order of runners to the order of times as they appear on the sheet.

A score card for comparison of the results of the test items is presented in a table that appears in Appendix V.

Appendix V

Norms for Fait Physical Fitness Test For Mildly and Moderately Retarded Individuals

25-Yard Run

Boys
(Score in Seconds)

		Trainable			Educable	
Age	Low	Av.	Good	Low	Av.	Good
9-12	7	6	5.2	6.2	5.2	4.4
13-16	6.5	5.5	4.7	5.4	4.7	4.2
17-20	6	5	4.2	5.1	4.4	3.9

Girls

9-12	7.4	6.3	5.3	5.8	5.4	5.2
13-16	6.7	5.6	4.7	6.1	5.2	4.3
17-20	7.3	6.1	5.1	6.4	5.4	4.7

Bent Arm Hang

Boys
(Score in Seconds)

		Trainable			Educable	
Age	Low	Av.	Good	Low	Av.	Good
9-12	2	10	16	3	19	33
13-16	11.2	22	30.2	5	25	43
17-20	23	23	31	8	30	50

Girls

9-12	2	8	12	3	9	13
13-16	4	14	22	5	15	23
17-20	3	9	13	4	12	18

Leg Lift

Boys

		Trainable			Educable	
Age	Low	Av.	Good	Low	Av.	Good
9-12	6	9	12	7	10	13
13-16	6	9	12	8	11	14
17-20	7	10	13	8	11	14

Girls

Age						
9-12	6	10	14	6	10	14
13-16	7	11	15	7	11	15
17-20	6	10	14	6	10	14

Static Balance

Boys
(Score in Seconds)

		Trainable			*Educable*	
Age	*Low*	*Av.*	*Good*	*Low*	*Av.*	*Good*
9-12	3	4.4	5.8	4	5	6
13-16	3.1	4.5	5.9	5	6	7
17-20	3.2	4.6	6	5	10	15

Girls

Age						
9-12	2.2	3.2	4.2	2.5	3.5	4.5
13-16	5.1	6.1	7.1	8.6	9.6	10.6
17-20	4.9	5.9	6.9	5.2	6.2	7.2

Thrust

Boys

		Trainable			*Educable*	
Age	*Low*	*Av.*	*Good*	*Low*	*Av.*	*Good*
9-12	4	8	10	6	12	14
13-16	4	8	10	8	14	16
17-20	5	9	11	8	14	16

Girls

Age						
9-12	4	8	10	5	9	11
13-16	4	8	10	8	12	14
17-20	5	9	11	5	9	11

300-Yard Run-Walk

Boys
(Score in Seconds)

		Trainable			*Educable*	
Age	*Low*	*Av.*	*Good*	*Low*	*Av.*	*Good*
9-12	145	115	95	105	80	60
13-16	111	86	66	95	75	55
17-20	104	79	59	74	59	39

Girls
(Score in Seconds)

Age						
9-12	198	148	108	143	113	83
13-16	158	108	65	125	91	61
17-20	159	107	66	142	102	71

Appendix VI

Food Values Chart*

*Jay S. Shivers and Hollis F. Fait, *Recreational Service for the Aging* (Philadelphia: Lea & Febiger, 1980), pp. 280-281.

	Measure or Weight	Calories	Protein gm	Fat gm	Carbo- hydrates mg	Calcium mg	Iron mg	Vita- min A I. U.	Vita- min B/ Thia- mine mg	Vita- min B/ Ribo- flavin mg	Vita- min B/ Niacin mg	Vita- min C/ Ascorbic Acid mg
Meats												
Chicken, broiled	3 oz	115	20	3	0	8	1.4	80	0.05	0.16	7.4	u
Cod fillet, poached	3 oz	89	20	u	0	11	0.45	0	0.07	0.08	2.5	2
Tuna, in oil, drained	3 oz	170	24	7	0	7	1.6	70	0.04	0.10	10.1	u
Shrimp, canned	3 oz	100	21	1	1	98	2.6	50	0.01	0.03	1.5	u
Ground beef, lean	3 oz	185	23	10	0	10	3.0	20	0.08	0.20	5.1	u
Ham, boiled	3 oz	203	17	15	0	9	2.4	0	0.38	0.14	2.3	u
Bacon, crisp	2 slices	90	5	8	trace	2	0.5	0	0.08	0.05	0.8	u
Bologna	2 slices	80	3	7	1	2	0.5	0	0.04	0.06	0.7	u
Frankfurter (8 per lb.)	1	170	7	15	1	3	0.8	u	0.08	0.11	1.4	u
Egg	1 large	80	6	6	trace	27	1.1	590	0.05	0.15	trace	0
Dry beans, cooked	1 cup	230	15	1	42	74	4.6	.10	0.13	0.10	1.5	u
Peanut butter	1 tbsp	95	4	8	3	9	0.3	u	0.02	0.02	2.4	0
Peanuts	¼ cup	210	9	18	7	27	0.8	u	0.11	0.05	6.1	0
Dairy Foods												
Skim milk, nonfat	1 cup	90	9	trace	12	296	0.1	10	0.09	0.44	0.2	2
Whole milk	1 cup	160	9	9	12	288	0.1	350	0.07	0.41	0.2	2
Chocolate drink	1 cup	190	8	6	27	270	0.5	210	0.10	0.40	0.3	3
Light cream	1 tbsp	30	1	3	1	15	trace	130	trace	0.02	trace	trace
Yogurt, part skim milk	1 cup	125	8	4	13	294	0.1	170	0.10	0.44	0.2	2
Ice milk	½ cup	100	3	4	15	102	0.05	140	0.04	0.15	0.05	trace
Ice cream, regular	½ cup	128	3	7	14	97	0.05	295	0.03	0.14	0.05	trace
Cottage cheese	½ cup	85	17	1	3	90	0.4	10	0.03	0.28	0.1	0
Process, Amer. cheese	1 oz	105	7	9	1	198	0.3	350	0.01	0.12	trace	0
Fats and Oils												
Butter	1 tbsp	100	trace	12	trace	3	0	470	u	u	u	0
Margarine, regular	1 tbsp	100	trace	12	trace	3	0	470	u	u	u	0
Lard	1 tbsp	115	0	13	0	0	0	0	0	0	0	0

Food	Measure	Calories	Protein (g)	Fat (g)	Carbohydrate (g)	Calcium (mg)	Iron (mg)	Vitamin A (IU)	Thiamin (mg)	Riboflavin (mg)	Niacin (mg)	Vitamin C (mg)
Corn oil	1 tbsp	125	0	14	0	0	0	u	0	0	0	0
Mayonnaise	1 tbsp	100	trace	11	trace	3	0.1	40	trace	0.01	trace	u
French dressing	1 tbsp	65	trace	6	3	2	0.1	u	u	u	u	u
Fruits, Vegetables												
Orange juice	½ cup	60	1	trace	15	13	0.1	275	0.11	0.01	0.5	60
Apple	1 med	70	trace	trace	18	8	0.4	50	0.04	0.02	0.1	3
Banana	1 med	100	1	trace	26	10	0.8	230	0.06	0.07	0.8	12
Peaches, canned	½ cup	100	trace	trace	26	5	0.4	550	0.01	0.03	0.7	3
Cabbage, shredded raw	½ cup	8	trace	trace	2	17	0.1	45	0.02	0.02	0.1	17
Carrot, raw	1 med	20	1	trace	5	18	0.4	5500	0.03	0.03	0.3	4
Tomato, raw	1 large	40	2	trace	9	24	0.9	1640	0.11	0.07	1.3	42
Green beans, cooked	½ cup	15	1	trace	4	32	0.4	340	0.04	0.06	0.3	8
Summer squash, cooked	½ cup	15	1	trace	4	26	0.4	410	0.05	0.08	0.8	10
White potato, baked	1 med	90	3	trace	21	9	0.7	trace	0.10	0.04	1.7	20
Peas, canned	½ cup	83	5	trace	16	25	2.1	560	0.11	0.07	1.1	11
Corn, canned	½ cup	85	3	1	20	5	0.5	345	0.03	0.06	1.1	6
Lettuce	2 large leaves	4	0.2	0	trace	12	0.2	324	0.01	0.01	0.04	4
Breads, Cereals												
White bread, enriched	1 slice	70	2	1	13	21	0.6	trace	0.06	0.05	0.6	trace
Whole wheat bread	1 slice	65	3	1	14	24	0.8	trace	0.09	0.03	0.8	trace
Corn flakes	1 cup	100	2	trace	21	4	0.4	0	0.11	0.02	0.5	0
Doughnut	1 med	105	3	5	22	147	0.7	0	0.12	0.07	1.7	trace
Angelfood cake	1/12	135	3	trace	32	50	0.2	0	trace	0.06	0.1	0
Yellow cake, choc. icing	1/12	366	4	13	60	68	0.6	160	0.02	0.08	0.2	trace
Sugars, Sweets, and Beverages												
Granulated sugar	1 tbsp	40	0	0	11	0	trace	0	0	0	0	0
Choc. fudge topping	2 tbsp	125	2	5	20	48	0.5	60	0.02	0.08	0.2	trace
Cola beverage	12 oz	145	0	0	37	u	u	0	0	0	0	0
Beer	12 oz	150	1	0	14	18	trace	u	0.01	0.11	2.2	u
Scotch, 80 proof	1½ oz	100	u	u	trace	u	u	u	u	u	u	u

u = unknown

Appendix VII (A)

Chart of Caloric Use in Various Physical Recreation Activities *

Mild to Moderate	Calories / Min.
Archery	3.4
Badminton (moderate)	6.1
Bowling	4.6
Calisthenics (stretching movements)	3.0
Calisthenics (lifting body weight, push-ups etc.)	4.9
Canoeing (moderate)	3.3
Cycling (slow)	4.0
Dancing (slow)	3.3
Dancing (moderate)	7.0
Fishing (sitting)	2.7
Gardening (moderate)	3.9
Hoeing, raking, planting	4.9
Horseback riding (walk)	3.1
Motorboating	2.7
Rowing (slow)	5.7
Sailing	3.3
Sitting (moving arms vigorously)	2.9
Sitting (moving arms and trunk)	3.1
Skating (slow)	5.7
Running in place (very slow)	6.3
Table tennis (moderate)	4.1
Table tennis (fast)	6.6
Walking (slow)	3.6
Walking (moderate)	6.1

Jay S. Shivers and Hollis F. Fait, *Recreational Service for the Aging* (Philadelphia: Lea & Febiger, 1980), p. 291.

Moderate to Vigorous	Calories / Min.
Badminton (vigorous)	10.0
Canoeing (vigorous)	7.3
Cycling (fast)	10.3
Dancing (fast)	10.0
Handball (vigorous)	11.2
Jogging (moderate)	15.3
Rowing (vigorous)	18.0
Running (moderate)	23.8
Running (full speed)	187.0
Skating (vigorous)	9.9
Stationary running (moderate)	12.0
Skiing (moderate)	21.2
Swimming, crawl (slow)	40.0
Swimming, crawl (fast)	80.0
Walking (fast)	9.9

Appendix VII (B)

Chart of Caloric Use in Exercises for Clients Confined to Wheelchairs*

	Minutes Performed	Calories Used
Warm-up Activities		
1. Rotate neck.	1	1.9
2. Rotate arms gently; start with small circles and gradually increase the size.	1	2.9
3. Bend forward at waist and return to original position.	1	3.1
Exercises		
1. Raise arms to shoulder height, bend elbow 90 degrees, swing elbows back four times.	1	2.8
2. With arms folded across chest, twist trunk to one side and then the other.	1	3.0
3. Lift one leg until it is straight, return to original position; repeat with other leg.	1	2.8
4. Lift both legs with knees bent and lower.	1	3.0
5. Cross right leg over left leg and then left leg over right leg.	1	2.2
6. With feet on floor, spread knees as far as possible and bring them together again.	2	3.8
7. With fist closed, push right arm out straight in front and return to original position; repeat with opposite arm.	2	3.8

*Jay S. Shivers and Hollis F. Fait, *Recreational Service for the Aging* (Philadelphia, Lea & Febiger, 1980), p. 293.

	Minutes Performed	Calories Used

Exercises

8. Place hands on knees and bend forward, sliding hands as far down on the outside of the legs as possible; return to original position. ½ 2.7
9. Reach with the right hand as far left as possible and then reach with the left hand as far right as possible. 1 2.8
10. Raise feet alternately. 1½ 5.7

Appendix VIII

Residents' Bill of Rights*

EACH RESIDENT has the right to considerate and respectful care and to be treated with honesty and dignity. It is recognized that every resident is an individual who has feelings, preferences, personal needs and requirements.

EACH RESIDENT has the right to be informed of his medical condition, unless contraindicated and so documented in medical records by his physician. Each resident also has the right to participate in the planning of his total care and medical treatment and to refuse treatment to the extent permitted by law and to be informed of medical consequences of such refusal.

EACH RESIDENT has the right to be informed of all rights and rules and regulations governing his conduct and responsibilities as a resident of the facility.

EACH RESIDENT has the right to be fully informed of all services provided by the facility and any charges for those services.

EACH RESIDENT has the right to manage his personal finances or at his request the facility will maintain an account and administer funds according to the resident's written authorization and instruction. Residents can expect an accounting at least quarterly or upon their request.

EACH RESIDENT has the right to privacy in treatment, in care, and in fulfillment of personal needs as well as during visits by his spouse, family, clergy, attorney and others. If a resident's spouse is also a resident and their physician approves, they may share a room provided accommodations are available.

EACH RESIDENT has the right to confidential handling of his medical or personal records. This information will only be released with the resident's prior consent except as required by law, or under third party contracts, or in case of transfer to another facility.

---

* Iowa Health Care Association, Des Moines, Iowa

EACH RESIDENT has the right to communicate, associate, and meet publicly and privately with any persons of his choice, unless to do so would infringe upon the rights of other residents, or if so indicated and documented by his physician (or if appropriate, a Qualified Mental Retardation Professional) in the resident's medical records.

EACH RESIDENT has the right to refuse to participate in experimental research.

EACH RESIDENT has the right to send and receive unopened mail and to have reasonable access to a telephone to receive and place confidential calls.

EACH RESIDENT has the right to be free of physical, chemical and mental restraints or abuse. Restraints will only be used under written physician's orders for a specific limited period of time, except in the case of an emergency as determined by qualified nursing personnel.

EACH RESIDENT is encouraged to participate in social, religious, and community group activities at his discretion, unless contraindicated by his physician (or if appropriate, a Qualified Mental Retardation Professional) and so documented in the resident's medical records.

EACH RESIDENT is encouraged and assisted to exercise his rights as a resident and citizen and may voice grievances and recommend changes in policies and services to facility staff and/or to outside representatives of his choice, free from restraint, interference, coercion, discrimination, or reprisal.

EACH RESIDENT has the right of continuity of care and is transferred or discharged only for medical reasons or for his welfare or that of other residents, or for nonpayment for his stay (except as prohibited by third party contracts). In the event discharge or transfer becomes necessary, residents will be given at least 5 days advance notice except in the case of an emergency.

EACH RESIDENT has the right to refuse to perform any services for the facility or other residents unless they are included as part of a therapeutic treatment plan which he has approved.

EACH RESIDENT may use and retain personal clothing and possessions as space permits, unless to do so would be contrary to his written plan of treatment or to do so would infringe upon the rights and safety of others.

EACH RESIDENT has the right to receive visitors at any reasonable hour or at times other than established visiting hours, particularly at times of critical illness.

In the event that questions cannot be resolved with the facility, the public is invited to submit to the Iowa Health Care Association, in writing, a request for Peer Review. Address communications to the Association, P. O. Box 236, West Des Moines, Iowa, 50265.

Index

A

Activity analysis, 49-51
Activity therapies, 62-63
Acute illness
  psychology of, 83-85
Adaptations, 130-135
Adapted, 6
Adapted recreational activities. See specific activities
Adapted recreational service, 7-10, 65, 68-75
  organization for, 68-70
Adaptive behavior, 154
Adjustment
  Problems of, 80-89
Advisory committee, 97
Affective disorders, 176-177
Aggression, 48-49
Aging, 192-200
  attitudes toward, 196-198
  mental capacity and, 194
  physiologic charges and, 193
  process of, 192-193
  psychologic changes and, 194-195
  recreational services for, 198-200
  senility and, 195
  social dimension of, 195-196
Ambulatory patients, 221-226
American Association for Health, Physical Education, Recreation and Dance, 6, 16, 19, 32, 227, 282, 286
American Association on Mental Deficiency, 155, 156
American Athletic Association of the Deaf, 273
American Psychiatric Association, 173
American Recreation Society Hospital Section, 16

AMESLAN, 149
Amputation, 113-114, 130-131
Anemia, 139
Angina pectoris, 136
Animal husbandry, 287-288, 292-294
Archery, 254-255
Art, 240-242
Art forms, 18
Arteriosclerosis, 139-140
Assessment, 90-108
  instruments for, 93, 95-96
  interviews and, 97-98
  inventories and, 99
  models of, 105
  observations and, 96-97
  questionnaire use in, 100
  SOAP, 105-106
  sociometric devices and, 100-101
Association for Mentally Retarded Citizens, 73
Asthma, 141
Attitudes, 80-89
Auditory impairments, 144-146
Auditory perception, 169-170
Austin, David, 49, 53, 98, 108
Avocational Activities Inventories, 99
Ayre's Southern California Motor Tests, 103

B

Badminton, 158-260
Bag punching, 265-266
Basic Skill Motor Profile, 102
Basketball, 262
Bedridden patients, 216-221
Behavior modification, 38-40
  reinforcement of, 38-40

Behaviorism, 38-40
  behavior modification and, 38-40
Billiards, 268
Body composition, 282
Body fat, 285-286
Bowling, 255-256
Boy Scouts of America, 73
Boy's Club of America, 73
Brain
  injuries to, 118-120
Bronchitis, 141-142
Bruininks-Oseretsky Test of Motor Proficiency, 103, 108

C

Camping, 313-323
  adaptation in, 321-323
  clientele served in, 318-320
  programming in, 320-321
  recreationist's role in, 315-318
  therapeutic adjunct of, 314-315
Canoeing and boating, 264-270
Cardiac disorders, 135-140
  causes of, 137-140
  symptoms of, 135-136
  treatment for, 136-137
Cardiorespiratory endurance, 280-281
  development of, 283-284
Catholic Youth Organization, 73
Cerebral palsy, 124-126, 133-134
CERT, 106-107
Certification, 30
  standards for, 327-329
China, 14
Client, 6
Client-centered organization, 69
Client-developed activities, 188-189
Clinical approach, 7
Combes, A.V., 317, 323
Community setting
  participant planning in, 76-77
Compensation, 40
Compentency based program, 23
Cong Fu, 14
Continuing education, 31
Continuum, 9
Coronary, 140
Correctional institutions
  recreational activities in, 207-211
Corrective therapy, 18
Councils, 77
Crafts, 127-240
Culinary arts, 294-298
  adapting activities for, 296-298

D

Dance, 243-244
Defense mechanisms, 40

Deformities, 120-121
Degenerative diseases, 132
Depth perception, 168-169
Deviant behavior, 201-211
  correctional settings and, 206
  criminal justice system and, 201-202
  halfway houses and, 206-207
  recreational programming for, 203-205
  security and, 205
  therapeutic program for, 202-203
Diagnosis, 8
Diagnostic and Statistical Manual of Mental Diseases, 173
Disabilities
  recreational programming for physical, 129-135
Disability, 6
  attitudes toward, 80-83
  defined, 6
  group attitudes toward, 81-82
  parental reaction toward, 81
  physical, 111-150
  self attitudes toward, 82-83
Discrepancy evaluation model, 105
Dissociative disorders, 177-178
Doll, Edgar, 155, 170
Drama, 246-249
Dunn, John, 108

E

Egocentricity, 89
Emphysema, 142-143
Enjoyment, 11-12
Epilepsy, 126-127
Evaluation, 90-108
  CERT, 106-107
  discrepancy, 105
  formative, 93
  instruments for, 93, 95-96
  item analysis and, 95
  models of, 105
  observation and, 96
  summative, 93
Exercise, 273-285
  body composition and, 276
  physical fitness and, 275

F

Fait, Hollis, F., 19, 38, 49, 101, 102, 108
Fait's Basic Motor Skill Test, 101, 156, 277
Fait's Endurance Ratio, 280
Fait's Physical Fitness Test for the Mentally Retarded, 155, 335, 336
  norms for, 337-338
Figure-ground perception, 168
Fishing, 269
Flexibility, 281-282
  development of, 284-285

Food values, 339-341
Fractures, 115-116
Freud, Sigmund, 40
Frostig's Developmental Test of Visual
    Perception, 103

G

Games, 251-272
    archery, 254-255
    badminton, 258-260
    basketball, 262
    bowling, 255-256
    box hockey, 269
    deck tennis, 270
    floor hockey, 269
    golf, 256-257
    horseshoes, 268-269
    pool, 268
    rope, 253
    shuffleboard, 261
    softball, 263-264
    table tennis, 260-261
    tennis, 257-258
    throwing, 252, 253, 254
    volleyball, 264
Girl Scouts of America, 73
Girl's Club of America, 73
Golf, 256-257
Graphic arts, 235-242
    activity selection in, 237-238
    adaptation in, 235-236, 239-240
    functional analysis and, 238-239
    safety and, 236-237
    therapeutic adjunct through, 240-241
    values of, 241-242
Gray, David, 4, 19
Greben, S., 4, 19
Group homes, 71-72
Group therapy, 41, 183
Groups, 42-43
Gunn, Scout L., 64, 79

H

Handicapped, 6
Heart failure, 136
Holahan, D. P., 161, 170
Home environment, 81
Homebound persons, 229
Homeostasis, 36-37
Horseshoe pitching, 268-269
Horticultural therapy, 289
Horticulture, 288-291
    adapting activities for, 290-291
Humanism, 37-38
Hypertension, 139

I

Identification, 40
Illness, 5

Imagery, 47
Individual Education Program, 17, 72, 104,
    162
Intelligence, 153
    measurement of, 153-154
    nature of, 153
Interview, 97-99
Involutional psychotic reaction, 184
Iowa Health Care Association, 234, 347

K

Kinesthetics, 167-168
Kinetics, 50-51
Kraeplin, Emil, 177
Kraus, R. G., 19
Krusen, Frank, 36, 53

L

Learning disabilities, 161-162
Legg-Calvé-Perthes, 132
Leisure
    counseling for, 51-52
    education for, 51-52,
Leisure Activities Blank, 99
Licensing, 30

M

Mainstreaming, 52, 159
Medication
    side effects of, 252-253
Mental health, 10-11
Mental illness, 172-190
    activity selection for clients with, 187-
        188
    attitudes toward, 179-180
    classification of, 172-179
    diagnosis of, 179
    drug therapy for, 180-181, 182
    individualized program for, 187
    mainstreaming and, 181-182
    medical practice and, 180-182, 185
    recreational activities for, 185
    therapeutic prescription for, 183-185
    treatment for, 182-183
Mental retardation, 152-170
    causes of, 156-159
    Public Law 94-142 and, 159
    recreational activities for, 159-161
Milieu therapy, 43, 183
Miranda's Leisure Inventory, 99
Motivation, 37-40
    behaviorirsm and, 38-40
    humanism and, 37-38
Motor fitness, 10
Multiple sclerosis, 127-128, 134
Muscular dystrophy, 128-134
Muscular endurance, 278-280

Muscular strength, 278
 development of, 282-283
Music, 244-246
Myocardial infarction, 137

N

National Association of Recreational Therapy, 16
National Association of Sports for Cerebral Palsy, 273
National Consortium of Physical Education and Recreation for the Handicapped, 33
National Council for Therapeutic Recreation Certification, 30, 327
National Easter Seal Society, 73
National Recreation and Park Association, 16, 30, 32
National Therapeutic Recreation Society, 9, 17, 32, 33
 philosophic statement of, 330-332
National Wheelchair Athletic Association, 262-272
Nerve injuries, 132
Nerves
 damage to, 116-118
Neurologic disabilities, 132-135
Neurologic disorders, 124-129
Normalization, 52

O

Objectives, 104-105
 behavioral, 104-105
 short-term, 104
Occupational therapy, 9
O'Morrow, G., 7, 20
Ortheses, 224
Orthopedic disabilities, 112-116
Osteoarthritis, 124
Osteochondrosis, 121, 132
Outpatients, 228

P

Parachute play, 271
Paranoid disorders, 176
Parental consent, 92
Parkinson's disease, 128-129, 134
Passive entertainment, 307-312
 games as, 310
 preparing clients for, 309-310
 special events and, 310-312
 structuring events for, 308-309
 therapeutic value of, 307-308
Patient, 6
Patients' rights, 223-234, 346-347
 access and, 273
 privacy and, 233-234

Perambulation, 226-228
 scooter boards and, 228
 wheelchairs and, 226-227
Perception, 145
Perceptual-motor learning, 162-170
Performing arts, 242-248
 adaption for, 243-244, 247, 255
 dance as, 243
 drama as, 246-248
 music and, 244
Personality disorders, 178
Pet therapy, 293
 adapting activities for, 293
Peterson, Carol, 64, 79
Physical activity, 342-345
 caloric use in, 342-343
 wheelchair-bound caloric use, 344-345
Physical disability
 broad values of, 85-86
 personality characteristics and, 89
 psychology of, 85-89
 respnonses to, 86-87
 social problems and, 87-89
Physical fitness, 10, 47-49
 concepts of, 48
 exercise and, 47
 stress reduction and, 48
Physical therapy, 18-19
Play therapy, 41
Prescription, 8, 43-45, 183, 229-232
 contents of, 44-45
Professional development, 21-34
Professional ethics, 29-30
Professional organizations, 31-34
Professional preparation, 26-31
Program evaluation, 189-190
Projection, 40
Prostheses, 224-226
Psychoanalysis, 40-41
Psychosexual disorders, 178
Psychotherapy, 41
Public Law 94-112, 17
Public Law 94-142, 6, 17, 22, 65, 72, 90, 91, 103, 152, 159, 162, 234
 due process in, 91-92
Public relations, 33-34
Pulmonary diseases, 140-141
 etiology of, 140-141
 pathology of, 141
Punishment, 39

Q

Quality assurance, 186
Questionnaire, 100

R

Rapport, 98
Rationalization, 40

Reality orientation, 46
Recreation, 4, 8
Recreation therapy, 5
Recreational activities, 8-13
    programming of 143-144, 148-150
    values of, 9-13
Recreational centers, 71
Recreational service, 4
    adapted form of, 65-66
Recreationist, 4-5, 21-34
    attributes of, 28-29
    competencies of, 23-26
    functions of, 23, 26
    professional development of, 21-34
Regression, 84-85
Rehabilitation, 35-53
    description of, 36
    homeostasis and, 36-37
    practices of, 37
    process of, 35-53
    responsibilities of, 22-23
    roles of, 22-23
Rehabilitation Act of 1973, 17, 66, 233
Rehabilitation team, 17, 22, 55
Reinforcement, 39-40
    extension and, 39-40
    negative, 39
    positive, 38
Relaxation, 46-47
    program for, 47
Remotivation, 46
Rheumatic fever, 138-139
Rheumatoid arthritis, 123-124
Roach's Purdue Perceptual Motor Survey,
    103

S

Schizophrenia, 175-176
Scooter play, 270-271
Screening, 91
Self-Leisure Interest Profile, 99
Senility, 195
Senior centers, 71
Sensory training, 45
Service activities, 304-306
    possibilities for, 306
    therapeutic value of, 304-305
Shivers, Jay S., 4, 19
Shuffleboard, 261-262
Skiing, 267
Skill analysis, 50-51
Sleator, Esther K., 233, 234
SOAP, 105-106
Social activities, 300-303
    prescription for, 303
    selection of, 302-303
    value of, 301-302
Social adjustment, 11
Sociogram, 101

Softball, 263-264
Solzhenitsyn, Alexander, 83, 89
Somatoform disorder, 177
Sontag, Susan, 196-200
Special, 5
    defined, 5
    needs, 5
    Olympics, 272
    physical education, 19
    population, 66-68
    program, 5
    recreational service, 55-79, 215-234
    services, 59-60, 62
Spina bifida, 121
Sports, 272-273
    associations for, 273
    organization of, 273
    safety in, 272
Sprague, Robert L., 233, 234
Stanford-Binet test, 155
Streptokinase, 137
Stress, 48
Stroke, 119-120
Sublimation, 40
Swimming, 267
Symptoms, 178
Syndromes, 178-179

T

Table tennis, 260-261
Tai Chi Chuan, 14, 47
Takata, Nancy, 97, 108
Tavar, S., 161, 170
Temple University, 23
Tennis, 257-258
Terminology, 1-19
Tests
    correlation coefficient in, 94
    criterion-referenced, 95-97
    motor performance, 101-103
    norm-referenced, 94-95
    perceptual-motor, 103
    reliability of, 93
    screening, 103
    validity of, 93-94
Texas Revision of Fait's Basic Motor Skills
    Test, 333-334
Therapeutic, 6
Therapeutic milieu, 43
Therapeutic recreational activities, 13-15
Therapeutic recreational service, 7-9, 56-
    58
    nature of, 56-57
    school programs of, 65
    type of, 57-58
Therapy, 6
Thomas, Dylan, 192
Thrombolysis, 137
Track and field activities, 266

Transportation services, 73-74
Trauma, 113-120
Treatment center, 55-66, 74-78
  administration of, 58-59
  classification of, 56
  equipment in, 75
  facilities of, 74-75
  organization of, 58, 59-65
  participant planning in, 77-78
  scheduling in, 75-76
  type of, 57-58

U

United Cerebral Palsy Association, 73
United States Association for Blind Athletes, 272
United States Civil Service, 5
University of Connecticut, 23, 102, 155
University of North Carolina, 23
Utah, 31

V

Value attainment, 12-13
Values, 9-13

Vineland Social Maturity Scale, 155
Visual disabilities, 146-148
Visual discrimination, 168
Visual perception, 168
Volleyball, 264
Volunteers, 70-79, 205-206

W

Weight lifting, 264-265
Winnick, Joseph, 277, 286
Witt, Peter, 7, 20
Wloodkowski, Raymond, 37, 53
Works Progress Administration, 7, 16

Y

Yoga, 47
Young Men's Christian Association, 73, 207
Young Men's Hebrew Association, 73
Young Women's Christian Association, 73, 207
Young Women's Hebrew Association, 73